T0281560

Only Dissect
Rudolf Klein on
Politics and Society

Edited by Patricia Day

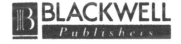

BLACKWELL
Publishers

First published 1996
Reprinted 1996

Blackwell Publishers Inc.
238 Main Street
Cambridge, Massachusetts 02142, USA

Blackwell Publishers Ltd
108 Cowley Road
Oxford OX4 1JF, UK

Library of Congress Cataloging in Publication Data
Klein, Rudolf, 1930–
Only dissect: Rudolf Klein on politics and society / edited by Patricia Day
p. cm.
Includes bibliographical references.
ISBN 1–55786–869–7 — ISBN 1–55786–132–8 (pbk)
1. Social policy. 2. Medical policy. 3. Policy sciences.
I. Day, Patricia. II. Title.
HN5.K54   1996   95–37532
361.2'5—dc20   CIP

British Library Cataloguing in Publication Data
A CIP catalogue record for this book is available from the British Library

Typeset by A M Marketing

This book is printed on acid-free paper

Contents

Preface

These articles and papers have been collected together under four separate, roughly chronological headings to illustrate the work of Rudolf Klein over almost four decades. The earliest papers in this collection were written in the mid 1950s when Rudolf was beginning his career as an observer of society and politics; it includes some of the articles he wrote as a leader writer and commentator on the national press in the 1960s and early 1970s and then a selection of research and policy analysis papers and books associated with time served (and still serving) in academic establishments in subsequent decades. But while the collected works are wide ranging over time, organisational associations and topics covered, the scholarship and analytic rigour are constant throughout. The contributions to obscure and long-gone periodicals, the mainstream journalism, the university researches and the books all display the hall-marks of sharp observation, intellectual breadth and a use of language we associate very specifically with Rudolf Klein.

One of the key reasons for making this collection, apart from celebrating Rudolf's 65th birthday, is to set out a stall of his wares for all to see. But apart from providing us with a gallery of good craftsmanship, it shows just how early on in his working life Rudolf produced the insights on politics and society that often made him a man ahead of his time; one has only to read a piece that he wrote in the 1970s and follow it immediately with one of his 1990s papers to experience the continuities in his themes and intellectual approach, straddling journalism and academic writing. For some possible explanations as to why Rudolf was able to maintain his distinctive style while working in different environments, we have to move outside of his collected works and look at his life before work: a brief biographical reconnaissance provides some clues.

Rudolf Klein was born in Prague in 1930 but left Czechoslovakia with his parents in 1939. All three lived variously in England and Scotland where Rudolf attended a number of schools in towns and cities where his father was working as a psychiatrist and neurologist in the NHS. After this peripatetic education, he went up to Merton College, Oxford in the early 1950s where he studied medieval history and was awarded the

Gibbs Memorial Prize. Oxford was followed by 20 years of leader writing and commentating in Fleet Street, divided equally between *The London Evening Standard* and *The Observer,* where he covered politics and football with equal enthusiasm. In the early 1970s he moved from journalism to academic research, keeping up his interest in politics but swapping football reporting for health services research. In 1978 he became, and remains, Professor of Social Policy and Director of the Centre for the Analysis of Social Policy at Bath University.

Acknowledgements

This book, and its companion, *The State, Politics and Health: Essays for Rudolf Klein,* began with conversations among the editors in the fall of 1993. The King's Fund and the Milbank Memorial Fund supported the project. Staff members of the two funds, especially Carmel McColgan of the King's Fund, and Gail Cambridge and Katharine Ristich of the Milbank Memorial Fund, managed editorial details. At Bath, Thelma Brown and Kathrine Wallis-King greatly assisted the editor in her task. The diplomacy of Rolf Janke, executive editor of Blackwell Publishers' North American branch, facilitated this transatlantic effort.

We also wish to thank the following bodies for giving permission to use some of Rudolf Klein's work which they had originally published: these articles and book chapters have been reproduced here in their original form, making no attempt to impose a stylistic uniformity.

British Journal of Political Science
Commentary
Encounter
Institute of Economic Affairs (Health Unit)
Heinemann
Journal of Health Politics, Policy and Law
Management Today
Milbank Memorial Fund Quarterly
New Universities Quarterly
Political Quarterly
Routledge
The British Medical Journal
The King's Fund Institute
The Lancet
The Listener
The Observer Newspaper
The Royal Society of Medicine
Threshold
Times Higher Education Supplement

Part 1

Spectator Sports

This section of Rudolf Klein's collected works is a miscellany of reviews and commentaries spanning 23 years from the 1950s to the early 1970s. It covers television, sport, books, theatre and opera and shows how he began learning his craft by observing things going on in a wide variety of public and social arenas, not least his beloved opera.

The content and tone of this section provides some insights into Rudolf's later work in which he has sometimes shown an unwillingness to assume the totally serious attitudes expected by academia. It starts with pieces he contributed as a 27-year old to a periodical called *Threshold* which was set up and published by the Lyric Players in Belfast in 1957. This small but valiant outfit was the brain child of the wife of an Irish psychiatrist exiled in Bristol whose object was to add to creative writing and objective criticism in Ireland.

But it would be misleading to imply that Rudolf's working youth was frivolously centred on the arts to the exclusion of the serious world of politics and government. In fact, this miscellany shows otherwise. Along with theatre and football there are several sharp political observations which serve as trailers for his later work. As further evidence of Rudolf's early inclination for hard work and a variable agenda, he was actually providing Threshold and others with his observations on the high arts in London at the same time as producing daily copy for *The London Evening Standard*.

The Gargoyle Theatre

THRESHOLD
February 1957

The London Theatre is remarkably resilient. It has to be.

For many of the critics seem to believe that they can only show themselves to be alive by shouting that the theatre is dead. Throughout the
1956 season the obituaries have been turned out in the Sundays and
weeklies with unfailing regularity. The solemnity of the occasion has
only been broken when some of the mourners dashed off to welcome
what they variously interpreted as either a resurrection or a new birth.

Looking down the list of London plays, with its plethora of second-
rate thrillers and third-rate farces, it is impossible not to sympathise with
the critics, condemned as they are to see every play which comes on.
But perhaps the professional view is too gloomy: it is rather as if a doctor
in an incurables' ward were to judge the health of the nation by that of
his own patients. Judged by its best productions, comparing its standards
with those of the theatres in other countries, the London stage does quite
well.

Certainly the reaction to the three foreign companies – two French
and one German – who visited London in 1956, supports this interpretation. Those who expected a new revelation, something on a different
plane from the English theatre, were disappointed. What they saw was
invariably competent and sometimes exciting. But it never had that extra
dimension which marks a new development in the evolution of an art
form.

The Brecht company, from East Berlin, was much boosted before its
arrival. Critics returned from forays to Germany congratulating themselves
on their acumen in discovering this new phenomenon. Charitably one

concluded, after seeing the company, that their enthusiasm was based on ignorance of the German language.

The company succeeds despite Brecht's theories, and despite Brecht's plays. That may seem a rather negative achievement, but, considering the theories and the plays, it is a considerable one. Brecht's language is deliberately flat, plodding and unemotional. His theory of the "alienation effect" debars him (except when he forgets it) from involving the audience in the action on stage.

Brecht's own failure as a dramatist and success as a producer was best illustrated by the company's showpiece, "Mother Courage" – a play of Wagnerian proportions. Mother Courage, a vivandiére, plods her way through the Thirty Years' War. By it she makes her living. By it she loses her children. She herself, the author explains in a footnote to the play "believes in the war to the last." Her sufferings are passive, she accepts them fatalistically. The masses, Brecht adds, "understand a catastrophe just as much as a guinea-pig understands biology." It is for the audience to draw the appropriate conclusion from the blackboard demonstration they have been given on the stage.

It is a theory for puppets, not for actors. A Hamlet or an Orestes consciously seeking to work out his personal destiny is beyond it. Play-writing becomes a didactic exercise. Playgoing becomes a visit to the lecture room. Catharsis becomes conversion.

Why, then, was it possible for anyone to regard "Mother Courage" as anything but a tremendous flop? Partly it is because of Brecht's own technical virtuosity as a playwright, despite his theories. But even more important is the virtuosity of his company.

It is not that the Brecht company has introduced a new style in acting. The performance by Helene Weigel – Brecht's widow – in the name part was "classic" in every sense. What does distinguish the company is the subordination of the individual actor to the whole. The result is an impersonal smoothness, a sense of the inevitable, a feeling of purpose-fulness which rescues the play from tedium. It is this, not the technical gadgetry (such as the scene where Mother Courage pulls her waggon on a revolving turntable, giving a wonderful impression of movement), which distinguishes the company.

Simplicity and directness were qualities also of Jean Vilar's Theatre National Populaire. This, too, aims to reach a large audience – as the name implies. But otherwise the company has no didactic purpose. Its London repertory – Marivaux, Moliére and Hugo – was limited to the classics. And interest was consequently concentrated on the style of production rather than the plays themselves.

To say that the style was crude would be an exaggeration, but an exaggeration based on fact. Jean Vilar relies on bold, simple strokes for his effects. He uses little scenery. He relies heavily on dramatic lighting. He does not use the curtain: when the audience comes into the theatre they at once see the stage set (what there is of it). The acting tends to be unshaded – in some of the smaller parts it was decidedly rough.

Partly, at least, this style has been forced on Vilar. The company's home is the immense and cavernous Palais de Chaillot in Paris: any delicacy of touch would be wasted in that giant auditorium. Vilar's budget is small: he cannot afford elaborate settings. His audience tends to be enthusiastic but unsophisticated: so the acting has to be full-blooded. Not surprisingly the company's most successful production was Hugo's unabashed melodramatic Marie Tudor which – rather than the mannered intricacies of Marivaux or the carefully designed manoeuvres of Moliére – allowed it to display its qualities most fully.

No one could call Jean-Louis Barrault's style of production unsophisticated. If Jean Vilar is a slightly slapdash impressionist. Barrault is a meticulous pointillist. Like Brecht he exploits every possible technical device. But, again like Brecht, he is never fussy. He never allows detail to obscure the shape of the play or interrupt its rhythm.

Barrault's showpiece in London was undoubtedly Claudel's "Christophe Colombe" – the only contemporary play in the repertory. This is not a good play. Columbus' search for America is interpreted as the search for another world, in the theological not geographical sense. The play is declamatory, rhetorical in the worst French theatrical tradition, the elaborately "poetic" language does not compensate for the poverty of its thought.

But once again the producer's virtuosity came to the rescue of the author. The relatively small cast was manoeuvred about with tremendous dash, creating a restless impression of movement. The scenery – mainly consisting of a large sail slung above the stage – was simple but evocative. From time to time the sail was used as a cinema screen on which short films, reinforcing the action on stage, were projected.

Different as their styles are in most respects, Brecht, Vilar and Barrault have this much in common as producers: a tremendous self-confidence, an assurance infectious enough to overcome any doubts the audience may have about the merit of the play, a personality strong enough to mould their actors to fit into the same over-riding pattern and so to infuse the whole production with their personality.

It is precisely this which the London theatre lacks. It may also lack good plays – but that is an affliction common to other theatrical centres. It is, however, the ability to make a commonplace play seem worthwhile which is most conspicuously absent in London. The London Theatre has lost confidence in itself. It is lacking in ambition. Too often it is tracing out a footpath on the map when it should be looking at the globe as a whole.

The Old Vic is a case in point. Accepting even its self-imposed handicap of producing all the Shakespeare plays, however bad, its productions are often lamentable. The company seems always to be searching for gimmicks. Iago has to be played as a Cockney barrow-boy. Emphasis is put on the minor characters. Endless pieces of business are invented for them. (Typically the only two actors of stature to have emerged from the Old Vic in recent years are character specialists, Paul Rogers and Michael Hordern.) An overall impression of fussiness is created. The "line" of the play is obscured by the detail. The gargoyles become more important than the cathedrals.

Another symptom of this loss of confidence, this inability to infuse old traditions with new life, is the relentless search for novelty. The new is welcomed not so much because it is better than the old, but simply because it appears to be different. It is this which perhaps explains the phenomenal success of John Osborne's "Look Back in Anger," hailed by some critics as the portent of a dramatic rennaisance.

John Osborne's language is violent. His characters are drawn from the intellectual no-man's-world of red-brick failures. Their emotions are pathological in their self-destroying intensity. Yet, for all this, his play is rather drably orthodox – curiously reminiscent of latter-day Coward, unlikely as this comparison may seem. Coward is the spokesman of those who feel resentful because they can no longer afford to keep servants. Osborne's characters are resentful because, unlike their parents, they have never even had servants. The target of both is the welfare state – seen from different ends of the telescope.

Colin Wilson has not yet written a play, although he is threatening to do so. But the success of the book, "The Outsider," only seems explicable in an intellectual, who puts the first emphasis on novelty. The novelty in his case is not the theme (for the central argument, that of the rebel against society, is platitudinous) but the author's age. He, like John Osborne, appears to be unable to distinguish between what is interesting as a psychiatrist's case history and what is of literary importance. Otherwise it is difficult to account for his pre-occupation with pathological cases like van Gogh and Nijinski, two of his prototype outsiders.

But this has not stopped the editors of literary magazines from canvassing Wilson's opinions on the future of the theatre (quite apart from pushing him forward as a general intellectual crystal-ball gazer). He has joined in the debate as to whether a "writer's theatre" or an "actor's theatre" or a "producer's theatre" is needed, a debate which has filled the pages of these same magazines.

It seems a pity that no one has bothered to point out that the theatre should be the meeting ground – not the battle ground – of writers, actors and producers. And that only when these join together, subordinating their individual interests to the whole, is London likely to see a theatrical revival.

2

London Opera

THRESHOLD
June 1957

Cooking apart, opera is possibly the most un-English form of art. No opera by an English composer has found a secure place in the international repertory; few singers from this country have achieved world rank. It is therefore all the more pleasing to be able to report a steady increase in both the quality and popularity of opera in London.

As yet opera is not as popular as either ballet or concert music. It tends to exist in a cultural no-man's land: despised by highbrows as a mongrel creation and, paradoxically, condemned by others as esoteric. But the resistance is breaking down. The B.B.C. has helped a great deal, particularly with its Third Programme broadcasts of opera. So has the sale of long-playing records. A social barrier seems to remain, though. Unlike Italian opera audiences, those in London still belong overwhelmingly to the intellectual middle-classes – as far as one can judge by their appearance.

This applies less to Sadler's Wells which, being outside the West End, attracts a partly local audience. It is certainly true, however, of both Covent Garden and Glyndebourne (which, despite its location in Sussex, is an essentially metropolitan institution and must be included in any discussion of opera in London). The appeal of Glyndebourne is inevitably limited: not everyone can afford to pay two guineas for a seat (the lowest price) or, for that matter, take an afternoon off to go into the country. Covent Garden's prices, in contrast, are very reasonable and anyone who can afford to buy tickets for the Crazy Gang should be able to go to the Royal Opera.

But if the total audience for opera is still restricted, enthusiasm compensates for lack of numbers. The opera seasons at both Covent Garden and

9

Sadler's Wells stretch over two thirds of the year. Glyndebourne is open for three months in the summer. Visits by foreign companies are frequent: in recent years London has seen those from Vienna, Zagreb, Stuttgart and Munich as well as a rag-bag of anonymous Italians. Empty seats are rarer than queues at the box-office. Lack of interest is the one problem of which opera impressarios cannot complain (though it could be argued that the interest is not discriminating enough).

The chief complaint of Covent Garden's administration is lack of money. With an annual public subsidy of about £250,000, it is the poor relation among the world's great opera houses. La Scala, Milan, receives a grant of twice that amount and yet charges far more for its seats. The financial problem is all the more acute because the Royal Opera is housed in an impressive but old building, expensive to run. At one time the administration was threatening to close the opera because of the shortage of funds.

The financial difficulties probably cannot be remedied. Solvent opera houses are as rare as handsome tenors. A change in Government policy, bringing an increase in the subsidy, is as unlikely as it would be desirable. But the lack of money adds a further complication in the choice of operas to present. How far is this choice to be dictated by box-office considerations and how far by the desire to have as wide and representative a repertory as possible?

Two recent productions illustrate this dilemma. When Maria Callas came to sing Norma – for two performances only – the house was packed out, although prices had been heavily increased. The streets leading to Covent Garden were lined with people pathetically jingling coins – beggars in reverse – hoping to buy tickets at black market rates. Norma was sung in Italian, and Callas was reinforced by three other Italian singers (among whom a tenor who looked a little out of place and seemed perpetually on the point of breaking into a Neapolitan love song). Janacek's Jenufa – a Czech opera written early in this century – was sung in English by Covent Garden's own resident performers. When I went, the Royal Opera was emptier than I have ever seen it. Financially Jenufa was a complete failure. In every other way it was a complete success. The critics were enthusiastic. So were the regrettably small audiences. Jenufa's lack of appeal is all the more curious because the opera is not at all difficult or unconventional. Its melancholy lyricism is most touching.

Traumatic financial experiences such as this may partly account for Covent Garden's rather restricted repertory. This, indeed, shows some astonishing omissions – including operas which, it might be thought, would have box-office appeal. In the 10 years of its existence the company has produced no Don Giovanni, no Falstaff, no Rossini opera at all and rationed its Beethoven and Strauss very strictly. (The last performance of Fidelio, for instance, is a very distant memory – though a painful one. This was one of Covent Garden's few really inexcusably bad productions.)

Perhaps, therefore, the public's caution reflects a certain lack of enterprise at Covent Garden itself. This timidity is seen not only in the choice of operas, but in their treatment. The average standard of the performances is remarkably high. But consistency is achieved at the expense of brilliance. Few productions are very bad – but equally few are very good. A visit to the Royal Opera can be relied upon to be enjoyable but (special occasions such as the visit of Callas apart) they do not excite – there is little sense of revelation. A routine Covent Garden performance will give a competent account of the opera as a whole, but it will rarely reveal new qualities in the work. Yet that, surely, is what is wanted if familiar pieces like La Boheme or Traviata are not to become bores.

This may seem a quixotic complaint – as if one were condemning the Promenade concerts for not being up to the Toscanini standard. But the atmosphere of conscientious plodding at Covent Garden can become infuriating: it would be easier to forgive the administration for experiments that fail than to praise it for the unadventurous, competent performances that successfully fill the house.

In 1949 Covent Garden commissioned Salvador Dali to design the sets for Salome. It was a disaster. Unfortunately this failure stopped the Royal Opera from repeating the experiment. Its sets and costumes are now impeccably conventional – pleasing but not exciting. The effects of Wieland Wagner's revolutionary changes in the production of his grandfather's operas have not yet percolated down to Covent Garden. The Royal Opera is still too literal, and is reluctant to exploit the powers of suggestion. Wood, canvas and paint are still more important than lighting. New sets may differ in style from pre-war ones but they remain of the same type.

Musically Covent Garden is more progressive. The quality of tameness – so evident in its production methods – is less evident. Rafael Kubelik, who was appointed musical director less than two years ago, is still relatively inexperienced as an opera conductor. He is not yet the equal of Karajan or Kempe. His range is limited: Carmen, which he conducted recently, was clearly outside it. But he has to his credit an exciting Otello and is particularly at home conducting the operas of his compatriots, Smetana and Janacek.

One reservation must, however, be made about Covent Garden's musical policy. The Royal Opera has imposed a quite unnecessary handicap on itself: the decision taken when the company was founded, to sing all operas in English. (There have been some exceptions: the Ring is put on in German every year and short Italian seasons crop up from time to time. But otherwise the rule is maintained.)

Ideally, of course, the audience should be able to understand the words – though this is a questionable pleasure in some operas. There is, therefore, a strong case to be made out for singing opera in English. But it is based on the assumption that the performers are available. And on the existing evidence this assumption is not justified. Nor is this either surprising or discreditable. The Covent Garden company has a short history. It has had little time in which to develop its own singers. It therefore does not have a team of resident performers strong enough to put on all the operas in the international repertory.

Other opera houses have the same difficulties. They, at least, do not have to find singers with the additional and rare qualification of being able to perform in English. Italian and German companies can afford to use Italian and German simply because singers able to use those languages are on tap. Significantly the only other great opera house in an English-speaking country, the Metropolitan, has not adopted Covent Garden's linguistic nationalism.

Covent Garden has some excellent singers, like Elsie Morison, Geraint Evans and Richard Lewis. The standard of vocal competence is high throughout the company. But inevitably occasions do arise when reinforcements are needed. And it is then that the disadvantages of singing in English are shown up. This season's new production of Wagner's The Mastersingers (better known as Die Meistersinger) is a case in point. Richard Lewis was to have sung the principal tenor part of Walther, but called off. No substitute could be found. So Erich Witte, a German character tenor, who was producing the opera, took over. The result was the musical equivalent of the Charge of the Light Brigade: one could admire Witte's courage but had to condemn the effects of his rashness. The massacre of the notes, particularly in the Prize Song, was appalling.

Yet otherwise The Mastersingers was a first-rate production, well conducted and sung. If the management had been able to find a top-class tenor to substitute, it would have been altogether magnificent. It would almost certainly have been able to do so had it not been for the language barrier: good Walthers may be scarce, but not nearly so scarce as good Walthers who can sing in English.

Occasionally Covent Garden has persuaded foreign singers to perform in English. The experiment has seldom succeeded; the result has often been embarrassing. The words might have been easier to understand if they had been in Italian or German instead of (nominally) English.

The tremendous advantages of being able to draw on singers of all nationalities is shown by Glyndebourne. The performers at this country house opera are not necessarily the most famous or the highest paid. Glyndebourne specialises in spotting singers before they become internationally known. But the over-all level of performance is probably the highest in the world. Consistency is not achieved at the expense of brilliance. The brilliance itself is consistently sustained. Long rehearsals and intensive drilling (by the Eberts, father and son, the two chief producers) does not destroy a sense of spontaneity, a feeling of high spirits. Perhaps the Sussex setting helps – as undoubtedly does the miniature size of the theatre which flatters small voices.

So high is Glyndebourne's reputation (and so well are its standards maintained) that it can afford to experiment. It specialises in resurrecting virtually unknown Rossini operas: Le Comte Ory the year before last, l'Italiana in Algeri this coming season. These are no better known than Jenufa, which proved so unsuccessful at Covent Garden. But the fact that they are being put on by Glyndebourne is guarantee enough for the audiences.

If Covent Garden would only abandon its English-only rule, it could build up a far stronger company. It could, like Glyndebourne, experiment far more in the selection of operas. It could use the talents of outstanding singers like Callas, Tebaldi, Milanov, Gobbi and Christoff more. It could put on now neglected operas like Don Carlos, Macbeth, Manon, Thais, and Boris Godunov. And the chances of attracting the public to unknown operas would be immeasurably increased if the performers themselves were well known. Rightly or wrongly London audiences would probably be ready to queue (and pay) to listen to Callas gargling or singing the scales. The cost of engaging such singers would be more than outweighed by the certainty of being able to sell all the seats.

Excessive nationalism at Covent Garden is accompanied by excessive parochialism. There seems to be absolutely no cooperation between the Royal Opera and Sadler's Wells – and both houses suffer through this. Both frequently and concurrently produce the same opera. Thus London has had two Traviatas, two Rigolettos, two Magic Flutes. It is an absurd state of affairs when two opera houses, both of whose finances are precarious, compete against each other.

Yet Covent Garden and Sadler's Wells could have complementary functions instead of competing, on the model of the Opera and the Opera Comique in Paris. As it is Covent Garden produces opera which would be far more suitable for the smaller house: notably Tales of Hoffman and Carmen. And Sadler's Wells stretches its resources by producing Don Giovanni, ignored by Covent Garden.

Sadler's Wells manages very creditably despite this. Its productions may sometimes be a little rough. But the company is enthusiastic – its spirits remain high even when the notes do not. Even the audience is more ready to unbend than at Covent Garden: applause comes more readily and cheerfully. Oddly enough, relatively few operas are tried out at Sadler's Wells. Thus it was Covent Garden which last year put on

Michael Tippett's Midsummer Marriage – an opera whose symbol-laden libretto (by the composer) destroys much of the musical effectiveness.

Now The Midsummer Marriage is in danger of fading out of Covent Garden repertory for lack of support. Yet at Sadler's Wells – a much smaller theatre with lower production costs – it could be given a much longer run at less risk. It might be sensible to use Sadler's Wells as a try-out theatre for new operas and new ideas in producing established ones. Experiments would be less costly there than at Covent Garden. And experiment is what the London opera scene most lacks.

3

A View from the Terrace

THE LISTENER
14 October 1965

The outside-right, his black hair slicked down and uncompromisingly parted down the middle, was short and stumpy with bandy legs like an overweight jockey. He had some difficulty in running at more than a stately trot. Occasionally, in a sudden illumination, his almost forgotten skill would flicker into life and the ball would float across to the goal menacingly and accurately. The outside-left, all curly hair and youthful enthusiasm, seemed intent only to break all Olympic sprinting records. In his frenzied dashes across the field the ball was an embarrassing encumbrance to be got rid of as quickly as possible to the jeers of the unadmiring crowd.

All this was twenty years ago when, as a schoolboy, I used to watch a struggling Third Division club in a small provincial town. Even now the names of the players stick in my memory. These days I patronize more aristocratic clubs in London, clubs whose players perform for their country and receive the final accolade of appearing in advertisements. The crowds are larger. The grounds are more grandiose. The football, undoubtedly, is far more skilled. But the excitement is missing. Of course I have changed. But so has the game of football. Its finances have changed. Its supporters have changed. Its players have changed. Its whole style has changed.

The key, perhaps, lies in the style. Twenty years ago football was a game, essentially if not exclusively, of individual skill. A good team would be like a combination of jazz soloists: the improvisations of its members blending together but never losing their individuality. Today the style of playing is more orchestral. There is a score: the team strategy laid down by the club manager. And the players are expected to subordinate their individual skills to it.

Much of the time, since a game involving twenty-two men who may lose their heads or tempers is even more subject to the laws of chance than a National Plan, the score is ignored or the music is played horribly offkey. But just occasionally, when everything goes right, when all the men run into the right positions at the right time, when the ball goes where it is meant to go instead of skidding off the grass at awkward angles, the effect can be as exhilarating as an orchestra launching into Beethoven's Ninth after the cacophony of tuning up.

For this is the paradox. At its best modern football provides a more satisfying spectacle when suddenly a pattern emerges from apparent chaos than the traditional game. But the traditional game was more consistently entertaining because it relied less on the ability of an entire team to achieve complete harmony and more on the ability of individuals to impose their own imprint on the game.

I don't want to push the contrast too far. Planning team tactics is not an invention of recent years: Arsenal owed their domination of the game in the nineteen-thirties to the adoption of a new defensive system. And there are still players today whose style of playing is unmistakably their own: for the memory of Tommy Lawton swivelling round with his back to the goal to shoot the ball into the net with insolent ease, I can trade the spectacle of Johnny Haynes's petulant disappointment when his team mates fail to anticipate the inward cunning of his passes. But the generalizations remain valid.

For the new style reflects new conditions. Players are no longer artisans, with wages corresponding to those of a skilled workman, whose highest ambition is to retire to manage a pub. They have become variety artists, with rewards to match, who have to submit to the demands of what is now an entertainment industry. Television has not only made football a national, rather than a local, spectacle. It has also helped to make the players the equivalent of the Tiller Girls – highly drilled, tightly disciplined performers.

The crowds tend to be smaller than in the past and less committed to their clubs. The expenses of the clubs tend to be higher. As a result the penalties of failure, and the rewards of success, are greater. Many clubs operate on the edge of bankruptcy. Managers often disappear overnight into some *oubliette* of football. While the spectators' expectancy is raised – by seeing international matches on television, for example – the difficulty of satisfying it is increasing. There is not an illimitable supply of football talent – and there will probably be even less in years to come as children from working class homes (the traditional source) find other ways of occupying their leisure hours than by kicking a ball around.

Britain's under-privileged areas, notably Scotland, now throw up a quite disproportionate amount of talent. And this source may well dry up with increasing prosperity.

If talent is in short supply, then most must be made of what is available. Hence the unrelenting search for new talent and the remorseless training. Boys are signed up by professional clubs before they have even left school. And a grinding training routine is imposed on the players in an attempt to make sure that they can run faster and longer than their rivals. The result has been to breed a new race of child prodigies. Some survive to become adult virtuosi. But very often their careers tend to be spectacular and short.

Moreover, the technical expertise of these child prodigies is often achieved at the expense of blunting their creative impulse. And football is, after all, a creative game – where the sudden, unexpected move, the spontaneous inspiration, can achieve more than any amount of planning. But today the game tends to be intolerant of eccentricity. For the point about eccentricity is its unpredictability. And how can managers afford unpredictability in their teams when it may mean giving away an unnecessary goal as well as scoring an unexpected one?

So when I look back nostalgically to the heroes of my school days what I am really regretting, probably, is the loss of a certain freedom: a tolerance of clumsiness and human failure, which is now increasingly missing from football. The tension nowadays is often extraneous to what is happening on the field and reflects, as often as not, the stresses of a big machine which has to succeed in buying success in the market if it is to survive. And while it is easy to identify with eleven men kicking a football about the field even when they are only playing for a lark on a Sunday afternoon in Regent's Park – to share in their exasperation when a pass goes astray, to join in the crowd's sigh of disappointment when a goal is missed – it is more difficult to have the same degree of empathy with eleven machine-turned athletes.

Even so, in one essential respect at any rate, the character of football does not change. The crowds, despite all the frustrations, still live in the expectation of that magical moment when everything goes right on the field, when the play suddenly seems to have been designed by some expert choreographer, and the ball goes into the net. Which is why, although we all think that things are not the same as they used to be, we are still to be found on the terraces come Saturday.

4

Chelsea Knock Down Ambitious Arsenal

THE OBSERVER
25 September 1966

Arsenal, a patchwork of reserves and new recruits, started out at Stamford Bridge yesterday as though determined to topple Chelsea from the top of the table. They played, if not with inspiration, at least with neat, unassuming efficiency. Within minutes they had scored.

While Chelsea were still in one of their moods of black introspection – trying to find themselves and their feet on the slippery grass – Arsenal sent a high ball into the penalty area. The Chelsea defence missed it and Addison nodded it into the net. It was a simple, pleasantly old-fashioned goal.

The man who sent the ball into Chelsea's penalty area was Ure, impeccably majestic in appearance but excessively mistake-prone at critical moments. Far from holding a rather fragile defence together, Arsenal's centre-half contributed to its disintegration as, slowly, the Chelsea attack found itself.

Teasing

Chelsea these days have, if anything, a superabundance of personalities. They are no longer the team of all-rounders trying to beat the record for

---

Chelsea – Bonetti; Kirkup, McCreadie; Hollins, Hinton, Harris (R); Boyle, Graham, Osgood, Cooke, Tampling.

Arsenal – Furnell; Simpson, Storey; McLintock, Ure, McGill; Coakley, Addison, Baldwin, Sammels, Walley.

19

perpetual motion. In Osgood and Cooke they have players who can tease opponents with ball and body, highly individualistic craftsmen.

Appropriately enough it was Osgood – a player I always think over-praised until I actually see him again – who scored first for Chelsea. After Cooke had appeared to lose himself in a maze of dribbling, the ball came to Osgood who, sidestepping a defender, sent it into the Arsenal goal with that ease which marks out a great player.

That was two-thirds of the way through the first half. Shortly before half-time an increasingly assertive Chelsea scored again. This time it was Tambling – the five-goal hero of Chelsea's win at Aston Villa last week – who scored after McCreadie had made one of his typically flamboyant forays into the Arsenal half.

In the second half with the sun sapping the players' energies, it was Arsenal who wilted – though occasionally even Ure appeared in attack in attempts to get his forwards going. And although Bonetti was forced to make some dramatic – if perilous – punching saves, Chelsea's supremacy was threatened only by their own arrogance.

It was Tambling – whose speed and relentless energy compensate for any lack of elegance – who scored Chelsea's goal, outpacing and out-witting Arsenal's defenders, by now in a state of jittery apprehension whenever they saw him. But it was Osgood who stuck in the memory – demoralising Arsenal's defence with his lazy body swerves and driving them to desperation: at one stage he disappeared under a Rugby-scrum pile of bodies.

Whether Chelsea will stay the course at the top of the table seems doubtful. They are still a team of fitful inspiration. But, at least, after all their domestic troubles, they are beginning to find themselves: to combine well-drilled efficiency with individual brilliance. As for Arsenal – one's heart goes out to their new manager.

5

Television

THE LISTENER
27 April 1967

The extent to which people are prepared to treat television as a public confessional is really quite extraordinary and, at times, even frightening. So, come to that, is television's readiness to exploit this particular human phenomenon. Watching *Whicker's World* (BBC-2, April 22) I found myself wondering just what obscure impulses had persuaded the six people taking part to talk about their marriages and divorces and precisely what the programme was trying to do. Wives talked about ex-husbands; husbands talked about ex-wives. All explained why they thought their marriages had broken down: some, like Elizabeth Jane Howard, with apparent detachment, and others, like Robin Douglas-Home, were bewildered and hurt.

It was, undeniably, gripping television. But it left me wondering whether this kind of psychological strip-tease is not far more distasteful – and perhaps even damaging – than the Soho variety. The exposure of human hurt when somebody breaks down crying in front of the cameras (as one of those interviewed in this programme did) seems far more stomach-turning than any exposure of human flesh. All the more so (and hence my comparison with strip-tease) since any psychological revelation on television is bound to be incomplete: five minutes of self-examination before the cameras, even with a shrewd interviewer like Alan Whicker, isn't going to peel away many layers of anybody's personality or get anywhere near the psychological core where the explanations for behaviour lie. The result is not a programme about a problem – divorce, in this case – but a new kind of peepshow: a circus with animals who have volunteered for the performance.

In defence of a programme like this, it can at least be said that it may help to break down traditional taboos. But not even this argument can be advanced in defence of last week's edition of *Man Alive* (BBC-2, April 19) – a programme which I always seem to see at its worst. *The Loved Ones* ostensibly set out to examine 'the British love of animals'. But in fact this theme turned out to be the excuse for showing us the pathology of deprivation: for using people who care obsessively about animals as fair-ground freaks for the viewers' entertainment. And a very mixed bunch they turned out to be: a twice-widowed woman with three dogs, a nineteen-year-old girl sharing her bed with a dog, a couple with thirty-four cats, and so on. Although John Percival, introducing the programme, tried hard to persuade us that he was investigating a general social phenomenon ('Vivisection is bigger news than starving children' in this country, he claimed with a fairground barker's exaggeration), all that he did in effect was to *expose* some personal neuroses.

Almost as remarkable as the readiness of so many people to confess their weaknesses in front of the cameras is the ability of others to conceal theirs. If anyone still believes the old myth that the camera exposes character, *Panorama* (BBC-1, April 17) should have exploded it with its interview of Jim Garrison – the New Orleans District Attorney who recently discovered the 'truth' about the Kennedy assassination. Asked whether this discovery had anything to do with his candidacy for higher office, Garrison replied, 'I would dislike myself if I started thinking how I'd profit' so convincingly that for fully half a second I found myself believing him. Handsome, unflappable, a master of the undisprovable assertion by innuendo, Garrison was a terrifyingly good TV performer. *Panorama* did its best to put him in the perspective of New Orleans politics and life – seedy, corrupt, violent – but Garrison's Galahad image proved remarkably untarnishable. So much for the ability of TV to 'show up' people.

The same edition of *Panorama* underlined the extent to which TV is taking over from the House of Commons as the forum for discussing the great issues of the day, by staging a debate on the Common Market between four Labour M.P.s A twenty-minute doubles match – Mayhew and Ashley *v.* Shinwell and Fletcher – it raised more issues than it had time to deal with properly. Even so, well worth staging if only for Mr. Shinwell's revelation of his reason for opposing entry: 'If I am going to be governed at all, I prefer to be governed by a British government – even a Tory one'.

After this, it was rather chastening to view the Common Market debate through the eyes of others in *Europa* (BBC-2, April 18) which showed a Danish TV film examining Britain's chances of entry. It did not dig very deeply; it used every visual cliché in the book – marching Guards and all. But it did raise awkward questions about whether the British people really want to go into Europe, if this actually means changing traditional ways of doing things. Difficult questions to answer – though if John Esmonde and Bob Larbey, the authors of the new comedy series *Room at the Bottom* (BBC-1, April 18), have their fingers anywhere near the pulse of industry, it's quite clear that Britain is not ready for entry into Europe. In this programme the class war is still being fought all out – with the workers, like an underground army, all out to beat the managers and in this particular episode succeeding with a mixture of fiddling and blackmail. A splendidly funny (though, one hopes, entirely inaccurate) picture of industrial anarchy, particularly notable for really good bad-taste jokes as when a coloured worker tells one of his mates who is afraid of being sacked: 'Don't worry, I can always get you a job on the buses'.

While *Room at the Bottom* went in for sly subversion, *A Brilliant Future Behind Him*, the Wednesday play by Thomas Clarke (BBC-1, April 19) tried a savage frontal assault. A journalist dealing in gossip and good-foodery writes a scandal-revealing paragraph about a politician, where-upon the political establishment seizes on his vulnerability both as a queer and an occasional dabbler in the milder form of drugs to have him framed, tried and convicted as a drug pusher and corrupter of youth. The journalist (acted by James Bree with just the right degree of shabby pathos) commits suicide. It would have been a convincing enough play about skulduggery in high places – though Mr Clarke ladles on sex interest as though it were icing for the cake – if it had not, quite deliber-ately, pointed up the similarities with the Stephen Ward case. This imme-diately raised what might be called the MacBird dilemma: either Mr Clarke meant his accusations to be taken seriously, and wanted us to believe that judges and policemen would deliberately join in a conspiracy, or he did not. If he did, he should have provided evidence. If he did not, then the whole exercise seems somewhat pointless. The whole Profumo affair – that moral Suez of the post-war period – showed society in a pretty disreputable light, with its mixture of hypocrisy, vindictiveness, and instant indignation. Which is why it needs a rather better play than Mr Clarke's to point the moral.

6

Soccer and Society

THE OBSERVER
28 January 1968

One of the more disconcerting experiences is suddenly to find oneself under the microscope: to discover that something one has been doing for years has overnight become a social problem. Here for years I have been going to watch football, happily booing players, shouting at referees, telling my neighbour on the terraces to stop talking nonsense, without once realising that I was contributing to that growing social menace: soccer hooliganism.

Now, however, I know better. I and the millions like me who make up the soccer crowds are the subjects of an inquiry into soccer hooliganism conducted by a Birmingham psychiatrist, Dr J. A. Harrington, and a 'multidisciplinary team.'

As their report points out, a football crowd – like any other crowd – is more than the sum of those making it up. A crowd is something new, with a personality of its own: –

'In the comforting anonymity of the terraces the young supporter finds relief from trying to be himself. No longer does he have to strive to be somebody. . . . The crowd makes him feel free of authority and other irksome social pressures that normally oppress him.'

Quite right. And this sense of being caught up in a tribal ritual – quite different from the more humdrum routine of work and family – isn't just limited to 'young supporter.' It is shared, I suspect, by everyone who watches football.

And it is here, I think, that Dr Harrington and his team have gone wrong: in under-playing the ritualistic element in football. Basically the crowd is *playing* at being savage, rather than indulging in atavistic sav-

25

agery. From the player rolling in agony on the ground (only to get up the next second to run about as fast as ever) to the spectator shouting insults at the opposing team, everybody is play-acting – and is seen to be play-acting – by everybody, that is, except Dr Harrington and his researchers.

There is, indeed, something exhilarating (if, perhaps, potentially dangerous) in finding oneself part of a crowd. As a society we are extremely short of tribal rituals. Coronations and State Funerals don't happen often enough, and in any case appeal mainly to the middle-aged and women. Pop concerts appeal mainly to the very young. For most of us, the opportunity to dip into a bath of shared emotion is very limited. Hence the appeal of soccer crowds.

But where Dr Harrington and his team go wrong is in arguing – as they tend to do – that violent partisanship, the chanting of slogans and all the rest of the paraphernalia of soccer has anything to do with hooliganism. Arguably (and since the whole report self-confessedly is only speculation, why not set one guess against another?) it is precisely this formalised partisanship which provides an outlet to emotions which might otherwise be expressed far more violently.

The report argues that 'there is some evidence that hooliganism may invade the home after the match. We have come across a few instances where wife-beating is said to be linked with a football game. If the local side loses a wife may fear her husband will return home the worse for drink and give her a thrashing to get rid of the anger he feels about the game.'

But if football provides an outlet for emotion why then try to have it both ways by arguing that it also *provokes* violence? Surely the only thing that is proved by the 'evidence' cited in the report is that some wife-beaters go to watch football. So, for that matter, do a lot of adulterers, income-tax dodgers, and criminals.

Unfortunately, this kind of intellectual confusion afflicts the report in a more important sense still. For what Dr Harrington and his team have conspicuously failed to show is that there is such a thing as the 'problem' of soccer hooliganism.

Of course there is hooliganism – though the authors tend to define it over-generously, to include the chanting of 'obscene' slogans, which, I would think has more to do with the generally permissive attitude towards language than with hooliganism. But then there always has, and the real question is whether it is on the increase.

Here the report, after having candidly admitted that the available facts and figures are extremely sketchy, goes on to assume that there has been such an increase. Here some intellectual referee should blow a loud blast on his whistle. Even if the number of prosecutions has gone up, does this mean an increase in the number of offences or a rise merely in the number of people caught? Is there more hooliganism or are we merely more sensitive than in the past? We can't be sure.

But the report's confusion goes deeper still. Even assuming that there is more hooliganism, this could mean one of two things. Either that soccer itself is a cause of hooliganism or that soccer simply provides the setting where hooliganism expresses itself.

Judging by the evidence offered in the report, the second explanation is by far the more convincing. Out of 497 cases of soccer hooliganism looked at by the team, 296 involved boys and youths with previous convictions. And most of the rest came from the kind of background which is usually assumed to produce delinquency: boys from the poorer parts of our cities in dead-end jobs. In this respect at least – as the report acknowledges, if only with a passing nod – there is no problem of soccer hooliganism. But there is a very real social problem.

So, perhaps, after all I can go back to watching football with a clear conscience – to participate in what the report calls that 'oceanic' feeling. Or can I? Or should I, as the report hints, be concerned that the modern trends in football – the tremendous financial stakes so often involved – are in fact putting a premium on violence?

I wasn't old enough to watch football 30 years ago, so I can't be sure. But there are some faintly alarming signs. A review of a book by Tommy Docherty (late manager of Chelsea, currently of Rotherham) cites the following passage: 'I told Kevan and Upton to harry Sunderland centre-half Charlie Hurley unmercifully, and manfully they carried out the task. From the kick-off Upton raced across and aimed a wild, hard tackle at Hurley, who had the ball. Poor Charlie went white. He wasn't used to this type of game.'

Maybe the only difference between the past and present is that, 30 years ago, managers didn't write books. Or maybe not. But I would like to know. And although like any self-respecting soccer fan I have been violently and unfairly partisan about the opposing side – in this case Dr Harrington and his team – I wouldn't at all dissent from their conclusion that more research is needed. But in the meantime don't let us worry ourselves into a tizzy over soccer hooliganism. Haven't we got enough problems already without inventing new ones?

Chelsea Cover Up Their Weak Spots

THE OBSERVER
1 September 1968

With Spurs trying to salvage a reputation dented by a lame start to the season and Chelsea trying to convince themselves that their advance to the top of the League table isn't an accident, it wasn't surprising that this match proved an even more frantically fought battle than usual.

Although the score-line accurately reflects the balance of the game, it could so easily have been four all or five all. It was a game of frenetic thrust and counter-thrust, of error and counter-error, rather than of thoughtful pattern making or tactical brilliance.

From the start, it was rather like Wimbledon: the crowds' heads swivelling from side to side as the play swung from end to end. Hardly had the game started than Baldwin just missed for Chelsea – one of the few occasions that Baldwin managed to elude the persistent Beal. Then it was the turn of Spurs: Jones fired over the goal after a muddle between the Chelsea defenders had cleared his path.

So it went on: fortunately too fast and furious to allow any reflections about the quality of the play. WHAM went the ball into the Spurs half – usually from the boot of Chelsea captain, Harris, who was as wild in his clearances as he was meticulous in his covering. BANG, it came back into the Chelsea half, usually from the dominating English. (The wham/bang language is irresistible: it was that kind of game.)

Disconcerted

With the Chelsea defenders covering up so neurotically that they were getting in each other's way, and with the Spurs defence rather too easily disconcerted, it was only a matter of time before the goals came.

After 24 minutes Birchenall, Chelsea's most persistent forward, snapped the ball into the net after it had run loose in the penalty area. Three minutes later Greaves took the opportunity presented to him by a tangled Chelsea defence. Coming from any other player, his acutely angled diagonal shot might have seemed like a happy mistake so finely calculated was it.

Then with half-time coming up, Beal either stomached the ball away from the Spurs goal (his own view, forcibly expressed) or fisted it away (the referee's view stoutly maintained despite pressure). After a sharp debate, the referee's view prevailed and Osgood scored from the penalty spot for Chelsea.

Finally, before either the crowd or the Chelsea defenders had settled down after the interval, Jones equalised for Spurs – Gilzean providing the crucial pass.

So much for the goals – almost incidental to a match spattered with incidents. There was Osgood, making his lunging runs from mid-field to pump the ball over the Spurs goal with such regularity that one began to assume that he was trying to hit some invisible target.

There was Chivers carving great holes in the Chelsea defence with his splendid acceleration. There was, above all, the frenzy and the desperately fast pace.

It was not that the players were lacking in skill. Indeed if they had not been so skilful, they could hardly have shown so many neat, controlled touches in this hectic atmosphere. But it was the kind of match where the Spurs backs were content at times just to kick wildly behind goal and where the Chelsea defence in one spell managed to push the ball three times in succession straight to a Spurs player.

Almost inevitably both the substitutes were required: Houseman replacing Tambling and Robertson coming on for Venables. Indeed, the main surprise at the end was that there were still 22 players on the field.

The risk of injury apart, there was at least one incident – a violent nursery tiff between Cooke and Kinnear – which suggested that the referee, Mr New, must be a man of exceptional charity and tolerance.

Left, Right & Other Stereotypes

ENCOUNTER
April 1969

The British tradition of political comment is one of sturdy, down-to-earth commonsense. Its practitioners, like their master Bagehot, tend to be wary of abstract ideas, rely for illumination on quarrying history for precedent rather than on principle, and are interested in what is possible rather than what is desirable. It is a complacent tradition. Its belief in the basic rightness of the British political system has been frayed but not destroyed by recent experience and its vocabulary belongs not so much to the world of intellectuals as to that of practical men of affairs.

Mr. Brittan, by contrast, is an intellectual. He is an economist who has ignored the demarcation rules – academic and journalistic – by writing about politics. When he sees that the Emperor is naked, he says so – instead of taking refuge in describing the processional route, the order of precedence among the courtiers and the intrigues that decided the date of the occasion. Moreover, he has the rare gift of indignation: rare in that those who write about politics professionally tend to take the pathological condition of their subject for granted.

Far from being the dispassionate intellectual looking at politics from somewhere on high in the clouds, Mr. Brittan is putting politics on the rack precisely because the system condemns the intellectual to playing the fool at the court of King Consensus: to being a half-comic, half-tragic figure on the margins of action, commenting on the proceedings rather than taking part in the drama. The book[1] is a cry of protest and is important

---

[1]*Left or Right: The Bogus Dilemma.* By Samuel Brittan. Secker & Warburg, 25s.

31

because Mr. Brittan's sense of exile is widely shared and equally widely resented.

The real starting-point of the book comes, I suspect, two-thirds of the way through. Here Mr. Brittan expatiates on the plight of what may be loosely called the classical liberal whose ideas cut across the symmetry of party politics. He is against the war in Viet Nam and in favour of libertarian social reform on matters like divorce and abortion: this brings him into line with the Labour Party. But he is also against paternalism in economic matters: this brings him into line with some Conservatives.

So the author (and Mr. Brittan, in this context, is something of an Everyman figure whose perplexities reflect those of a great many "liberal intellectuals") is forced to exist in a kind of political no-man's-land. He cannot identify wholeheartedly with either party, and indeed suspects organised parties as such because in the last resort they are based on authority rather than the free play of ideas; as a result he feels himself to be something of a political outsider:

> There are, for example, many gatherings attended by those interested in economic policy, from private parties to formal meetings, where there is a predominantly right or left-wing flavour in the room. The real embarrassment arises not for someone known to be on the other side, but for someone whose loyalty is felt to be uncertain or ambivalent.

It is a view which, as a political journalist without party allegiance and as someone who would probably agree with Mr. Brittan on most issues, I find only too easy to understand. But the temptation to adopt an anthropomorphic approach to politics, to evolve a political system designed to resolve one's personal moral or emotional dilemmas, is as dangerous as it is comprehensible.

Mr. Brittan, for his part, embraces the temptation joyously. For the aim of this book – an unconscious aim, no doubt – is to describe a political society fit for intellectuals to live in. (I hope this does not make him sound arrogant. On the contrary: his attitude seems to spring from the generous assumption that other people are as clever as he is.) While he has little difficulty in demonstrating the extent to which both politicians and those writing about politics are the prisoners of their own clichés, he is less successful in claiming conviction for his own alternative.

The book's central argument – which provides the title – is that the stereotypes of "Left" and "Right" are not only meaningless but positively damaging. To describe a man as belonging to the "Left" or to the "Right," Mr. Brittan argues, is to pin a label on him which provides little guidance as to his likely position on specific issues.

So far it is difficult to quarrel with the thesis. Every political journalist must be guiltily aware that he often uses "Left" and "Right" as a kind of lazy shorthand which may imply more to his readers than he actually intends – since he himself is usually conscious that this apparently neat classification can conceal a swarming horde of significant differences.

Again, Mr. Brittan's attempt to devise a new system of pigeon-holing is illuminating if not entirely convincing – though, to be fair, he himself doesn't claim that it is much more than an intellectual parlour game. Developing Professor H. J. Eysenck's ingenious scheme for classifying political attitudes by their *radicalism/conservatism*, on the one hand, and their *tender-mindedness/tough-mindedness*, on the other, he proposes a still more sophisticated system. Politicians, he suggests, should be classified by their leanings towards liberalism or authoritarianism, égalitarianism or élitism, radicalism or orthodoxy.

In lots of ways this is more illuminating than the conventional *Left/Right* classification. It brings out the finer shades. It shows that Harold Wilson and Edward Heath – though some way apart on égalitarian/élitist scale – have more in common with each other than they have with the extremists in their own parties – whether these be authoritarian-minded Marxists or authoritarian-minded Conservatives.

But it still isn't very satisfactory. Indeed as an instrument of prediction it is, in many ways, less satisfactory than the political correspondent's crude *Left/Right* classification. For example, in Mr. Brittan's system of classification, Roy Jenkins and Michael Foot appear to be first cousins as far as their attitudes are concerned. This is convincing up to a point, since on libertarian issues the two men tend to be on the same side. But it doesn't explain the fact that on a great many other issues dividing the Labour Party, they generally hold diametrically opposed views.

The weakness lies, I suspect, in the failure to cope with what may be the most significant dimension of all: the historical dimension. Even if two men share the same temperamental bias – even if they are both dedicated liberal, radical égalitarians – the expression of that bias is liable to be shaped by historical experience. Michael Foot is a man of the 1930s, just as Roy Jenkins is a man of the 1940s. Clearly someone whose views were shaped by the Spanish Civil War and mass unemployment is likely to behave differently from someone whose views were shaped by the Cold War and the problems of full employment.

But whatever the weakness of Mr. Brittan's own system – and he doesn't claim very much for it anyway – his main indictment remains: the accepted stereotypes of Left and Right have a distorting effect on the whole political system. Not only does this way of looking at politics, Mr. Brittan argues, encourage the easy, automatic dismissal of ideas simply because they are held by men at the extremes of the conventional spectrum. As a result, the intellectually soft-centred compromise views of the Centre are often accepted merely because they happen to fall between the extremes. But the *Left/Right* stereotypes encourage the parties to live up to them, to assume the roles which the words seem to imply for them. As a result, there is the frequently farcical pretence that policies themselves must conform to the stereotypes, that a policy is self-evidently wrong because it has come from the other end of the spectrum.

Once again there is a great deal in Mr. Brittan's indictment, but rather less than he claims for it – if one allows for the historical dimension. It's perfectly true that the Pavlovian reaction of political parties is, when an issue first comes up, to reject the view of the other side – or, for that matter, to reject the views of their own "extremists." Far too often policies are condemned not by argument but by pinning a *Left/Right* label on them.

But this, after all, is only the first reaction. What Mr. Brittan does not allow for is the gradual permeation of ideas. In practice, although immediate reactions may conform to the stereotypes – and may be influenced by them – long-term policies are not shaped by them to anything like the same extent.

To take only a couple of contemporary examples. The Labour Government, after recoiling with horror from the idea of "selectivity" in the social services, has in fact accepted it: the introduction of higher family allowances counter-balanced by lower tax allowances is at least a form of back-door selectivity. Equally it now looks as though the consensus of the Centre in favour of an incomes policy is being undermined by both the "Left" and the "Right."

Mr. Brittan, for his part, is contemptuous of such intellectual drift. Consensus, in his vocabulary, is almost a dirty word – a way of fudging issues and avoiding the need to face up to difficult decisions (*e.g.*, the front-bench consensus that devaluation was the ultimate betrayal). As he sees it, the Labour and Conservative Parties both exaggerate irrelevant differences between them and avoid argument about real issues:

> This reluctance to engage in general argument, combined with the issuing of shopping lists of unrelated policy points, has its roots in the two-party system and the mass electorate. Indeed it is a characteristic feature of duopoly in a market characterised by imperfect information. (Two rival department stores are more likely to be adjacent to each other in the High Street, rather than at opposite ends; and they are likely to copy each other's best-selling lines.)

The comparison is telling, and it's tempting to echo Mr. Brittan's conclusion: that the two-party system should be broken up and that there should be a more fluid political system – and leave it at that. It is certainly a view which has been encouraged by the failures, hypocrisies, and ritualistic battles of the present party system.

Unfortunately, Mr. Brittan is better at analysing weaknesses than at prescribing remedies. Some of these belong to the realm of wishful thinking: such as his hope for a crossbench coalition which would allow more freedom of voting to the ordinary M.P. (though he can quite legitimately reply that this is to fall into the political commentator's habit of dismissing the desirable simply because it is unlikely to happen – a sure-fire recipe for never advocating anything at all).

Some of Mr. Brittan's other prescriptions could be directly counter-productive: notably his sponsorship of the proposal for primary elections to choose parliamentary candidates. This assumes that the result would be to produce cross-party voting by the enlightened. In fact it is just as likely to produce cross-voting by the unenlightened. The evidence of the public opinion polls suggests that there is a permanent, all-party majority *against* the kind of libertarian social reforms which Mr. Brittan himself thinks desirable.

But these are only quibbles. The real objection to Mr. Brittan's approach cuts deeper. It is that he seeks to impose a subjective view of political rationality on a system shaped by historical and social forces which cannot just be dismissed simply because some of their consequences prove to be unpalatable.

Here the single most important fact is surely that, for the great majority of people, politics is a very marginal activity. The level of information of the average voter is abysmally low; so is the level of interest, elections apart. Moreover, this is a perfectly rational attitude (however patronising it may sound to spell the point out). For most people the cost of obtaining the extra information needed to cast an informed vote is not matched by any likely gain he can make – as Anthony Downs, another economist to have turned his attention to politics, argues in *An Economic Theory of Democracy* (Harper & Row, 1965).

To acknowledge this is also to acknowledge the "two-audiences" problem. There is the *élite* audience which, by and large, wants the kind of open dialogue which Mr. Brittan wants to promote; and is resentful of a basically paternalistic process of decision-making which often reflects inherited historical patterns. And there is the "mass electorate" which lacks the knowledge, sophistication and, in all probability, the desire to join in any kind of open-ended dialogue.

In the past the *élite* audience was, in a very real sense, part of the governing system – socially and educationally. The new phenomenon – which accounts for much of the current sense of dissatisfaction and the attacks on what used to be called "The Establishment" – is that of the extra-mural *élite*: the growing number of those who feel themselves, by right of their educational or professional status, entitled to a place among the governors but find themselves, instead, among the governed. Hence, perhaps, the vogue cry for more "participation" – essentially, I would guess, the aspiration of an expanding, frustrated *élite*.

It is obviously a perfectly legitimate aspiration which cannot be ignored. But the danger is that, in seeking to satisfy it, the requirements of a minority may be projected on to a majority which has quite different needs. To deny the faults of the party system would be foolish. But it has more virtues than its critics are prepared to concede. Party labels are, admittedly, a crude form of shorthand and can, at times, be positively misleading (as the history of the present Government has amply demonstrated). But, as I have suggested, the historical and social experience which has shaped the parties has also shaped the attitudes of voters. Hence there is a kind of rationality, though not Mr. Brittan's, in voting for parties because of their prejudices: for abjuring the free-play of intellectual argument in favour of settling for the animal you know and whose instincts you share. Paradoxically, too, the politics of the "stereotype" may even increase the scope for the kind of policies which Mr. Brittan favours: a great many Labour voters, for example, were in favour of the Suez enterprise – but accepted their party's opposition to it because the "stereotype" as a whole satisfied them.

For the minority of intellectuals (including some who would recoil from this description) the politics of the stereotype are distasteful. But they are not perhaps quite as damaging as Mr. Brittan implies, though it would be insufferably complacent to pretend that much of his criticism doesn't stick. Opinions and policies do change. They often change painfully slowly and sometimes too late. Indeed this is probably inevitable, given a profoundly conservative society. If the intellectual is condemned to be the fool at the court of King Consensus, he can at least console himself with the thought that he is an influential fool (at least in the long run). Mr. Brittan has certainly been influential in his role as an economic commentator. Perhaps he will be equally influential in his new role as a political commentator: for he has written a book which is always illuminating even if it is sometimes wrong-headed, and which should command respect for its generosity of mind even if its conclusions are rejected.

9

Ministering to Britain

COMMENTARY
February 1972

There are two basic stereotypes of politicians, with a great many variations on each. The first is what might be called the "politician-as-conspirator" stereotype: this sees politicians as pursuing deviously their own long-term ends, wirepullers and intriguers ruthlessly bending events and manipulating people to their own purposes. The second is the "politician-as-weathervane" stereotype: this sees politicians as men without principles, adjusting their policies to events, changing even their public personae to make them more acceptable to the voters, ready to abandon any long-term aims they may happen to have in order to maintain themselves in office. In the context of the United States, Lyndon Johnson would probably fit the first stereotype and Richard Nixon the second. In the British context, Harold Macmillan emphatically fits the first while Harold Wilson represents the second.

The recent publication of the fourth volume of Macmillan's "memoirs"* and of Wilson's "personal record" of his premiership† provides a good opportunity to examine how well such popular ideas about politicians, their style and motives, stand up. For certainly, to approach either of these two volumes with any hope of *historical* illumination would be to insure disappointment. Both books are examples of verbal inflation: too many words chasing too few goods. There are precious few "revelations." There is nothing which will cause us to look at past events in a new

---

Riding the Storm: 1956–1959, Harper & Row, 786 pp., $15.00.

†*A Personal Record: The Labour Government 1964–1970*, Atlantic-Little, Brown, 836 pp., $15.00.

light. There is, instead, a self-indulgent torrent of self-quotations from old speeches and a disregard of the reader's boredom threshold. As historical contributions these volumes provide footnotes for the specialists; as literary efforts they are non-events.

The two volumes do have a certain fascination as involuntary self-revelations: the psychoanalyst's case notes which provide new insights into the nature of politicians and, indeed, into the nature of the British political system. Macmillan, long since retired from active politics, is writing for posterity; Wilson, still active as the leader of the Labour party, is addressing the voters at the next general election. Macmillan's world is largely peopled by the dead: John Foster Dulles, Khrushchev, Adenauer; Wilson's world is that of those with whom he has to live, negotiate, and bargain.

As for our two basic images of politicians, Macmillan, as I noted above, seems type-cast as the devious conspirator-politician. When his book begins he is Chancellor of the Exchequer, with Eden still Prime Minister. When it ends Macmillan has been Prime Minister for more than two years, having successfully held together the Tory party in its retreat from Suez although he was among the most fervent and unrepentant advocates of this adventure in the first place. Chosen as leader of the Conservatives precisely because he appeared to be a traditional tough Tory – an anti-appeasement man in the 30's in contrast to his rival for the leadership, the elusive R. A. Butler – he completed the liquidation of the British Empire which had been started by Attlee's postwar Labour government. In this volume the process is only beginning but the trend is already clear, as Macmillan prepares to pull out of Cyprus and sheds the leading Tory diehard, Lord Salisbury, from his Cabinet. On the knowledge of Macmillan's past record as an enthusiastic European (the previous volume) and his future as an applicant for entry into the European Economic Community (the next volume, presumably), it seems reasonable to conclude that all his policies formed part of a grand design, and that when he was acting the traditional Tory statesman it was a charade carried out for the benefit of his party, a cynical exercise in deception calculated to give him greater freedom of maneouver.

This sort of explanation, though it is generally accepted and fits in well with the stereotype, does not to my mind survive a reading of the Macmillan memoirs. What really destroys the stereotype, as applied to Macmillan at any rate, are the unconscious revelations. These suggest that, while he was a ruthless politician and shrewd tactician, there was also a romantic side to his character, attracted by the chance to play the historical roles of British statesmanship. If he acted out what now appear to be political charades – notably the attempts to play the middleman between Washington and Moscow – it was because he enjoyed doing so and because he was able to suspend any disbelief about their efficacy (and, to be fair, they may well have had some marginal value).

In other words, Macmillan's memoirs underline that being a politician means playing what is often an inherited role – and that it is virtually impossible to act it out successfully in a spirit of cynicism; self-deception comes before the deception of others. Macmillan, in those days of reflected if ebbing Churchillian glory, behaved in the way a British Prime Minister was still expected to behave; this, rather than conscious play-acting, is the simplest and most convincing explanation.

But if Macmillan was a traditional romantic in his postures, he was also realistic enough to recognize a brick wall when he met it face to face. It was the romantic in him which made him an advocate of the Suez adventure to the point where he ignored the warning signals from Eisenhower and Dulles. (Interestingly enough, even now Macmillan considers that it was United States opposition which caused the failure of the expedition, rather than the unrealistic nature of his hope of being able to install a friendly, pro-Western regime in Egypt.) But it was the realist in him which caused him to liquidate the policy which had led to disaster. In many ways, this volume suggests that Macmillan was emotionally on the side of those diehard Tories who throughout the 50's bitterly fought the disengagement from imperial grandeur; intellectually, though, he knew that the policy did not make sense. It was this quality of imaginative sympathy, rather like a novelist thinking himself into the mind of one of his characters, which made him so successful a politician for so long, not the cynicism and calculation of the stereotype. Indeed, the Macmillan memoirs, despite their ponderous orotundity of style, suggest that one of the key qualifications of a successful politician is precisely a quickness of intuition, a readiness to imagine the hitherto unimaginable – for example, to consider, as Macmillan did when he became Chancellor of the Exchequer but as Wilson refused to do when he became Prime Minister, devaluing or even floating the pound.

Wilson conveniently provides a counterpoint to Macmillan. Although he reputedly modeled himself on the Tory master-tactician, as he saw him, Wilson seems much nearer to the "politician-as-weathervane" stereotype: a model of the politician who, lacking convictions of his own, is prepared to trim his sail to whatever wind happens to be prevailing, concerned only to keep himself in office. The record of the Labour government from 1964 to 1970 – the subject of his book – is the story of policies abandoned and reversed: of the long struggle to defend the pound which ends in devaluation, of the determined attempt to maintain Britain's East of Suez position which ends in withdrawal, of the dream to keep on playing a world role which ends in the application to join the European Community. While Macmillan appeared to be leading his party, Wilson seemed to be led only by events.

This view of Wilson is certainly more convincing than the picture of him – widely accepted in 1964 but destroyed by his actual performance in office – as the archetypal political tactician: unlikable perhaps and certainly not to be compared to Hugh Gaitskell with his moral commitment to policies, but to be admired, if only reluctantly, for his adroitness and dedication to survival. In the event, Wilson turned out to be not Mephistopheles but Micawber, not so much the unscrupulous schemer as the euphoric optimist. Wilson's record (the "memoirs" for the period are presumably reserved for a later date) does, on the whole, fit the weathervane stereotype reasonably well – with one very important reservation, however. The stereotype assumes that politicians who act without principles necessarily have none; the Wilson volume suggests that an apparently shiftless drift from expedient to expedient is perfectly compatible with what seems to be a genuine, even a deep-rooted, attachment to principles.

Looking at the events chronicled by Wilson himself, one gets the impression more of excessive stubbornness than of excessive suppleness. The reversals of the Labour government's policies tended to be violent precisely because Wilson was reluctant to modify or abandon them until left no option by events. Wilson was weak precisely where Macmillan was strong: the apparently down-to-earth, commonsensical, numerate Labour politician – with his elaborately constructed public facade as the first British Prime Minister with his feet firmly in the age of technology (this was before technology got a bad name for itself) – turns out, on inspection, to have had a less firm grasp of reality than the apparently anachronistic Tory leader whose manners and style often seemed to be a deliberately theatrical parody of the Edwardian.

Again, the crucial element in Wilson's performance as Prime Minister seems to have been his own private vision of himself in this role. Macmillan, as I have argued, saw himself still in the Churchillian mould – which is why he carried so much conviction even while he was reversing the historic policies which he had inherited together with his role. Wilson, I suspect after reading his book, was concerned primarily to establish himself as a moral figure: the man of principle, the inheritor of the Labour tradition based on an ideology of doing good. It was a role which perhaps he pursued with all the more energy because of its being suspect in the first place; it was as though he were, if only unconsciously, trying to live down his reputation as the man who had refused to stand up and be counted while Hugh Gaitskell successfully fought and fought again to prevent the Labour party from going neutralist. His career as Prime Minister suggests that no politician is more stubbornly attached to his principles than the one who is publicly suspected of having too few.

This sort of psychological overcompensation mechanism helps to explain a lot about Wilson, and perhaps also about other politicians. For example in this book Wilson tries to present his commitment to defend the parity of the pound as a practical, not a moral, decision; this is not convincing to anyone who remembers the emotion with which he used to denounce those of us who dared to use the word devaluation in print at a time when a change in the parity would have saved years of deflation, stagnation, and rising unemployment. Precisely because of this moral, emotional investment in the pound as a symbol of financial integrity and virtue, devaluation happened at the worst possible moment – when it was forced on Wilson by events, and there was no alternative. In all this, Wilson certainly showed himself a man of high principle who put country before party in his own view of things: after all, his policy probably cost Labour the 1970 election. Unfortunately he also showed himself a disastrous Prime Minister because – unlike Macmillan – he proved to be an insensitive politician who did not recognize the signals warning him to change direction.

A recurring theme throughout his volume is the emphasis on the unexpected event which somehow robs Wilson of the credit which his intentions ought to have won him. Domestically there is the stress on the various strikes which weakened the pound and therefore helped to defeat Wilson's economic strategy; in Britain, at any rate, this is rather like complaining that the climate prevents tropical fruit from being grown. Abroad, there is the lament that he was betrayed by the hawks in the Johnson administration in February 1967 when on the point of successfully negotiating a formula with Kosygin in London which would have allowed the start of negotiations between the United States and North Vietnam (though no recognition, despite subsequent events, that getting negotiations going is a pretty meaningless and futile exercise while there is not a shadow of agreement as to the possible outlines of a settlement).

So, once again, a stereotype needs revision. Like the politician as devious conspirator, so the politician as weathervane is not a psychologically convincing type. It lacks shade and subtlety. For to think in terms of such crude caricatures – implicit in many current attitudes toward politicians which tend to range from tired cynicism to brutal contempt – is to forget that even politicians have mirrors. It may be the mirror of their own personal code, in which they have been brought up. It may be the mirror of their own parties or friends. It may be the mirror of the media, press, and television. Whatever it is – and whether one tries to explain it in terms of reference groups or role playing, as the psychologists and sociologists might – the very distortions and inaccuracies of political memoirs and records are a tribute to its existence. The way in which politicians try to justify their actions is significant precisely because it reveals what their own ideals are – an attempt to fit events into the patterns of what they would have liked to do instead of what they actually did. Thus the ideal Prime Minister of the Tory Macmillan – implicit in his account of his own actions – is a very different sort of political animal from the ideal Prime Minister of the Labour Wilson.

The Wilson self-portrayal is a reminder that political parties of the Left tend to be parties of morality: that some of the Labour party's roots, for example, go back to the Levellers and other Puritan sects of the 17th century. As a result, lurking invisibly but omnipresently in the book is the specter of the ideal Labour leader – something of a Calvinistic Old Testament character, strong on good works, hard on moral lapses, intolerant of slackness. Hence perhaps the curiously defensive character of *A Personal Record*, the constant emphasis on how hard Wilson tried and worked, the endlessly boring chronicles of ceaseless activity. This need for self-justification may, of course, simply reflect the fact that the book was written in the wake of an election defeat, or some personal psychological quirk peculiar to Wilson. I suspect, though, that it is also indicative of the attitude of left-wing parties toward their leaders, who are made to feel perpetually on trial and assumed to be corrupt unless they prove the contrary by their actions (leading logically to the Chinese habit of public self-confession).

Right-wing parties, on the other hand, at least of the moderate, non-ideological sort represented by the British Tories, expect their leaders to be successful rather than morally spotless, if Macmillan's memoirs are anything to go by. The memoirs suggest a relaxed sense of superiority, as well they might given Macmillan's astonishing political achievement in pulling together a dispirited and disunited party after Suez and leading it to a triumphant election victory in 1959. Unlike Wilson, he does not fight a retrospective running battle with his newspaper critics, nor does he conduct long inquests on his own failures in order to secure a verdict of "not guilty." There is a deliberate if deceptive air of patrician nonchalance about the writing. It is deceptive in a double sense, because Macmillan is no patrician (though he married into the dukeries) and because in practice he was anything but nonchalant in his style of running his government. For instance, he was far more ruthless in getting rid of ministers than Wilson; those who disagreed with his policies, as his memoirs show, went down the political oubliette.

These books do more, however, than illuminate the differences between the British political parties and the personalities of their authors. They are also revealing about the problems involved in exercising political power. This is particularly true of Wilson's book. It is interesting in this respect precisely because of its stylistic ingenuousness. Unlike Macmillan, who chops up his material into chapters each of which deals with a specific issue, Wilson's account of his premiership is strictly chronological – day by day, hour by hour. As a result, it gives a vivid sense of a political leader besieged by events, with important international occurrences taking their place in the same queue as the small change of party political disputes. And although this sort of timetable makes the book dreary reading it also makes it one of the best case-studies ever written of the pathology of power, of the incredible physical and psychological pressures which events can impose on politicians, and of the consequent need for an effective filtering system to distinguish the key messages coming in from mere background noise. (This, in turn, points to the difficult question of who should control the filtering process – and the importance of those chosen by the political executive to select the key messages on his behalf.)

Given Wilson's obsessive memory, the omissions from his book are all the more interesting. They suggest that for a politician, the capacity to forget may be almost as important as the ability to remember: that if he cannot reinterpret events to his own satisfaction, he must diminish their importance to the vanishing point. The politician cannot afford to have the pea of intellectual self-doubt under his mattress. Characteristically Wilson dismisses Britain's once famous National Plan in a brief half-page; no one reading this book would realize that the Plan was the centrepiece of the Wilson government's economic strategy – an attempt to emulate French-style planning which, it was hoped and promised, would introduce an era of smoothly accelerating economic expansion.

Equally these books suggest that politicians develop another psychological defense strategy: this is to narrow their interests (always assuming, of course, that they are not successful politicians precisely because of a monomaniacal interest in politics). The years covered by the two memoirs were an exceptionally interesting period in Britain's history, and not just because the country was trying to find a new international role, indeed almost a new national identity. Behind the crises of imperial disengagement, behind the crises of economic readjustment – faithfully recorded by the two ex-Prime Ministers – the country was undergoing rapid social and cultural changes. While politically the Macmillan-Wilson generations were still in power, culturally a much younger generation was taking over. In turn, there was a shift in public morality reflected in changes in public policy. Of this, there is hardly any hint in these memoirs. Macmillan openly shrinks from the subject, while Wilson simply omits any mention of what was after all one of the great achievements presided over by his government. Between 1964 and 1970, homosexual conduct between consenting adults in private was legalized, the divorce laws were liberalized, and publicly-regulated abortion was introduced. So anxious throughout his book to salvage credit even from disaster, Wilson refuses to take it in this instance. Is it that he thinks there are no votes to be gained from this kind of issue? Or is it because he himself is just not concerned, or even hostile?

Conceivably the stylistic coarseness of these two books – the reach-me-down 19th-century style of Macmillan and the computer prose of Wilson – reflects a coarsening of the perceptions in a more general way. The intriguing question is whether this kind of coarsening is the occupational hazard of politicians, or whether there is some process of natural selection whereby only those capable of taking a one-eyed view of life come to the top. Macmillan's story suggests the first explanation: enough hints of a once-sensitive intellectual come through to suggest that he was at least partly stunted by his environment. Wilson's book suggests the latter explanation: of a man who in politics has found his natural, inescapable vocation.

10

Crumbling the Barricades

COMMENTARY
August 1972

A specter is haunting the world – the specter of failed socialism. In the century and a quarter since Karl Marx wrote the words parodied in that sentence, as the opening of the Manifesto of the Communist party, socialism has attracted the idealism of millions and provided rallying cries for countless political movements. Even those who have betrayed it most brutally – Stalin, Hitler, Mussolini, among many others – have usually done so in its name. All that is missing is an example of socialism, uncontaminated by totalitarianism, actually working. There are plenty of examples of collectivist dictatorships and well-intentioned social-reform movements. But socialism – a system which, in the eyes of its disciples, seeks to reconcile the requirements of democracy, social justice, and liberty and to create a society in which men and women respect each other in their diversity and develop, at work or at leisure, their full potentialities – remains a secular vision: respected by all, adopted by none.

The attraction of Michael Harrington's book* is that he is a socialist who is clear-eyed and honest about this predicament. He does not fall into the trap of wish-fulfillment – of hailing the latest hero-figure of the Left, whether he be Castro or Mao Tse-tung, as the Moses who has led his country into the promised land of socialism and so set an example to the rest of the world. Equally he is sceptical about the tactics of the Western European social-democratic parties: he argues that the welfare-

---

*Socialism, Saturday Review Press, 436 pp., \$12.50.

state policies of the European Left, whether of Harold Wilson's Labour party in Britain or of Willy Brandt's Social Democrats in West Germany, have failed to deliver the goods of socialism – and that the distribution of wealth and power in these countries has not greatly changed.

So in this book Harrington goes back to the drawing board in an attempt to design a doctrine of socialism relevant to what Daniel Bell has called post-industrial society. Rejecting both what he regards as the ineffective reformism of traditional liberalism and the utopian anarchism of New-Left revolutionaries, he tries to present an alternative analysis. The starting point of this analysis is Marx. But it is what might be called the "real-Marx" as distinct from the "pseudo-Marx" – that is, Harrington's own interpretation of Marx's writing, not the popular, simplified version of Marxism. In line with recent fashions in Marxology, the emphasis is put on Marx the humanist as distinct from Marx the revolutionary authoritarian – the Marx who had a vision of man emancipated from the tyranny of machine-dictated work routines, fulfilling himself as a complete human being instead of being frustrated by the social superstructure of a capitalist economy.

This is a perfectly fair, if not exactly novel, reinterpretation. However, in historical reinterpretation as in picture restoration, there is always the danger that in removing the old varnish and overpainting done by other hands, the restorer may also remove some of the original as well. So, since Harrington himself attaches much importance to his version of the "real Marx" and devotes a large section of the book to this theme, it is worth looking at the restorer's technique in some detail. Take the question of Marx's attitude toward democracy, which is crucial, as I shall argue later, to the whole question of the role of socialism today. Harrington justly points out that the much-quoted, notorious phrase about the "dictatorship of the proletariat" is usually taken out of context. It should be seen, he argues, in the wider context of Marx's general attitude toward democracy. Thus he quotes Marx writing approvingly of the 1870 Paris Commune and in particular its introduction of universal suffrage for the election of officials, who were also subject to immediate recall by the people. From this Harrington concludes that dictatorship for Marx "does not mean dictatorship but the fulfillment of democracy."

But does it? And if it does, is not the implication that Marx's idea of democracy may have been rather special? For Harrington's argument cuts a lot of corners. In the first place the unsuspecting reader may assume from Harrington's interpretation that Marx approved of the Commune. He did not. He thought it was (to quote Isaiah Berlin's classic biography) "a political blunder." It was dominated by the various left-wing revolutionary sects for whom Marx reserved his very special hatred and contempt: those whom he once described as the advocates of "mutton-headed, sentimental, utopian socialism." However, he gave the Commune his blessing because it gave the international socialist movement its heroic martyrs: fodder for the propaganda machine. Secondly, it is not at all clear what either Marx or Harrington understands by "democracy." I suspect that in fact – all honour to Harrington – their definitions would have very little in common. For Marx and the Commune must be seen in their historical perspective: the perspective of Rousseau and the French Revolution, the intellectual and historical influences which did so much to mould 19th-century socialist thinking.

Rousseau disliked the word democracy and thought the ideal unattainable. The ideologues of the French Revolution, the link in the intellectual chain between Rousseau and the Communards, believed not in democracy but in the will of the people. This almost mystical concept could be used – as J. L. Talmon has shown in his *The Origins of Totalitarian Democracy* – to justify almost any act of crowd tyranny or the dictatorship of an elite claiming to speak for the collective mind. It is a concept which is the antithesis of democracy if by democracy we mean (among other things) the toleration of dissent and respect for minority opinions. For to tolerate dissent is to betray the general will (or the party).

In other respects, too, Harrington does not explore sufficiently the complexities and contradictions of Marx. The popular picture of Marx as the man who claimed to have discovered the "iron laws" of history may be an oversimplification. But to underplay this element is an equally misleading oversimplification. For psychologically, surely, Marx's appeal largely rests on his identification of the desirable with the inevitable. This goes a long way toward explaining Marx's reputation among the millions who have never read a word of him. Others may have had equally subtle and rewarding insights into social processes, but no one else used those insights with such force and imagination as the basis of a secular prophecy. Indeed, there is considerable evidence to suggest that this was Marx's view of himself: for example, he wanted to dedicate *Das Kapital* to Darwin – the man who had discovered the law of revolution paying homage to the man who had discovered the law of evolution.

Although Harrington rightly points out that Marx gave much greater emphasis to human freedom than the popular version of his doctrine would suggest, he ignores the other side of Marx, which was the authoritarian welder of a revolutionary movement. The early history of the International is largely the history of Marx's complete intolerance of disagreement; like Freud, he had no time for disciples who strayed. His concern was to build an effective instrument of revolution, not a debating society for educating the masses – which is what I suspect Harrington, as a gentle and humane man, would like. If democracy means a willingness to put up with dissent, Marx was not a democrat.

Harrington's attempt to reinterpret Marx is an essential part of a more ambitious exercise still: to square the ideals of humane liberalism with those of traditional socialism. It is a courageous attempt which, I think, in the end fails, just as his attempt to redraw the portrait of Marx is not convincing, despite many shrewd touches.

For what, after all, distinguishes liberalism from socialism? On the whole it is not their ideals. Most liberals and socialists would probably find little difficulty in agreeing on a common platform of general aims. To a large extent they draw on a shared vocabulary – social justice, racial equality, and all the rest. It is this which has so often made it easy for dictatorships of the Left to appeal to the more unsuspecting liberals. The difficulties come, and the splits appear, when rhetoric has to be translated into action. There may be conflicts among different aims, all desirable in themselves: the redistribution of wealth may be highly desirable on grounds of social equity but undesirable inasmuch as it limits individual liberty. Equally, there may be cases where the means chosen – the actual programme adopted – may threaten some of the ends, and liberals may then part company from socialists.

The weakness of Harrington's book is that his argument tends to peter out before reaching this crucial point. Take the example, much stressed by Harrington himself, of the power exercised by private corporations. Harrington makes a twofold indictment of this power. First, he cites the example of Britain and other European countries to argue that corporate power is used to block effective measures to redistribute wealth and eliminate poverty. This argument, when applied to Britain, is certainly an oversimplification, if not without some basis in fact; the failure of Wilson's Labour government was caused predominantly, though not exclusively, by its ineptitude in handling economic policy. To argue that it was the power of the bankers which sabotaged the Wilson administration, as Harrington comes close to doing, is to invite the counterargument that it is the trade unions who are sabotaging the Conservative government of Edward Heath which is now being forced to abandon Tory policies quite as much as Wilson was obliged to abandon socialist policies; the balance of power is perhaps not quite as one-sided as Harrington's argument requires. Second, Harrington rightly stresses the social implications of business decisions. He argues, quite fairly, that the slogans about market forces insuring freedom of choice are empty rhetoric in that these forces may block as many choices as they open up: my freedom of choice is diminished, for example, when my favorite brand of biscuits is taken off the market.

From this double-pronged argument, Harrington concludes that the European social democrats have been wrong to abandon their traditional emphasis on the social ownership of industry. And he puts forward instead a program for socializing industry by taking over control – though the liberal in Harrington insists that this socialist aim can be achieved gradually and painlessly, for instance by introducing inheritance taxes. The trouble is that if Harrington is correct in putting so much emphasis on the power of the corporations, then surely the conventional Communist emphasis on revolutionary tactics must be right as well. If the European social democrats are wrong in believing that the aims of socialism can be achieved without changing the power structure of society (as Harrington thinks), then why assume that the power structure itself can be changed with the consent of those who are currently in control of it?

As so often happens, Harrington here is betrayed by his own niceness. He is a revolutionary who believes in good will. But he really cannot have it both ways. If those wielding power in Western capitalist societies can be persuaded to give up that power – and this is what Harrington's scheme for more social ownership implies – then presumably they could more easily be persuaded into accepting the less painful measures involved in a programme of social engineering. Even income redistribution is less threatening than property redistribution. However, Harrington is pessimistic about the chances of successfully carrying out such a programme of social engineering – despite his diagnosis of an emerging social-democratic mass movement, represented by social-reform-conscious trade-unionism, in the United States. So it is all the odder that he should be hopeful about his own, far more radical programme of political action. Indeed it is difficult to take Harrington seriously as an analyst of the political situation. Either he ought to be urging the people to storm the barricades of privilege and power, or he ought to rally to those who, despite defeats and disappointments, pursue the tactics of gradual melioration. As it is, Harrington gives the impression of a man who hopes that the barricades will gently crumble away under the pressure of his eloquence and the faith of the masses. He is too much of a liberal to urge revolutionary tactics and too much of a socialist to settle for liberal-reformist policies.

Again, it is worth being pedantic on some points of detail. For there is a danger that Harrington's book may reinforce the legend that the welfare-state tactics of gradual social improvement have failed. This is certainly not true of Western Europe, from which Harrington himself takes most of his examples. It is true that welfare state policies have admittedly failed – as in Britain, frequently mentioned in the book – to *eliminate* poverty, slums, and inequality. But it is the successes of the welfare state which have largely sensitized us to these failures: every advance reveals new requirements of social action which in the past would have been ignored because far more rampant evils were claiming our attention. One might even argue that one of the characteristics of a welfare-state society should be a permanent state of dissatisfaction and a continual search for improvement in social conditions – by constantly raising standards it will always fall short of its own expectations – and paradoxically, this will provide ammunition for those who want to argue that the entire approach has failed. Harrington's argument also assumes that we know how to deal with social problems, that our failures are those of will, not of comprehension. In many areas of social action, this is simply not true; we often create new social diseases in our attempts to deal with old ones. The failures of urban renewal cited by Harrington are often the result not of a lack of social planning but of planners' *hubris*: the assumption that we are in a position to calculate the consequences of all our actions.

To be fair, Harrington fully recognizes the fallacy of equating social planning with bureaucratic planning. He is aware that bringing industries into state ownership may simply mean the emergence of a more powerful bureaucracy. But, as so often in this book, after having defined difficulties with precision, he relies for their solution on verbal incantation. What does social control and social planning mean in practice? What social criteria are to be applied, and by whom? A brief reference to "cooperative and neighborhood forms of ownership" hardly answers questions like these. It is pretty clear that Harrington is as flummoxed as the rest of us when it comes to giving precise, specific meaning to the rhetoric of good intentions, and is original chiefly in his optimism.

The British experience suggests that it is easier to place industries under social ownership than to run them on any principle of social accountability. As Harrington points out in a pained sort of way, the Labour government's renationalization of steel "left many of the previous managers in control of the public enterprise." Why the surprise? Given the increasing technical complexity of industry, rightly stressed by Harrington in another context, it is precisely the "previous managers" who have the required know-how – even when the nominal exploiters, the stockholders, have been expropriated, to use the Marxist jargon. The problem of accountability has exercised a number of committees of the British Parliament. The result is a shelf of reports and a series of unanswered questions. But the main conclusion, paradoxically, has been that the best form of social accountability is financial discipline: the rate of return on investment and similar capitalist indices of performance. Although Harrington advocates moving toward a moneyless economy – and is scornful of economists who insist on the importance of costs – the British experience points in the opposite direction. It is easy enough to provide some services – like health – free of charge. However, as was pointed out by Aneurin Bevan, one of the great figures of the British Labour party's left wing, priorities are the language of socialism. And determining priorities in turn means measuring the cost of alternatives. Even though Harrington sees socialism as the outcome of economic growth rather than as its cause – indeed for Harrington socialism is made possible only by affluence – it seems unlikely that any society, however prosperous, can shrug aside this sort of problem.

To talk about priorities is also to admit that there may be conflict about aims. Different groups in a society may have different demands. Somehow any social system – capitalist or socialist – has to address itself to the resolution of conflict. One man's gain in freedom may be another man's loss of liberty. Further, a balance has to be struck between what Isaiah Berlin has called negative and positive liberty; very crudely put, this means freedom from interference (the ability to do one's own thing) on the one hand and freedom to carry out certain activities (which may require publicly-provided facilities) on the other. Issues like these are absolutely crucial to any discussion of what social control means in practice, but they are left untouched by Harrington. Perhaps his assumption is that conflict is a product of capitalism, which is certainly the traditional Marxist doctrine. But this is overly simple. Take the issue of a factory which is polluting the atmosphere and rivers, an example of market forces imposing extra social costs on the community. This seems a clear-cut case for limiting the freedom of the factory owner in the interests of the freedom of the community as a whole. But what if the result of curbing this freedom to pollute is to increase the cost of the product – and the product is consumed by only one group in the community? Again, a classic clash of freedoms is involved in the current American debate over school busing: how far is the freedom of whites to be curbed in the interest of extending the freedom of blacks?

Harrington's implicit assumption in neglecting this whole area – the crucial area of political institutions and choice – seems to be that socialism in itself eradicates conflict and produces a harmonious community of interests, a latter-day version of Rousseau's general will. And it is at this point that liberals will probably part company with Harrington – despite the generous humanity of his vision. He has succeeded in demonstrating yet again that even modified capitalist societies are far from eradicating freedom from hunger, social and cultural deprivation, and a sense of powerlessness in the face of technological complexity. But he has not demonstrated, what is indeed far more difficult to demonstrate, that his brand of affluent socialism can bring all the advantages of collectivism and none of its disadvantages. The dilemma of the liberal reformer who may well share Harrington's indignation about present evils but who cannot relax on his featherbed of optimism about a socialist future remains unsolved; the prospect still seems to be that of a dogged, long-drawn-out campaign of change – less enticing than Harrington's leap but more realistic.

11

Orthodox Unconventionality

COMMENTARY
January 1974

Success must be very frustrating for Professor Galbraith. He has now spent a lifetime attacking the "conventional wisdom" of society, criticizing his fellow economists for clinging to outmoded ideas, and advocating a variety of heterodox policies. He has done so with wit, elegance, and passion. But what happens? He ends up not as a prophet in the wilderness but as the pet intellectual of the mass media. His fellow citizens send him abroad to represent their country. His fellow economists elect him as the president of their association. His ideas about changing the balance between private consumption and public investment have become everyday slogans of political discourse.

For someone who appears to pride himself on being unorthodox, who takes so much pleasure in trying to shock his audience, this must be a disconcerting experience. And much of the interest of Galbraith's latest book* lies in the stratagems he adopts to meet the challenge of success and acceptance.

The starting point of Galbraith's argument, following on *The Affluent Society* and *The New Industrial State*, is that any resemblance between the traditional market model of the economy and reality is coincidental. Far from the consumer calling the tune, decisions are made by the "technostructure" of managers, technocrats, and bureaucrats straddling the worlds of the big corporations and government. This technostructure is primarily interested not in maximizing profits but in maximizing its own

---

Economics and the Public Purpose, Houghton Mifflin, 334 pp., $10.

security and growth. To this end, it plans its own progress by limiting competition, by manipulating the consumer through advertising, and by harnessing the expenditures and policies of government to its own ends.

Much of this is familiar, if only because it repeats what Galbraith has been writing over the years. How, then, can it be given a gloss of unorthodoxy? The answer is by presenting Galbraith's fellow economists as a band of fuddy-duddies – subscribing to the "neoclassical model" of the economy, worshipers at the shrine of Adam Smith and other false prophets, so deluded by their theories that they cannot see what goes on in the world around them, and consequently indoctrinating their students with at best irrelevant, at worst damaging, notions.

Galbraith's fellow economists can, no doubt, take care of themselves. If his picture of them is a caricature, they are capable of saying so. More serious is the price Galbraith pays for his insistence on distinguishing his own views from the professional consensus (although he does admit that a few converts have gathered around him). This leads him to adopt an inflationary verbal rhetoric of exaggeration: just as in Gresham's law bad money drives out the good, so in Galbraith's case the exaggerated arguments drive out the good ones.

Take, for example, his central argument that in the planning system the power of the producer has replaced the power of the consumer. In a weak form, this argument would command widespread agreement: Galbraith's point that employers and trade unions share a common interest in raising wages and prices, rather than adjusting both to consumer demand as the classic model demands, has been given added point by the inflation of the past year. But he is not satisfied to argue, with the majority of economists, that the traditional model is imperfect. He wants to demonstrate that it is irrelevant. And that involves him in some curious verbal slitherings.

Galbraith's argument demands that the consumer be presented as the passive victim of the planning system. At one point we read that the "admirable vision of the ultimate power of the user cannot be sustained, however, if his tastes and needs fall under the authority of the producer." But a few lines later this thundering phrase appears in a minor key, and becomes "a measure of authority." Subsequently, there are further variations still, with producers having "effective power over the users," "the power to influence the individual consumer," "the power to manage the individual consumer," and so on. Later Galbraith concedes that the process of consumer management by producers is imperfect and incomplete. But if it is, and if for "authority" and "power" it is better to read influence and persuasion, what is left of Galbraith's model? Classic economic theory is held up to ridicule by him for holding that the consumer is sovereign. But why, then, should we accept Galbraith's antimodel of producer sovereignty? Why substitute one inadequate model for another?

In any case, Galbraith himself now clearly realizes that this is an incomplete picture. So in this book he introduces and develops a further idea: that alongside the planned system of the technostructure, there exists also a market economy – "the world of the farmer, repairman, retailer, small manufacturer, plumber, television repairman, service-station operator, medical practitioner, artist, actress, photographer, and pornographer." This fragmented market economy is, in Galbraith's view, where the traditional model of cut-throat competition still applies, with the consumer dictating to the producer. As a result, he argues, the market economy is exploited by the planning system. This exploitation is all the worse for often being self-induced: the farmer and his family, and the others, are so deluded by the work ethic – such slaves to the conventional wisdom of society – that they voluntarily work longer hours for smaller rewards than do those employed in the planning system.

Obviously, there is an implicit contradiction between this theme and Galbraith's insistence, when discussing the planning system, that the consumer is a sort of idiot child. If the consumer is so manipulable by the technostructure, why does he become the conventional figure of the economic textbooks in pursuit of his own self-interest when he deals with a repairman or shopkeeper? Galbraith's answer would seem to be that the big corporations can spend millions brainwashing the public while small firms cannot. To this, though, there is a very simple reply, if one adopts one of Galbraith's own strategies for dealing with inconvenient criticisms and for giving an appearance of bold unorthodoxy: this is that Galbraith himself has been brainwashed by Madison Avenue's claims for its own products – advertising. For one of his most irritating habits is to present himself as the one man who sees the truth behind appearances – who can distinguish (like the Marxists) between false and real consciousness or (like the Freudians) between rationalizations and real motives. If one disagrees with him, one therefore stigmatizes oneself as conventional in thought and conformist in one's views; if one agrees with him, one becomes part of the select band of those who are not deceived by the "socially convenient virtues" and who sees them for what they are – the values propagated by the planning system in order to further its own purposes.

Irritation is compounded by the fact that Galbraith is right to question conventional wisdom, then spoils a good case by his intellectually arrogant assumptions about the motives of other people. Underlying much of his thesis is the belief that most people simply do not know what is good for them, but that Professor Galbraith does. It is just conceivable, after all, that the real power of the technostructure rests not on its ability to control the consumer but on its readiness to adjust its activities to the self-interest of the majority of the public. This does not necessarily make those activities any more admirable: it is still possible to argue, with Galbraith, that too little emphasis is placed on social activities like the arts. But it does make them comprehensible in a way Galbraith's assumptions do not. As he correctly points out, the common interests of managements and unions frequently outweigh their differences; however, he fails to draw from this the appropriate conclusion – that the technostructure now has a constituency measured in millions, and that its power rests on the concordance of its self-interest with that of a very large section of the population. The values of that population may not be Professor Galbraith's (or mine, for that matter); that does not mean that they can be dismissed as artificial or corrupted by advertising.

Altogether there are a number of odd features about Galbraith's line of reasoning. Implicit in his whole argument is the idea that there is some sort of "right" or "appropriate" standard of living – rather like the medieval just wage – beyond which consumers can only be induced to go by persuasion and manipulation. But this is too crucial a point, surely, to be left implicit and unargued. If this is indeed Galbraith's view (and it is difficult to see how it cannot be), then the onus is on him to specify what the right standard of living is. It is clear that he thinks too much is spent on cars and too little on mass transit; but what, in this context, is too much? Again, in referring to innovations which are produced to satisfy the desire of the technostructure to expand rather than real needs, he can do no better than cite plastic grass and genital deodorants – which hardly make a significant dent in the GNP, I should imagine.

More fundamentally still, there is a contradiction at the root of Galbraith's argument. The technostructure, he rightly points out, is concerned to maximize its own satisfactions, not profits. Its members want security for themselves, opportunities to exercise their own expertise, and chances of promotion. Hence, he concludes, the emphasis on economic growth, irrespective of social considerations about pollution and so on. But he fails to notice, oddly enough, that the values he imputes to the technostructure may have a wider appeal. After all, it doesn't need an advertising campaign or any great effort of persuasion to make people value security, opportunities, and promotion prospects. In short, the technostructure may well be delivering the goods – in a general, not specific, way – that most people want.

There remains Galbraith's other indictment of the planning system: that it involves the exploitation of the market economy. Here there is a very real problem in following his argument: its imprecision is such as to make it difficult to discuss in detail. (At one point Galbraith says: "In assessing the public influence of the planning system, there is danger in being too specific. Its greatest source of such power is subjective." This sort of assertion seems to put Galbraith's thesis beyond rational proof or disproof.) About the only evidence cited by him is that in 1971 average hourly wages in durable-goods manufacture were $3.80, while in services, retail trade, and agriculture the equivalent figures were respectively $2.99, $2.57, and $1.48. All this suggests to me that the workers in these industries were underpaid, perhaps because the unions are weak in these sectors; it does not tell me anything about the income of the owners of small businesses, farms, and so on – or, perhaps more important, about the range of income distribution as among different sectors and different parts of the United States. In any case, since Galbraith includes medical practitioners and pornographers in this category – not conspicuously exploited occupations – it is impossible to know just how wide an application his generalization has.

But, then, Galbraith tends to be contemptuous of those who dare to ask for such precision. In doing so, I am again in danger of stigmatizing myself. For as a footnote points out, "the standard (and highly effective) weapon of the defenders of established belief is to argue that any challenge is deficient in scholarship and therefore intellectually disreputable. . . . Scholars of the most mediocre mind are often the most vehement." To argue with Galbraith over facts is therefore to label oneself as both conventional and mediocre, and what could be more terrible than that? Still, accepting the risk, I think it worth citing one example of Galbraith's belief that the reiteration of assertions is an adequate substitute for reasoned arguments.

This comes out most clearly in his discussion of the position of women (a new departure for Galbraith: women do not feature in the indices of his two previous books and for once he seems to be following rather than setting fashions). Women, he writes, have become a crypto-servant class: sacrificing their careers on the altar of economic growth. "In few other matters has the economic system been so successful in establishing values and molding resulting behavior," he concludes. So one would naturally expect that as the planning system has developed, the number of women imprisoned in their own households and occupied in promoting consumption will have increased. In fact, as Galbraith could have discovered by consulting the Brookings Institution's *Setting National Priorities. The 1973 Budget* – a not altogether inaccessible or obscure publication – precisely the reverse has happened. In 1940 less than 10 per cent of all mothers with children went out to work. In subsequent decades the figure rose steadily, and by 1970 it was above 40 per cent. Yet oddly enough, consumption rose steadily over these decades. Using Galbraith's methods, one is almost tempted to diagnose an inverse relationship between economic growth and the role of women: growth increases as women emancipate themselves from their crypto-servant role.

The same sort of disdain for facts is evident elsewhere in the book. The interests of the technostructure, Galbraith argues, tend to promote expenditure on defense rather than on social purposes. Again, this is less than self-evident. Expenditure on defense fell from 41.8 per cent of the federal budget in 1950 to 33.0 per cent in 1974 (*Setting National Priorities: The 1974 Budget*), while expenditure on cash income maintenance rose from 15.2 per cent to 30.3 per cent. These figures are far from conclusive, even though they seem to point in the opposite direction from that assumed by Galbraith's argument. Still, at the very least, they need discussion.

Given the flimsy foundations, it is not surprising that Galbraith's superstructure of proposals for reform is ramshackle. These fall into two categories. First, he proposes more public ownership – both in the planned system of the big corporations (where control has long since passed from the nominal owners of the capital in most cases) and in the market sector (where some form of public monopoly, as in medical care, may be preferable to the chaos of the market). Second, though, he concedes that transferring control from corporation managers to government bureaucracies leaves the technostructure untouched – and, if anything, reinforces its grip on power. So there follow a number of political proposals. Congressmen, for example, should not serve for more than one term, since otherwise they themselves become sucked into the technostructure. Above all, "the all-important question in choosing a President must henceforth be whether the candidate distinguishes the planning from the public interest and is committed to the latter."

Writing this review from Britain, I find it possible to take a fairly detached view of the proposals for greater state ownership and control. Once, this might have been denounced as socialism; now it is practiced even by conservative governments. While the U.S. government underwrote the Lockheed company, the Tory government in Britain actually took Rolls-Royce into public ownership. But the British experience has not only shown prophecies of catastrophe to be wildly wrong; it has also shown unexpected difficulties. Most people would probably agree that the British National Health Service is vastly preferable to anything found in the United States. But one of the hallmarks of its success has been its ability to provide a reasonable service, while keeping costs down: it absorbs a much smaller proportion of the national income than medical care in the U.S. This suggests a very different conclusion from that drawn by Galbraith, who always quotes medical care as one of his examples of under-spending on social services in the United States. It is not so much the level of spending which – above a certain minimum – determines the quality of the service provided, as the way in which the resources are distributed geographically and used by the professional running it. Even in the British NHS, the medical technostructure plays a large – and distorting – role in determining the distribution and use of resources: so far, at any rate, doctors have managed to prevent anything like political control over the policies of the NHS, though the battle is still being fought.

Here we come to the central weakness of Galbraith's whole thesis: the absence of politics. It is central because it stems directly from his analysis of the problem. If one assumes, as he does, that there is such a thing as *the* public interest – as distinct from shifting coalitions of self-interest – and that this has been corrupted by the planning system, then Galbraith's search for a philosopher-king-president makes some sort of sense. But if one assumes that the public interest is constantly being redefined in the light of changing ideas (including those of Galbraith) and changing self-interests, then this St. George slaying the dragon of the technostructure looks remarkably like Don Quixote. Who, after all, would be the constituency and supporters of Galbraith's ideal President – if not those poor, deluded consumers? What is the alternative power base – if not the technostructure and its allies, the unions?

Galbraith's ideas are too influential to be treated as nothing more than entertainment. It would be a pity if he continued to take the view that oversimplification is the soul of wit, and that neat generalizations are an adequate substitute for sustained, rigorous argument.

12

Inequality and Politics

POLITICAL QUARTERLY
January-March 1980

The current debate about inequality and poverty, to which all these books* contribute in varying ways, has a significance which goes far beyond technical arguments about the adequacy or inadequacy of the social policies that have been pursued over the past 30-odd years. It is, in effect, a debate about the nature of Britain's political system: a post-mortem on the post-war consensus – the commitment of both the Labour and Conservative parties to the creation of a more fair society. The nature and degree of that commitment has, of course, varied both as between the two parties and over time. Still, disagreement was constrained within the framework of widely shared views about the general direction of policy.

Now, however, there are signs that the post-war consensus is breaking up. The Right increasingly see the Welfare State as a threat to the market economy – the engine of economic growth. The Left, conversely, increasingly see the market economy as a threat to the Welfare State: the idea that the market economy, by generating growth, creates the necessary conditions for the achievement of greater equality is being questioned. What both sides have in common is disillusion with the achievements of the post-war era – a disillusion not unconnected perhaps with Britain's gloomy economic prospects.

---

*Peter Townsend, *Poverty in the United Kingdom,* Penguin; John H. Goldthorpe, *Social Mobility and Class Structure in Modern Britain,* Clarendon Press; Nick Bosanquet and Peter Townsend, eds., *Labour and Equality,* Heinemann.

The significance of both Peter Townsend's study of poverty and John Goldthorpe's study of social mobility is that they allow us to take stock of what our society looks like: what the post-war consensus actually did or did not achieve. Both authors are committed to the achievement of greater equality; both conclude by rejecting, from the perspective of the Left, the post-war consensus. The interest of their books therefore lies in both what they describe and what they prescribe for future policy.

If poverty has become a major political issue, Peter Townsend can claim a large share of the credit for this. Informed by a generous sense of outrage, his work has over the years helped to dispel complacency and to create a constituency for reform. His latest book is his *magnum opus* in every sense of the word (not least in its forbidding physical bulk.). Although primarily based on a survey carried out in 1968/69, it is also an attempt to bring together the various strands of the poverty debate: to present, at is were, a comprehensive account and theory of poverty.

The first problem with Townsend's book is, of course, the central question of how helpful or accurate it is to talk about "poverty" as distinct from "inequality". Is this more than an emotive label? Townsend argues that it is, and that it can logically be distinguished from inequalities in the distribution of resources. "For example", he argues, "the 20 per cent. with the lowest incomes in Sweden are not so badly placed as the corresponding 20 per cent. in the United States": this is because the bottom fifth in Sweden have a larger command over resources – as measured by their share of total income – than the bottom fifth in the U.S.A. But this is simply another way of saying that there is more inequality in the distribution of income in the U.S.A. than in Sweden. Poverty, in the last analysis, can surely be best defined as that degree of inequality in access to resources which is deemed to be socially unacceptable. And Townsend's book should be seen as an attempt to push out the frontiers of the socially unacceptable: as much an exercise in persuasion as an exercise in measurement.

Conventionally, inequality tends to be measured in terms of income. But, as Townsend rightly argues, this is inadequate. There are many dimensions of inequality: in terms of command over capital, in terms of job satisfaction and security, in terms of working conditions and in terms of social environment. And perhaps the most important evidence Townsend draws from his survey findings is the extent to which inequalities of income tend to be associated with, and reinforced by, other kinds of inequalities. But there remains the problem of devising criteria for the "cut-off point" between acceptable and unacceptable degrees of inequality. The practice of using the Supplementary Benefits scale as a baseline is unsatisfactory; it means, for example, that the numbers in poverty increase whenever the Government of the day decides to improve the scale. It can, conversely, lead to the paradoxical conclusion that the more parsimonious governments are, the less poverty there is.

So perhaps the most ground-breaking aspect of Townsend's book lies in his attempt to devise independent measures of relative deprivation: to define poverty, or unacceptable inequality, as an inability to share in the "style of living which is generally shared or approved" in any given society. Unfortunately, the deprivation index used is somewhat unsatisfactory. It includes such items as the lack of indoor lavatories which (we would probably all agree) suggest that people are falling below the "style of living which is generally shared or approved" in our society. However, it also includes some other items where a majority of the population turn out to be deprived: this would seem a logical nonsense if the shared or approved standard of living, which provides the norm for the whole exercise, is to be based on the actual behaviour of the population as distinct from Townsend's own sense of what is right or proper. For example, the deprivation index includes "has not had a cooked breakfast most days of the week" (67.3 per cent. of the population) and "has not had a week's holiday away from home in the last 12 months" (53.6 per cent. of the population). Such indicators may tell us a great deal about *prevailing* standards of living in Britain; do they tell us anything at all about the minimum *acceptable* standards of living as defined by actual lifestyles?

Townsend's deprivation index is therefore more than a little problematic. Even though the number of items on which deprivation is recorded increases sharply once income dips below a certain level, this does not really help us – given the heterogeneity and ambiguity of the indicators in the first place. So the final conclusion, that more than a quarter of Britain's households fall below the deprivation standard, must be treated with caution: no figure can be better than the measuring rod used, and this seems to be a particularly elastic one. Indeed, throughout, it is important to read the fine print of the definitions used before accepting the figures of deprivation. For example, to elicit information about poor housing, the survey asked whether the house had "rising damp, damp walls or ceilings, loose brickwork or plaster, roofs which leaked, windows or doors that fitted badly or did not open or close, and floorboards or stairs which were broken". On these criteria my own Grade II listed house would show me to be living in very poor conditions indeed. Similarly, the "need" for better housing is derived from questions about people's "wants" for more rooms: an unpardonable intellectual confusion, surely.

Now all this is not to suggest that we can complacently dismiss the problem of inequality. There is, as Townsend shows, a great deal of cumulative deprivation. There are, as his case-histories document, a great many families living in disgracefully miserable conditions. But it is to suggest that the kind of figures which hit the headlines and, at second hand, fuel political discussion – so many millions in poverty, so many millions deprived – must be treated with scepticism. After all, the fact that inequality appears to have so little salience as a political issue does have to be accounted for: why, if a quarter of Britain's households are indeed deprived, is it so difficult to get up steam for measures of reform?

One answer might be variations on the theme of "false consciousness" or the ability of the policy-making elite to screen out certain demands. But there are other answers as well. For example, there is Townsend's own finding that objective and subjective deprivation are not the same: of those whose incomes are only 50 per cent. of the mean of their household type, 49 per cent. consider themselves to be either better off or the same as the average for the country as a whole. Partly this may reflect low expectations and limited frames of reference; partly, however, it may also reflect differential capacities to cope (an issue which tends to get neglected in the somewhat paternalistically-orientated poverty literature). Again, it may not be helpful in trying to explain the politics of inequality to lump together, in the same figure of total "poverty", those whose circumstances mean that they may be permanently condemned to multiple deprivation (*e.g.* the handicapped) and those who move in and out of whatever parameters are set for defining the category of the deprived. Aggregation may help to produce figures with emotional impact; disaggregation may be necessary to produce a sensible debate about policy options.

There is a further problem stemming from taking a cross-cut look at deprivation at one point in time. The continued existence of relative deprivation at one point in time is quite compatible with a reduction of total deprivation in absolute terms over time. The point can be illustrated by taking one of Townsend's deprivation indicators: lack of basic amenities. In 1951, for instance, 38 per cent. of households were without the use of a fixed bath; by 1977, only 4 per cent. lacked a bath. The conventional response to such figures is to assume that such improvements are the automatic product of greater prosperity. But why assume an automatically even distribution of improvements in living standards? Why ignore the possibility – perhaps indeed probability – that, but for political decisions to spend more on various forms of social policies, large sections of the population might actually have not shared in the by-products of growth? Given the changes in both the demographic and the industrial structure of society, it cannot be taken for granted that there would have been no widening of inequalities in the absence of redistributive public policy. To show that there has been little or no decrease in inequality –

as measured by the distribution of income – does not necessarily prove the failure of such policies, although it may tell us a great deal about the excessive expectations invested in these policies. The sense of things improving may therefore help to explain Townsend's otherwise seemingly puzzling finding that continuing statistical inequality is compatible with a surprising degree of subjective satisfaction: when people actually get a bathroom, they may not be too worried about the Gini co-efficient.

There may, of course, be a further explanation of why a high degree of deprivation fails to generate political demands. This is that the experience of deprivation is limited to a relatively small section of the population: that in Britain (as in other advanced industrial nations) there is now a permanent majority of "haves". Alternatively, it could be argued that even if the experience of occasional deprivation is widespread, the chances of upward mobility are now such as to encourage an ethos of individual competitiveness rather than collective solidarity. In other words, if people feel that they can escape from the threat of deprivation through their own efforts, they may not be particularly interested in solidaristic social policies.

Here the study of Goldthorpe and his colleagues is of central relevance. This is an investigation of social mobility patterns, based on a large survey carried out in 1972 and carried out with great technical elegance. Two crucial findings emerge from this. First, the study shows that Britain is a relatively open and fluid society. The "service class" – of professionals, managers, company directors – is in no sense self-recruited: of the men in this category in 1972, as many had fathers who had been manual workers (28.5 per cent.) as fathers who had themselves been members of the "service class" (28.4 per cent.). So in effect, there has been a great deal of upward movement. Secondly, however, the study shows that over time there has been no change in the relative chances of members of different occupational groups moving to the top: that is, the odds on someone born into the "service class" remaining there are very much higher than the odds on someone born of a working-class father moving into it. So, in practice, there has been no change in the inequalities of opportunity. The circle of persisting inequalities and high mobility has been squared because the "service class" itself has been expanding rapidly (largely because of the kinds of jobs created by the growth of the Welfare State, it might be added).

Two bits of conventional wisdom take a knock from these findings. First, it is clear that there is no closed ruling elite (unless that elite is defined much more restrictively) of the "service class". Secondly, mobility is not fragmenting the working class: on the contrary, the working class is becoming increasingly a self-recruiting group of the population. So, in effect, there is a very heterogeneous "service class" and an increasingly homogeneous working class in terms of their members' social origins.

All this might suggest increasing working-class support for solidaristic social policies: a collective enterprise designed to attack inequalities, whether of opportunities or access to resources (and the two, of course, largely go hand in hand). And this is, indeed, the conclusion drawn by Goldthorpe and his colleagues – although with many cautioning reservations. But there are a number of difficulties about such a proposition. First, the evidence used by this study about attitudes is quite different in terms of quality and rigour from that deployed about mobility patterns: I would describe it as journalistic if, in my vocabulary, this was not a term of praise and if it did not flatter the prose style of the book. Secondly, and perhaps more crucially, there is no analysis of those falling into the very wide categories used for describing the working class – which includes skilled as well as unskilled workers. These may well be homogeneous, as the study shows, in terms of mobility. Are they necessarily homogeneous in other respects as well? Specifically, can it really be assumed that there is homogeneity of interest or attitude as between those in the "corporate" sector of the economy (the most unionised and best protected) and those who are in the "competitive" sector of the economy (the least organised and the most vulnerable), between the skilled and the unskilled?

Now it may be that the policies of the present government will smudge the difference between these two sectors: that it will be as risky to work in the corporate sector (such as British Leyland or British Steel) as in the competitive sector, where bankruptcies and redundancies tend to have less political visibility. But, on present evidence, it is tempting to argue that the problem of deprivation is largely that of the competitive sector. In which case, the persistence of the present structure of inequality – in all its many aspects – becomes explicable in terms of the present power structure of society: for all the big battalions, including the trade unions, have a stake in the *status quo*. On this assumption, even the present defence of the Welfare State by the trade unions falls into place: it can be interpreted not so much as an altruistic gesture of support towards the deprived as a straightforward defence of jobs.

If, in fact, this assumption is rejected – if the explanation of inequality as the product of a majority stake in the preservation of the existing order is dismissed – then, logically, only two reactions are possible. The first is to interpret the failure to deal with deprivation through the lenses of a conspiracy theory. This, indeed, tends to be the view taken in the Bosanquet-Townsend volume on the record of the 1974-79 Labour Government. As with all multi-author books, there is a great variety of perspectives, just as there is a wide range of quality. But the prevailing – though not unanimous – view taken is that the Labour Government failed to deal with inequality: a verdict which seems to ignore the staggering change in the economic circumstances of the Western world in this period – when, it might be argued, simply preventing inequalities from getting worse was something of an achievement. And the reason for this, put most forcibly by Townsend in his introductory chapter, was a conspiracy by the civil service – notably the Treasury. Social policy, he argues, cannot be left to the "private machinations within the Treasury" but must be dealt with by a "Social Development Council" – apparently by-passing the normal machinery of Parliamentary and Cabinet Government. Even Townsend himself seems to recognise the inadequacy of this, whether as a diagnosis or prescription, when he says: "I would not wish to imply that a piece of machinery can solve deep-seated problems". So it is perhaps kindest to pass to the second kind of reaction to frustrated expectations: that of Townsend in his book on poverty.

This reaction consists of acknowledging that inequality is rooted in the social and economic structure of society, but to conclude from this that consequently it is the entire social and economic structure which needs changing. In short, if piecemeal social engineering appears inadequate, take the whole machine apart and start anew. So Townsend concludes his study of poverty with a manifesto for total reform. Among other things, this calls for the "abolition of unemployment" and the "introduction of an equitable income structure": by this is meant, in effect, the abolition of market-determined wages and salaries, and their replacement by "tax-free incomes according to a publicly agreed and controlled schedule". This last point recognises, of course, that one of the problems of financing more generous social policies lies in the resistance of trade unions to higher taxation.

The reason for spelling out Townsend's manifesto is that there is a certain logic in this. Just as the demonology of the Right leads to seeing the trade unions as the cause of all evils, so the demonology of the Left sees the market as the enemy. So if we do not like certain aspects of our society – if we are frustrated in our hopes of reform (which may tell us more about the naïvete of those hopes than about actual social change) – then, quite consistently, we may well believe that abolishing the market will solve everything. But consistency is the only merit in this argument, and it is the consistency of utopianism run amok. The paternalistic centralism implied in designing a "controlled schedule" of wages and salaries is really somewhat frightening in its implications, and it is unfortunate that the Left's reading does not seem to extend to the literature on the Communist bloc: State Socialism, this would suggest, does not get rid of either inequality or deprivation (and when the Left talks about the inequities of capitalism, it should more accurately be talking about the problems of all advanced industrialised societies).

Equally, theories of poverty tend to demonstrate the poverty of theory in this area. There is a basic fuzziness in its terminology. What is "excessive" wealth or income? What criteria are we to use in determining the extent of acceptable inequalities? More seriously still, if Townsend is right in his assertion that poverty can be distinguished from inequality, then it could well be argued that the best way of dealing with poverty is by increasing inequality: this, of course, is the view taken by Sir Keith Joseph and, although I happen to think that he is wrong on empirical grounds, it is difficult to see on what theoretical grounds such a strategy could be opposed by the poverty lobby. Assuming that a policy of incentives – widening inequality – could indeed produce economic growth, which in turn would produce vast improvements in any deprivation index, why should it not be pursued? Again, the relationships – actual and desired – between different kinds of inequality need to be teased out. Assuming that progress were to be made towards achieving more equality of opportunity (in Goldthorpe's sense of perfect equality of chances in obtaining the most desirable "positional goods" in our society) would this make existing inequalities of income more or less tolerable? Can the two aims of policy be separated?

But, quite apart from the need for more clarity about objectives and possible trade-offs, there is also an urgent need for more discussion about strategies. If one rejects utopian reformism as a desperate flight from reality, there still remains the need to think through the strategy options that remain; and in particular the problems created by a stagnant economy. And this requires, I would suggest, the creation of a new consensus around the recognition that the trade unions are part of the power structure of Britain and that many of the problems of adopting social policy to an era of non-growth stem from the consequent rigidities of the Welfare State (mirroring rigidities in society as a whole). In turn, this would seem to imply – as Goldthorpe and his colleagues hint – a move towards corporatism: the inclusion of the trade unions within the policy-making machinery, and a willingness to offer them participation (at all levels of decision-making) in return for a readiness to reform themselves. In the mid-1970s, there were signs of a consensus forming around such a concept – although in the event the trade unions were not able to deliver the goods and took refuge in anarchic opposition to change. Since then, it has been rejected by both Left and Right. Hopefully, however, the consensus may re-emerge again – when the full, appalling, logic of both Left and Right strategies becomes apparent.

Part 2

Government Observed

This selection of newspaper commentaries covers the years from 1965 to the early 1970s and comes exclusively from Rudolf's time at *The Observer*. But although it covers highly productive years of his life in journalism, it does not include any of the output from the ten years hard labor he did on *The London Evening Standard*: unfortunately these pieces have been lost from his personal archives. But although this period is missing from the written records, it cannot be overlooked. Rudolf would like it to go on record that the hard hack days on *The Standard* were not only highly productive but an important training ground for him. He was working, so he says, with "one of the most talented bunch of journalists around at the time." These writers covered everything going on in the universe from politics to theatre under the direction of Lord Beaverbrook. But if energy and talent were lavishly spread at The Standard, there was no doubt about the single source of control; all opinions printed reflected the owner's.

If the owner of *The London Evening Standard* had to be negotiated carefully by the writers, so too did the editor of *The Observer* who had an idiosyncratic line on items of political interest which Rudolf especially did not always share. David Astor's interests were divided between the meta-politics of nuclear disarmament (and similar global issues) and the micro-politics of psycho-analysis; the nitty gritty of how governments run themselves and manage the economy left him unmoved. Rudolf meanwhile persevered with his developing enthusiasm for public expenditure and other public policy issues, interests not always shared by the editor. However, this was the period of the first Wilson Government, when *The Observer* was much concerned with the modernization of Britain and of the Labour Party, so giving Rudolf the opportunity to write about the kind of issues that were to dominate the political agenda in the 1980s and 1990s.

13

Shame and Prejudice

THE OBSERVER
22 August 1965

It has been a shaming and disillusioning experience – shaming for what it has shown us about ourselves and disillusioning for what it has revealed about our politicians. Five years ago the issue of coloured immigration was the monopoly of fringe politicians. Now the major parties are competing to see who can go farthest to conciliate the extremists.

For the Government's White Paper on Immigration – slipped out during the dog days at the end of the parliamentary term – has managed to make the worst of every possible world. It has set a new limit on immigration – low enough to incur the charge of discriminating against coloured immigrants but too high to conciliate the extremists. And it has perpetuated the pretence that colour doesn't come into the whole question – so absolving the Government from the need to do anything bold or difficult about discrimination against the immigrants already in this country.

Smethwick

Having started to conciliate the extremists, the Government has abandoned the only weapons which would have allowed it to fight them: political courage and honesty of principle. Hardly had the White Paper been published than Mr Peter Griffiths, the victor of Smethwick, was proclaiming that it had vindicated him – as indeed it had.

Naturally Mr Griffiths thinks that the White Paper does not go far enough. Inevitably he, and those who think like him, will now press for

71

still tighter controls. And what will the Government be able to say in reply to such demands?

There is a perfectly respectable case to be made for limiting immigration. Every nation has a right to control immigration. And in the case of Britain there is now a pressing reason for exercising this right – a reason we mostly prefer to ignore.

This is that British society is far less tolerant than we had thought and hoped. Colour and race prejudice exist – exacerbated by some politicians and condoned by many of the Conservative Party leaders who are prepared to profit from it politically while shrinking from accepting responsibility for the activities of their own extremists.

But to acknowledge the existence of prejudice is also to accept our responsibility for dealing with it. Unfortunately, the Government, after its White Paper, cannot take up this position without incurring a charge of hypocrisy. The limit it has set to immigration – 8,500 voucher-holders a year, plus the relatives of those already here – is entirely arbitrary. Why 8,500 rather than 5,500 or 10,500? If the Government knows, it isn't telling.

Moreover, it is quite clear that the coloured countries of the Commonwealth will be hit particularly hard. No one country will be entitled to more than 15 per cent of the total quota. And it is only the coloured Commonwealth nations which have an unsatisfied queue of would-be immigrants who will be kept out as a result.

No Need

But even this would not matter so much if the restriction were clearly meant as a temporary expedient to gain time for measures to deal with the causes of prejudice and discrimination to take effect. If this had been the intention, there would, in any case, have been no need to introduce new legislation – since the existing system of controls gives the Government quite enough power to regulate the flow in accordance with social and economic conditions.

But how effective will the Government's positive measures be? Alas, the White Paper substitutes wishful thinking for action. If everyone were as sensitive and well-intentioned as the White Paper assumes them to be, there would be no problem.

Housing

Take the central problem of housing for immigrants. This is to be left to local authorities in the expectation, apparently, that the immigrants will be all right when the millennium arrives and there are plenty of houses for everyone. But local authorities are often most subject to pressure and frequently guilty of discrimination themselves: Deptford, for example, designed a slum-clearance scheme so as to skirt areas occupied by immigrants in order to avoid having to give a council house to coloured families.

A policy of positive discrimination towards immigrants of the kind adopted in America towards Negroes – to give them the special favoured treatment in housing and education which alone can put them on equal terms with the rest of the community – will require considerable political courage. But this is all the more reason why the Government should accept responsibility for the task, instead of trying to shuffle it off on to others, whether voluntary organisations or local authorities.

Nor do the Government's professed aims of ensuring that immigrants are not treated as second-class citizens ring true in the light of the White Paper's policies. They are, for example, to be subject to deportation without appeal to the courts. Immigration officers will be able to turn them back at the ports without any right of a hearing. It may be said that this merely brings the immigrants into line with aliens. But if aliens are badly treated (as the Labour Party tirelessly pointed out while in Opposition) is this an argument for extending the same system to Commonwealth citizens, instead of reforming it?

The political calculation behind the Labour Government's desperate attempts to square the circle is obvious: to conciliate the extremists while still clinging to its principles. But it can't be done. And the Government runs the risk of losing out on both flanks.

If the Government doesn't move in the direction of greater restriction, it may well lose votes at the next general election. But if it moves closer to the Tory position, the chances are that the Conservatives will trump its ace: already Mr Selwyn Lloyd has hinted that the aim should be to prevent *any* overall increase in the immigrant population. Inhibited by its traditions and professions of principle, the Labour Party (to its credit) will always be out-bid in any auction of illiberalism.

Vain Hope?

But In the attempt to reconcile expediency and principle, Labour may antagonise still further that large section of opinion – in all parties – which has been increasingly unhappy about the attitudes of politicians to race and colour. Is it too much to hope that, come October, the Government will announce that it has had second thoughts about the White Paper?

14

The £6,000,000,000 Question

THE OBSERVER
20 March 1966

Quite possibly the 1966 General Election may go down in history as the most boring campaign ever fought. With issues which ought to be in an old people's home being marched into battle, with Mr Wilson himself almost apologising on television to the voters for inflicting the whole dreary business on them, with public opinion polls making the whole thing appear a foregone conclusion, it certainly looks like it. However, the campaign may turn out to have been memorable in one respect: as the election which made the Welfare State a key political issue.

If so, it will not be before time. By far the largest item in the nation's accounts – lumping together all forms of public expenditure – is the money spent on providing cash social benefits: about £2,500 million this year.

There are more than six million old-age pensioners. There are more than three and three-quarter million families drawing family allowances. There are the widows, the sick, the disabled and the unemployed.

And all this on top of the services provided by the State as part of the welfare system. The £1,600 million-plus spent on education; the £1,300 million-plus spent on the various health services; the £730 million-plus spent on public housing and subsidies. In all, the cost of the Welfare State, taken in its broadest sense, accounts for over £6,000 million, or more than half the total of public spending.

This seems a breathtaking, rather frightening, sum. But after spending the 20 years since the Second World War congratulating ourselves on building the finest Welfare State in the world, we have suddenly woken up to find that it is in fact a down-at-heel, patched-up job which doesn't stand up well to comparison with more modern, streamlined models elsewhere.

Despite all the benefits and services, large pockets of poverty remain. More than a fifth of all pensioners rely on National Assistance – though even this figure flatters the adequacy of the pension, since there are at least 500,000 (and possibly one million) old people who would qualify for such help but don't ask for it.

But then, as Peter Townsend and Brian Abel-Smith pointed out in a recent study, there are those who live in poverty because they simply do not earn enough to keep their families. There are something like 250,000 households with an average of three children whose *earnings* are less than they would be entitled to under the National Assistance scales (which don't exactly allow for luxurious living, anyway). With one million men earning less than £11 a week the size of the problem hardly needs stressing.

On all this there is unanimity between the parties. Indeed the rivalry between them is to see who can produce the more radical-sounding proposals of reform. Thus, Mr Crossman, in his best indignation style, accuses the Tories of wanting to replace the Welfare State by the "means-test State." Mr Hogg immediately denounces this as a "poisonous smear." The Tories attack the Government on wasting the country's resources by giving indiscriminate benefits. And Mr Callaghan ripostes by accusing the Conservatives of fiddling the costs of their pension proposals.

It is all good fun, if a little confusing for those not qualified in accountancy and not equipped with a slide-rule as we watch the television spots. But underlying the quarrels of the politicians is, in fact, a theological dispute about the Welfare State which has been quietly rumbling away for years, long before erupting in the present campaign.

This is the dispute between the collectivists (or the outside-left of the Labour Party) and the individualists (or the outside-right of the Conservative Party). It is between those who believe that the community should take full responsibility for its citizens and those who believe that the State should do only the minimum necessary to prevent suffering. It is between those who believe that the Welfare State should (to put it very crudely) look after people from the cradle to the grave, and those who argue that it should act only as a safety net for social casualties.

There is a further argument between the outside-left and the outside-right. This is between the universalists and the selectivists. The former believe that it is of the essence of all State benefits that they should go to everyone – that as soon as you start tailoring benefits and services to the needs of the worst-off, they will degenerate in quality (since the better-off will have no incentive to insist on higher standards). Selectivists argue that since there will, for the foreseeable future, be a shortage of resources, the only way of making sure that the worst-off get the help they need is by concentrating efforts on them: after all, to make the present old-age pensions big enough for everyone to live on would be so prohibitively expensive that no one would even dare suggest it.

These propositions have been put forward most boldly, not by the politicians themselves but by academics. The outside-left's spiritual home has been the London School of Economics, where Richard Titmus, Tory Lynes, Peter Townsend and others pioneered the study of the Welfare State and its defects. The outside-right, a less-well defined group, which includes as many Liberals as orthodox Conservatives, has found a platform in the Institute of Economic Affairs, which has published a series of pamphlets by Arthur Seldon, Alan Peacock, Jack Wiseman and others urging the case for changing the whole approach to the Welfare State.

The emotional attitudes of the two parties – if not their actual policies – tend to reflect the views of their ideologues. Thus Labour goes into the election committed to introducing a universal pension scheme, where both contributions and payments would be related to earnings. And the Tories are committed to maintaining a flat-rate State pension scheme, with the butter in their case being provided by private occupational schemes.

Both are, in effect, an attempt to get round the central weakness in the original Beveridge-based system. Which was that this was conceived essentially as a scheme for *subsistence* payments: for a man and wife, 13s. a week on food, 3s. on clothing, 4s. on fuel, light and sundries, 2s. margin and 10s. on rent at 1938 prices, as his report calculated. It did not allow for the natural demand of people to share in the nation's rising prosperity and to have pensions related to their earnings.

Labour's sliding-scale pension proposals would get round the problems of inflation and rising standards by tying contributions to earnings – which will automatically rise. In fact, of course, the best guarantee of a State scheme keeping pace with expectation is simply political pressure.

The Tory proposals aim to deal with this problem by encouraging private saving, in the shape of occupational pension schemes. They criticise Labour's scheme for being so expensive that no one would have the money left over to make their own provision for old age; they themselves are criticised in turn for not offering enough protection against inflation. Oddly enough, though, they are nearer in spirit to the original Beveridge Report, whose stern contention was: "Management of one's income is an essential element of a citizen's freedom. Payment of a substantial part of the cost of benefit as a contribution irrespective of the means of the contributor is the firm basis of a claim to benefit irrespective of means."

So far, the policies of the two parties fall neatly into the universalist v. selectivist, collectivist v. individualist pattern. There is, for once, a clear division of principle. But, as always, it is easier to be principled about what is distant in time than about immediate problems.

For whatever new pension scheme is introduced will not come into full effect for another 20 to 40 years. In the interregnum, the real problem will be how to make the best of the scheme we have got now. And it is at this stage that principle tends to get somewhat blurred. When it comes to the point, everyone is in favour of some degree of discrimination.

At present the main instrument of discrimination is the National Assistance Board. This year it will distribute some £280 million. It is extremely efficient at doing its job: which is to distribute the minimum amount of money to the minimum number of people.

Both parties are pledged to abolish it, and to incorporate it in a new Ministry of Social Security which would be charged with positively seeking out poverty and social misery. But, having ceremonially dropped the means test overboard, it would promptly be smuggled in again – perhaps disguised (in Labour's case) as a minimum-incomes guarantee. The emphasis now is that people should be assured of help *as of right* and not be made to feel that they are the objects of charity. But the idea of a test to determine need remains.

In fact, when it comes to the point even Labour is not prepared to stick to the principle of the same benefits for everyone or free services for all. It may have abolished prescription charges with a great flourish. But it has kept dental charges (are teeth supposed to be dispensable?).

Similarly, the Conservatives are notably more cautious in their policies than in their speeches. They certainly show no sign of accepting the arguments of their outside-right in favour of extending the fee-paying principle in education or in the health service.

Again, both parties are in something of a dilemma over family allowances. Even to bring these up to the level recommended by Beveridge, adjusted to today's earnings, would cost something like £300 million a year. Some form of discrimination therefore seems inevitable.

In all this, there is a danger that the real problem may be overlooked: the problem of finding the *resources* needed to cure the Welfare State's deficiencies. The proportion of gross national product devoted to welfare cash benefits (pensions, etc.) has been creeping steadily, and in particular leapt up in the past 10 years. It now stands at about 7 per cent – as against roughly 10 per cent in Germany, 9 per cent in Sweden and 8 per cent in France (though these countries are less generous in providing free services, like health).

Even Labour's National Plan despite its optimistic assumptions about the rate of growth doesn't allow for any massive increase in the proportion of our wealth devoted to welfare. So how best can we tap the nation's resources, ideology apart, to catch up?

One obstacle is simply our system of accounting: whenever pensions go up, there is great outcry about an increase in public spending. In fact what happens is that contributions also go up – and the resources have been transferred from those working to those who are not. It doesn't mean that the nation faces bankruptcy because of an orgy of extravagance.

The other obstacle is that both parties have skirted round the real issue. As Beveridge put it "both social insurance and children's allowances are primarily methods of redistributing wealth." To what extent are we prepared to, or do we want to, change the distribution of wealth in favour of the young, the poor and the old?

15

Egoists of the World

THE OBSERVER
28 August 1966

Mr Wilson's decision to put his head in the lion's mouth is less foolhardy than it looks.

A Tory Prime Minister who dared show his face at a Trades Union Congress after doing what Mr Wilson's Government has done – introducing a compulsory wage freeze, interfering with the sacred right of free negotiation, deliberately adopting policies designed to induce more unemployment – would risk being tarred and feathered and set alight to join the other illuminations on the Blackpool front. But a Labour Prime Minister can at worst be sure of a respectful hearing, and at best hope to persuade the conference to support his Government's policy.

For the unions still feel that a Labour Administration is, somehow, *their* Government – historically their creation, financially their dependant and spiritually their blood-brother. The tie is as much emotional as institutional.

Sentiment

But although it would be a mistake to underestimate the power of sentiment – and no doubt Mr Wilson will go all out to exploit it at Blackpool tomorrow week – it would equally be wrong to think that it is immune to erosion by events. In practice, the relationship between the unions and Labour – however special – is increasingly being frayed under the pressure of circumstances. In particular, two long-term trends are transforming the entire labour movement.

The first is that the role of the trade unions themselves has changed. From being the outsiders, representing the interests of the oppressed and the under-privileged, they have entered not just the corridors but the drawing-rooms of power. The Bevin-Citrine revolution, begun in the thirties and pushed to a successful conclusion in the war years, is an accomplished fact. The unions are part of the machinery of government.

Whichever party is in power, the unions are consulted by Government departments, invited to sit on official committees and represented on advisory policy shaping bodies like Neddy. They have their own private hot-line not just to a Labour Government, but to the whole State machinery of government.

But this very success has created an entirely new problem. To the degree that the unions are becoming mixed up in the whole process of government, they are also becoming instruments of government. They may be able to convey their views to Ministers and civil servants more forcibly and intimately than ever before; but, in return, they are also expected to sell the Government's policies to their own rank and file. The wage freeze policy is a case in point.

Indeed the greater the activity of Government – the more it reaches out to regulate prices, pay, and so on – the more important becomes this new role of the unions. For the Government apparatus by itself simply lacks the capacity to sort out all the multitudinous wage claims, for example. Hence it looks to the TUC (as it does to the Confederation of British Industry over prices) to co-operate in checking the flood.

Is this what the unions really want? Do they want to become one of the limbs of the State colossus? The question poses itself in a particularly sharp form when a Labour Government is in power because such an Administration can exert the kind of moral blackmail which Tory Ministers cannot: it can ask, are you going to let us down, brothers? But the problem exists even when the Conservatives are in office.

As the full implications of this trend sink in, the unions may come to doubt whether it is entirely to their advantage. Indeed this is already becoming apparent in the attitude of Mr Frank Cousins and some of the other opponents of the wage freeze. Paradoxically even left-wingers like Mr Cousins are asking that unions should be allowed to behave more like free enterprise animals – making the best bargains for their members not serving some abstract "national interest."

More Money

Indeed there is a lot to be said for such purely commercial approach to union affairs. For in the last resort the most compelling arguments in favour of productivity agreements for instance is not that they serve the national interest but that they give the workers involved a chance to earn more.

But if the unions come to accept that this is the real line of advance for the future then they are likely to rebel against the trend towards involvement with the Government: which often means accepting restrictions on their liberty of action in return for pats on the head. They may evolve more in the direction of the American unions, hard-headedly selling labour and forgetting sentiment about class solidarity and so on. Indeed, even as it is, many unions are more concerned to maintain differentials than to help their struggling brothers.

If this trend continues, the unions will drift farther apart from the Labour Party. For once they come to accept that their prime purpose is to look after their own members (the practice already, even if the rhetoric is all about the brotherhood of workers), they will inevitably be less concerned to look after the interests of the Labour Party – particularly since the two are not always identical.

The second new factor in the situation is the change in the whole political climate since the links between the Labour Party and the unions were forged. Labour has moved away from the politics of fraternalism towards the politics of egoism (to adapt a concept launched by W. G. Runciman in his recent book on Relative Deprivation and Social Justice). The politics of fraternalism rested on class solidarity: the idea that the workers could achieve a better life only through common action. The politics of egoism rests on the belief that what people want is a chance to rise out of their class, not necessarily with it.

Although the Labour Party is still a working-class party – in that it draws most of its support from that class – Mr Wilson has quite deliberately switched the appeal from fraternalism to egoism. He himself epitomises the egoist approach (and I am not using the word in a pejorative sense): he is the bright grammar-school boy who has risen in the world as the result of his own abilities and believes that others should have the same chance as he had.

The 1964 and 1966 elections made it clear that Labour can only achieve power by repudiating its exclusive working class image and by stressing its independence of the unions. Mr Wilson set out to reassure and appeal to the "egoists" – to the white-coated workers, technologists and so on who seek not so much an equal society as one in which they will be given more scope. Efficiency and competence were the watchwords. But efficiency is not necessarily compatible with fraternity. Fraternity demands that work should be shared out in bad times, but efficiency demands that men should move to other jobs.

Last Triumph?

The implications of these trends for the future relationship between the unions and the Labour Government are considerable. Tomorrow week Mr Wilson may be able to triumph by playing on sentiment. But this is a rapidly diminishing asset. In future, the relationship between the unions and the Government may have to be put on a more business-like basis.

If so, it will be all to the good. The worst way to run a country is by appealing to people to do what they don't want to do because of what happened 50 years ago.

16

Planners Who Leap into the Dark

THE OBSERVER
13 September 1966

The trouble about most politicians, even child prodigies like Mr Wilson, is that they come to office much too late. Just as Mr Macmillan spent his Premiership trying to tackle the problems of the thirties – when he was a rebel against Tory orthodoxy – so Mr Wilson is now girding himself to tackle the problems of the fifties, when he was a left-wing heretic.

The Government's policy for "planned growth" has failed. The July 20 measures – whose effects, in terms of growing unemployment and declining industrial activity, are only now beginning to be felt – wrote the final epitaph to Labour's high hopes. So what is the Government's reaction? It is not to change the medicine but to give the patient a bigger dose: *more* planning is the new slogan.

That, at any rate, is the theme of Mr Richard Crossman, Mr Wilson's self-appointed court philosopher. The National Plan is contemptuously described as a Mark I model. Indicative planning – that is, planning which sets industry targets but does not compel firms to achieve them – is dismissed as inadequate.

The new Crossman orthodoxy (and it is familiar to anyone who remembers the arguments of the Labour Left 10 years ago, when both Mr Wilson and Mr Crossman were in the wilderness) appears to be that the Government must intervene directly to give effect to its targets: we must have planned investment, planned incomes – and no nonsense about a free for all.

The Muddle

The danger of this approach is not that it will lead to a totalitarian society: one can probably rely on Mr Wilson's political sense not to push Mr Crossman's arguments to their logical conclusion. After all, he wants to win the next General Election.

More acute, and more immediate, is that Mr Crossman's approach will divert attention from the real problems of how to plan effectively. It will tend to polarise the argument between the non-planners (like Mr Enoch Powell) and the all-out planners (like Mr Crossman).

But this, of course, is an entirely artificial and meaningless choice. The fact is that we are stuck with planning – and that planning in a free society based on a mixed economy must always be a muddled compromise between compulsion and persuasion. The Powell and Crossman models may be intellectually enticing because of their logical coherence. The only trouble is that they don't correspond to the circumstances that face any Government, Tory or Labour.

Any Government nowadays wields enormous power over the economy – and must plan ahead if it is not to trip over its own decision. With the Government controlling something like 40 per cent of all expenditure, its own domestic housekeeping plans inevitably merge into a national plan (whether it is called that or not).

The difficulty is that any plan is only as good as the information on which it is based. And – as the Labour Government has discovered to its cost – the information at present available is often ludicrously inadequate.

Take the incomes policy. It is all very well Mr Crossman talking grandly about using this as an instrument of socialist planning – about using it not just to restrain excessive growth in incomes but to distribute wealth justly. How is this to be done?

Poverty

The Government has announced that it wants to give special preference to the poorest workers – an admirable aim. Unfortunately, the Ministry of Labour doesn't even know how many lower-paid workers there are. No statistics exist to show just how many men earn less than, say, £12 a week or less than £15. So, to begin with, we don't even know the scale of the problem – which suggests that talk about ways of curing it is premature, to say the least.

Then there is the question of planning investment. One can see Mr Crossman's point: which is that economic growth will be retarded if private industry doesn't invest enough (though he forgot to point out that if this happens it will be mainly because the Government's economic strategy has induced a mood of apprehension and gloom).

But it is difficult to see how compelling firms to invest more – whether by direct controls or by administrative arm-twisting – will help. Would it help to force the motor industry, say, to invest money on plant to produce cars which cannot be sold? Would it improve the economy to persuade ICI to invest even more in spare capacity beyond the demand for its products?

Obviously, there will always be firms who invest either too much or too little. But at least their mistakes of judgment may cancel one another out. A Government error of judgment (and, after all, even Mr Crossman wouldn't claim that Governments are infallible) tends to cause far more damage.

Again, to take the very urgent issue of the "redeployment" of labour. This is supposed to differ from earlier periods of growing unemployment in being a "planned shake-out" (though whether those who lose their jobs will be able to tell the difference is another matter).

But how planned is the redeployment? In 1956, when the Midlands car industry sacked 6,000 men, more than half of them returned to their previous jobs after the recession – as a survey by Dr Hilda Khan showed. Other firms were reluctant to take them on, because they knew that the men would return to the highly paid motor industry at the first opportunity.

So there is very little evidence that unemployment automatically equals redeployment – in the sense of switching men from industry making goods for the home market to firms making goods for export. Indeed, no one in Whitehall even knows for certain whether cutting the home market of, for example, the car industry encourages exports – or whether it makes exporting more difficult by sending up costs.

Yet this is precisely the kind of information on which intelligent Government planning – indeed action of any kind – depends. To talk about extending the scope of planning while the machinery is so preposterously inadequate is simply to risk increasing the scale of mistakes.

The Risk

To make excessive claims for planning is to risk excessive disillusion when the promised vision fails to appear. To centralise decision-making may give effect to a Government's policies. But it also gives effect to – and magnifies – Government mistakes.

The need at the moment is not so much for more planning as for better planning. The planners need to admit that at present they are often groping in the dark – and that lack of information dictates caution.

We need to admit that we cannot transform society by planning, but can use planning only as an instrument in a cautious process of social engineering. We need scepticism, not an appeal to faith. We need more information and less exhortation. We need, not to concentrate, but to diffuse decision-making – albeit within a framework which allows those in charge to relate their own decisions to those of others.

This may seem a timid doctrine. But if the Labour Government rejects it – in favour of the chest-beating all-out approach favoured by Mr Crossman and the party's ideologues – the result may well be to discredit the whole idea of planning. For Tories, like Labour politicians, tend to live in the past – in their case the period of reaction, in the fifties, against Labour's postwar controls and restrictions. A still more spectacular Labour failure now might increase Tory temptations to reject planning altogether.

17

Callaghan's Dilemma: to Tax or Not to Tax

THE OBSERVER
11 December 1966

The whirring of pledges coming home to roost in the corridors of Whitehall is becoming increasingly loud. For the Government is up against it. In two elections, Mr Wilson persuaded the voters of one simple proposition: Labour, possessing as it did the secret of maintaining a fast rate of economic growth, could increase Government spending without also increasing taxation.

Now the first part of this proposition has exploded in Mr Wilson's face. The National Plan, with its ambitious growth target, is today only an embarrassing memory. The Government no longer has the soft option of painlessly paying for rising social expenditure out of the extra wealth created by a fast rate of economic expansion.

So the Chancellor is on the rack. On the one side, he is under pressure to contain Government spending – to cut back the estimates of the spending departments, many of whose plans were based on false assumptions about growth. On the other side, he is being nagged by his party's Left. In a recent lecture to the Fabians, Professor Brian Abel-Smith pointed out that the National Plan's target of a 28 per cent rise in social expenditure (health, housing, education, pensions and so on) between 1964 and 1970 compares badly with the 34.5 per cent increase achieved by the Conservatives in the previous six years.

Of course, Mr Callaghan can cut out the odd school or hospital from the programme, delay the starting date of a road or two, keep his fingers crossed and hope that no one will notice. Meantime, Ministers can trot round the country assuring everyone that when things are better they will be able to make up for lost time.

Challenge to Ministers

But this won't do. For what is really alarming about the present situation is not only that the Government's plans have gone awry. It is that Ministers have, in public at any rate, burked thinking through the consequences of this failure – a failure which represents a basic challenge to the Government's entire philosophy.

The first question facing Ministers is whether maintaining the existing level of taxation has priority over maintaining the existing plans for expanding the social services. For the simplest way out of their present dilemma would be to raise taxes.

To some extent this is, of course, what they have done already. The shift in the balance between private and public spending – with the State disposing of a higher proportion of the nation's resources – is bound to become more pronounced in the coming financial year. For it looks certain that Government expenditure will rise much faster than the nation's income.

Can this process be allowed to continue? There is nothing immoral about Government expenditure as such although Governors of the Bank of England have an occupational weakness for thinking so. During a period of economic difficulties, public spending is the most effective way of preventing stagnation turning into recession.

Similarly, there is no magic formula which tells us what the right level of public spending or taxation should be. Thirty years ago the present level would have seemed quite unacceptable. Even now we are groping our way through a fog of guesswork.

Soaking the Rich?

For instance, the level of taxation in Britain (measured as a percentage of national output) is significantly lower than in most West European countries. But the pattern of taxation is different and so, therefore, is its social and psychological impact. Although France has a higher level of taxation, direct taxes on income are lower: a man with a wife and two children earning £2,500 a year there keeps 92.8 per cent of his salary, as against 79.1 per cent here.

Quite conceivably taxes here could be raised without damaging the economy. We simply don't know. Even on the much-debated question of whether high taxes discourage effort there is much strong feeling but little hard evidence. Politically, however, financing the Welfare State by increasing taxation is going to be very tricky – for it is bound to hit large numbers of voters. For higher taxation is not just a matter of 'soaking the rich'; even if they were bled dry, the amount raised wouldn't begin to meet the need.

There is a further consideration. This is, that as the share of the nation's wealth taken up by the State increases, so the opportunities for private choice in the disposition of wealth narrow. Is this desirable? Do we want such a concentration of economic power? The United States may be an example of private affluence and public squalor. But it is also a country where decision-making is dispersed – where private affluence allows private initiative.

But is there an alternative to raising taxes? Is there any other way of raising the money needed to finance the adequate expansion of the social services? This is the second challenge to Labour Ministers.

A survey conducted last year by the Institute of Economic Affairs – which argues that the social services should be financed out of private contributions rather than taxation – produced some interesting results. It showed that while between 30 per cent and 40 per cent of those interviewed were prepared to accept higher taxes in return for improved services, the rest preferred to make individual contributions – to buy their own services, in effect.

There are a great many objections to switching to a market economy in the Welfare State. The fundamental one is that to do so would introduce a double standard: one for the well-to-do, another for the poor. If the middle classes were allowed to opt out, the result might be to take out of the Welfare State precisely those who are now most anxious to raise standards.

Scaring Off People

But what the institute's survey did show is that it might be psychologically easier for the State to raise more money by charging fees rather than by increasing the general level of taxation. The real resistance is to higher taxes; it is not to paying more for State services from which people benefit directly – like better schools or hospitals.

The objection to such a policy is that it would involve a means test to decide who should be exempt from payments. And it is perfectly true that the means test – in its present form – often scares off the people in greatest need.

But this objection could surely be removed if half the energy which has gone into arguing about the principle of the means test were devoted to devising ways of making it less offensive and more acceptable. Is it necessary to have detailed and frequently humiliating inquisitions into family income? Would it not be possible to devise a scheme under which all citizens make a single declaration of income – and all subsidies they receive and all the taxes or charges they pay were determined by this?

But, of course, while changing the methods of financing the social services may ease the problem it does not solve it. The Government still has to face up to the fact that there will never be enough money to sustain the social services. Even if the nation's wealth does increase – as it will, despite the squeeze – the demands of the services will go up even faster. The revolution of rising expectations means that there will always be unsatisfied demands.

A much more hard-headed approach will therefore be needed in the use of the available resources. When we build a new motorway, we first (in theory, at any rate) try to decide where the investment of a given sum of money will yield the biggest results. A similar 'cost-effectiveness' approach is needed in the social services.

Labour's Lost Image

Is it sensible to build expensive halls of residence for new universities? Or would the money be better spent on expanding the universities themselves more rapidly? Again, is the best way of dealing with anomalies in the system of housing subsidies (in the way of help to council tenants and tax allowances) by adding yet another layer of concessions? Would it not have been wiser for the Government, before it launched yet another scheme of concessions to mortgagees, to have looked at the whole system of subsidies to decide where their application would yield the best results? Certainly the present system doesn't help those in most need.

Not so long ago it would have been easy to catalogue the features that made up Labour's conventional identikit. It was the party of full employment. It was the party of efficient planning. It was the party that would get rid of Britain's nuclear albatross.

All this now belongs to the past. But there also remained – however many words Labour was forced to swallow, however much its ideology had to be watered down – the feeling that it was the party which would put first the interest of the old and the sick, the young and the crippled. It was this emotional commitment which remained to reassure loyalists at times of disillusion and to attract middle-of-the-road radicals.

If Labour fails to carry conviction on this score – as it will, unless it thinks its policies on the social services out afresh – Mr Wilson will be revealed as a kind of political Peer Gynt: who, as he looks back on his life, stripping one skin after another from the onion, finds that in the end he is left holding – nothing.

18

New Deal for Incomes

THE OBSERVER
8 January 1967

The Government's march for a long-term incomes policy is beginning to resemble a parade of circus elephants. Ministers are plodding round and round the ring, holding on to one another's tails, uncertain of where they are going but content as long as they continue to give an appearance of purposive progress.

With the New Year, we left the era of the pay freeze and entered that of 'severe restraint': which means that some people may get some rises some of the time. But even this period is supposed to last only until 30 June. And long before then the Government will have to show its hand.

But the longer we wait, the more apparent it becomes that the Government has no hand to reveal. Mr Woodcock, of the TUC, goes to see Mr Stewart at the Department of Economic Affairs and emerges looking even more puzzled than usual. Mr Gunter, at the Ministry of Labour, is forced to deal with earth-shaking issues like the case of 28 artificial-limb fitters.

In this kind of situation, Mr George Brown could always be relied on to assure the doubters that faith was more important than deeds. But now that Mr Brown is practising this technique on the less receptive ears of Hanoi, there is only dour Mr Stewart – who doesn't fit into the role of revivalist preacher.

Probably this is just as well. If ever there was a time when a cool look at the whole question of an incomes policy was needed, this is it – particularly now that a new supporting cast has taken over at DEA. For at the root of the Government's apparent success in freezing wages lies a paradox. In the past, the main justification for an incomes policy has always been that the only alternative is massive unemployment. But we have now got ourselves into a situation where the main reason why the Government has managed to restrain wage and salary rises is because there is an unpleasantly high number of unemployed.

Jones's Test

So the Government's policy has proved very little except that when Ministers put the fear of God into people about impending national bankruptcy – and reinforce their exhortations by knocking hell out of the economy – it's possible to restrain incomes. The real test, as Mr Aubrey Jones has pointed out, is what happens when the economy starts reviving.

What indeed? Will the Government continue to maintain legal sanctions to give force to the Prices and Incomes Board's recommendations? Will a Ministry of Labour man sit in on all wage negotiations? The questions echo round Whitehall, but as yet no answer comes rumbling back.

Given this general perplexity, here is a counter-suggestion. This is that we should scrap our incomes policy and launch out with a wage bill policy.

To go back to the beginning. The idea of an incomes policy was born, not because anybody thought that the State should determine individual incomes, but because of the need to ensure that the total wages and salary bill would rise roughly in line with national productivity.

Advantages

But if this is the aim – rather than some vague notion that we somehow know what wages and salaries *ought* to be (which we don't) – then isn't it possible to work towards it more directly? Isn't it possible to devise some framework which will keep the overall wage and salary bill in check, but which will dispense with the elaborate apparatus for scrutinising individual claims or settlements? Instead of planning wage levels, couldn't we plan wage totals?

Let's assume, very roughly and very crudely, that the Government decides that incomes can go up by 3 per cent in 1968 (by which time the economy ought to be reviving). Let's assume that it then tells all employers that it doesn't care what wages or salaries are paid out, so long as their *total* bill goes up by no more than 3 per cent.

The advantages are obvious. Unions would have a direct incentive to abandon restrictive practices. At present they often feel that wages come out of a bottomless purse. But if the total were fixed they would know that higher wages could be obtained only if fewer men were employed. Unions would still preserve their traditional bargaining roles; and employers would know that a concession to one union could be made only after making certain that this would not encourage other unions to make claims above the limit of the money available.

Moreover, it wouldn't matter whether Mr Smith got a rise of 20 per cent while Mr Robinson got a rise of only 10 per cent – provided always that the total paid out in wages and salaries did not rise above the permitted figure (which could be kept down by paying some people no increase at all or sacking others).

But if the advantages are obvious so, to be candid, are the snags. The basic difficulty to be overcome is that such a system would tend to perpetuate the existing state of the economy. It would not allow for the fact that one industry is declining (e.g. the railways) and another expanding (e.g. engineering). It would not, for that matter, allow for the fact that even within the same industry one firm may be doing well and taking on more men while another is heading towards ruin and laying off its labour force.

Non-Starter

An essential element, therefore, would be some device for reviewing, say once a year, the allocation of wages as between different industries and (if possible) between different firms. It is here, surely, possible to adapt the idea of the Trades Union Congress that it and the Confederation of British Industry should decide incomes policy.

The proposal that the TUC and CBI should settle individual wage claims always was a non-starter: to begin with neither has any power to make its decisions binding on its members. But it might be far more feasible if the two bodies – under the chairmanship of Mr Aubrey Jones, representing the public interest – were to settle the overall target figures. For then individual employers and trade-union leaders would still keep their traditional role of deciding on the share-out of the available money.

One of many objections is that any such targets would reflect assumptions about the future which are only too likely to be proved wrong by events. But since this applies to any 'guiding light' (remember Mr George Brown's $3^1/2$ per cent norm?), it does not seem insurmountable. No one, after all, can expect incomes or wages policy to be absolutely foolproof; it certainly isn't in Sweden, the country usually held up as an example, where earnings regularly go up by as much as double the norm.

Penalties

In any case, since I am dealing in the currency of long-term hopes, isn't it possible to envisage a time when wage and salary rises are treated like dividend increases? That is, rises should reflect the financial achievements of the past year, not hopes about the future.

Finally, there is the question of sanctions. How would such a system be enforced? Rather than a cumbersome machinery of legal sanctions, I would suggest financial penalties: an excess payments tax (EPT) to be paid out on all wages and salaries above the fixed norm. If this were fixed at, say, 50 per cent it would be large enough to discourage employers flouting the system light-heartedly, but not so prohibitive as to eliminate all flexibility.

Something along these lines could provide a framework of national planning within which individuals would be left free to make their own decisions (and mistakes). At present it looks as though we are stumbling on with our present incomes policy, without knowing quite where we are heading, for no better reason than that there isn't an alternative in sight.

19

Labour Moves Closer to Tories on Welfare

THE OBSERVER
15 January 1967

There will be plenty of scope for Mr Patrick Gordon Walker's special talent of looking lugubrious in the months ahead. Having emerged from the Government reshuffle as Minister without Portfolio, he has now to prove that this title does not mean Minister without work.

His predecessor, Mr Douglas Houghton, was the invisible man of politics. Eleven years younger than Houghton, hopefully looking forward to a long political career to come, Gordon Walker can't afford to inherit this reputation with the office. Like Houghton, he is ostensibly supremo of the social services. Will he also, like Houghton, fade away into limbo?

The question is worth answering, not least because Houghton's own career illustrates one of the most remarkable – if, understandably, least talked about – changes in Labour's policies since the party took office in 1964.

In October 1964 Houghton became co-ordinator of the social services. It was the first time that such a post had been created – a symbol of the importance Labour attached to social policies.

A special Cabinet committee, chaired by Houghton, was set up to deal with the social services, to coordinate policies and decide financial priorities. It was backed by another committee of civil servants. The great age of revolution in social security was about to dawn.

At the Mercy of Ministers

The dawn never came. It was not that Houghton lacked drive or expertise. Probably no one in the country knew more about taxation and insurance. But although he knew what should be done, he was never allowed to do it.

It was partly that Houghton found himself a commander-in-chief without an army. Ministers nominally subordinate to him – like Miss Peggy Herbison at Social Security – complained bitterly if Houghton so much as mentioned their plans in public.

Houghton himself, without a penny of his own to spend, without any civil servants of his own to command, was at the mercy of the departmental ministers. The overlord became the prisoner of his subjects.

So, deprived of political authority and lacking a platform in the House of Commons, Houghton made himself useful chairing Cabinet committees. It was important. It was essential. But it wasn't what he had been appointed for.

But although Houghton never produced the promised social charter he did preside over what in the long term may turn out to be rather more important: a basic shift in Labour's attitudes towards the social services.

It was a change imposed by events. As financial crisis followed financial crisis, it became clear that Labour's hopes of paying for all social benefits out of economic growth were doomed.

Houghton fought hard. Pensions, he argued, should be exempt from the squeeze on public expenditure. If contributions were raised at the same time as benefits, he reasoned, there was after all no net increase in public spending.

But the Treasury won. By July 1965 it was clear that Labour's cherished plan for a guaranteed minimum income was as good as dead. From that time on, economic – not social – considerations dictated policy. Earnings related unemployment benefits, for example, were introduced largely at the insistence of the Department of Economic Affairs worried about job mobility.

With the grand scheme for a completely new approach to social security benefits which would eliminate the need for any kind of means test mouldering in the files, it became a question of making do and mending. Family allowances are now on the agenda (again, as much because the DEA is concerned about lower paid workers as out of humanitarian motives). Help for the disabled is next.

It is, in effect, an unspoken revolution. The emphasis has switched from 'universality' (across-the-board-help for everyone) to 'selectivity' (help for those in greatest need).

Indeed, in private conversation it becomes clear that there has been a remarkable convergence between Labour and Conservative thinking. Some Labour Ministers now actually welcome the growth of private pension schemes – which raise benefits without imposing a new burden on the taxes (which can lead to demands for higher wages).

There is a limit, they are heard to mutter, to the extent to which you can use the tax system to achieve social advance. Moreover, private contributions represent genuine savings. It's not so very different from the Conservative line that State benefits should represent the bread, with private schemes providing the butter.

Precisely Why He Was Appointed?

The rethinking goes farther still. Not so long ago any suggestion that State schools should make charges to parents would have been anathema. But last week Professor A. J. Ayer (long a Labour sympathiser), Dr. Michael Young (once head of Transport House research department), Professor David Donnison (extremely influential in shaping Labour's housing policy) and Dr I. C. R. Byatt (about to take up a post as senior economic adviser at the Department of Education) put their names to a minority recommendation of the Plowden Committee in favour of charges at State nursery schools.

The extent to which this rethinking will be carried through is in doubt now that Houghton has left. Lacking his predecessor's seniority and expertise, Gordon Walker may find it difficult to impose any kind of coherent pattern on the Government's social policies.

Which, as some cynics have been quick to point out, may be precisely why he was appointed. For to have a strong Minister representing the social services could be a source of embarrassment to Mr Wilson at a time when there is so little money to dole out.

20

What is Wrong With Housing

THE OBSERVER
12 February 1967

Any word association test starting with 'housing' would almost certainly end up with producing 'scandal.' A few years ago we had the scandal of Rachmanism. More recently we had the 'Cathy Come Home' scandal of the homeless. Now we have the scandal, as the Conservatives see it, of the Government's failure to achieve its target of 400,000 new homes a year. There are few issues on which the Pavlovian reflexes of indignation work more overtime.

But if there is a real scandal, it cuts deeper. It is that the housing policies of successive Governments, Labour and Conservative, have produced a mish-mash compounded of ideological prejudice and political expediency which doesn't even begin to meet the country's needs. To sum up the muddle in one sentence: we have now got a housing policy which might deliberately be designed to give least help to those who need it most.

The housing problem is not just a reflection of an overall shortage of homes. That does exist, and is likely to go on existing for the foreseeable future even if the Government achieves its 1970 target of 500,000 homes a year. It's not only that we need 150,000 houses a year just to keep up with an expanding population. It's not just that there are a million houses already condemned as slums, with another two million well on the way.

The problem is more intractable still. The demand for better houses is never likely to be satisfied. For standards are rising the whole time with incomes, and in another 20 years' time people may regard as utterly inadequate homes which meet today's needs quite adequately. There is always the danger that, in our anxiety to cure today's housing shortage we may be building tomorrow's slums.

Immigrants

But if we accept that there is no quick cure to the problem created by the overall shortage of housing, it is all the more essential to concentrate Government help and effort where it yields the biggest results. And this is where successive Ministers of Housing have failed so conspicuously.

For the housing shortage does not affect all parts of the country and all citizens equally. It is, in essence, the problem of a handful of big cities and of a relatively small minority. It is the problem of London and Birmingham, of Glasgow and Liverpool, among others. It is the problem of the immigrants from Jamaica and Ireland, of the young people who move into the big cities in search of work, of the newly married couples with a family on the way.

As the Milner Holland report on housing in Greater London concluded: 'The people who suffer most from housing stress are those with average incomes and large families, and many of the newcomers to London.' This is where the real hardship lies, though other people are also affected if a shortage of homes drives up prices and rents.

But although this is where the real hardship lies, this is not where the real help is given. The Government is just putting a Bill through Parliament which will greatly raise its housing subsidies to council tenants, now running at the rate of £83 million a year (quite apart from another £25 million found out of the rates). The Government has introduced its mortgage option measure which will give another £13 million a year to people buying their own homes, in addition to the existing tax concessions which help owner-occupiers to the tune of £125 million a year.

Unfortunately, the worst-off families do not live in council houses nor can they afford to buy their own homes. It's not simply that most councils give low priority to newcomers. In many cities the waiting lists are so long that newcomers would have to wait for years even if they were allowed to join the queue.

But the difficulties of those who have to rely on renting accommodation from private landlords, far from being eased by Government policy, are actually increased by it. Again, as the Milner Holland report emphasised (in a section which Mr Crossman, then Minister of Housing, chose to ignore), taxation policy discriminates against the private landlord. In contrast to the United States, France, Norway, Germany and most other Western countries, there are no subsidies or tax reliefs for privately owned flats or houses to let. Landlords, unlike other businessmen, cannot even set the depreciation of their property against tax.

Rent Control

The result is that private landlords have little incentive to build new homes to let, and the supply of such accommodation is shrinking at a time when the demand for it is, if anything, increasing. The Government's new rent control measures – even though they do allow rents to go up in certain circumstances – may help to ameliorate some of the worst effects of this situation. But they may, by discouraging the private landlord, do so at the cost of aggravating it in the long term.

One much-canvassed solution is to charge economic rents to all council house tenants who can afford to pay them, in the hope that they will then move out to make way for the less well-to-do. But though there is an overwhelming case for doing so, this is no solution. Although there are some council tenants who could well afford to buy their own houses, they are only a minority.

The real solution will have to be more radical – this is to subsidise directly those in need, whether or not they are council tenants, whether or not they are buying their own houses. It is to scrap all the existing subsidies and tax concessions and to use the £250 million thus saved to help every family whose income is inadequate to meet its housing needs. It is to think of housing subsidies, not in terms of particular forms of home ownership or occupation, but in terms of the needs of particular families.

Inevitably this means some form of means test. But there is no reason why such a test should be more shaming than the incomes declaration most of us fill in for the Inland Revenue. The only valid objection to the means test is to the form it has taken – which can easily be changed.

Fresh Start

Quite apart from the means test argument, there is a further objection: that subsidising the private tenants means subsidising private landlords. But what is wrong with that? There are strong social arguments in favour of such a course. The policy of the Tory Governments between 1951 and 1964 was to encourage a 'property-owning democracy.' The policy of the present Labour Government is to encourage more council building. The result is that 46 per cent of all houses and flats are owned by their occupiers, while another 28 per cent are owned by local authorities.

It is a situation unique to Britain which could well have serious social disadvantages. Not only does it discourage mobility from place to place and from job to job – which the Government wants to promote – since no one lightly gives up squatter's rights in a subsidised council home or incurs the costs involved in buying and selling. It is also likely to lead to social stratification: with the council house tenants (working class) glaring over invisible walls at the owner-occupiers (middle class). We might even be in danger of developing a new form of class structure based on forms of home ownership or tenancy.

This, then, is the case for scrapping all our existing housing policies and making a fresh start. It means acknowledging that, at a time when our resources do not begin to match our housing needs, it is essential to concentrate our efforts where they will yield the biggest social dividends.

21

Jay as Wilson's Secret Weapon

THE OBSERVER
19 February 1967

On the face of it, Mr Douglas Jay's conduct could only be explained by a sudden, suicidal impulse. Here was the President of the Board of Trade quite deliberately challenging the Prime Minister, just as Mr Wilson was engaged in extremely tricky negotiations in Bonn, by questioning the wisdom of Britain's entry into Europe. Short of putting his head on the block, Jay could hardly have done more to court instant axing.

For Jay's action was quite deliberate. As a rule, Ministers are invited to address the Labour Party's economic affairs group. Jay invited himself. As a rule, Ministers talk only about the affairs of their own departments. Jay addressed himself to the much wider problem of the Common Market. As a rule, too, Ministers let it be known in advance what they are going to talk about. Jay didn't – which is why only about a third of the group's 60 or so members bothered to turn up.

As it was, Jay took the group's chairman – Mr Robert Sheldon – and the assembled MPs entirely by surprise when he opened a bulky departmental file and began to expatiate on the tribulations Britain could expect to suffer if she entered the Common Market.

Bored with It

Not only would there be a 4-per-cent rise in the cost of living (Wilson had earlier given a figure of $2^1/_2$ per cent). But Britain would face an economic crisis every three years (though, as someone irreverently pointed out, this would be better than the recent record).

It wasn't an unfamiliar theme for Jay. His Cabinet colleagues say they have long been bored with it. The new element was that he should choose to voice it publicly – for although he was addressing a private party meeting, everyone accepts that such speeches are automatically leaked (and if they aren't their authors tend to put the omission right as soon as possible). 'It was as good as putting out a Press release,' one Labour MP said afterwards.

So why did Jay do it? The answer perhaps lies in Wilson's reaction to his speech – or rather, the lack of reaction. The axe didn't fall. Jay is still President of the Board of Trade. And all this despite the quite obvious embarrassment his little charade must have caused the Prime Minister.

Hence the Machiavellian explanation which some Labour MPs now have for Jay's move. Jay, they argue, has been a failure at the Board of Trade: although no one disputes that he comes in the upper half of the Cabinet in terms of sheer IQ and intellectual ability, he has been the conservative head of a conservative department. Apart from anything else, he allowed himself to be surprised by a series of nasty insurance scandals.

So, continues this line of reasoning, Jay's life expectancy at the Board of Trade is strictly limited. To everyone's surprise he was left at his post during the last reshuffle; but no one would be in the last astonished if, say in the autumn, he were dropped. Jay, although a far more amiable and lively figure in private than his rather austere and prim public appearance would suggest, has no personal following among back-bench MPs to provide any kind of political bodyguard.

What, then, did Jay have to lose by his outburst? At worst, if Wilson had decided to sack him, he would have brought the date of his retirement forward by a few months. Moreover, he would have gone as a martyr in a great cause instead of fading out. At best, this argument concludes, Jay has made it far more difficult for Wilson to get rid of him, since the Prime Minister doesn't after all want to alienate the anti-Marketeers in the party more than necessary.

The trouble with this theory is that, while it fits all the facts, it doesn't quite fit Jay's own character. Not even his best friends have ever accused him of being a consummate political tactician. On the one earlier occasion when he did engage in kite-flying – in 1959 he suggested that Labour should drop its commitment to wholesale nationalisation – he did so in a transparently direct, not to say clumsy, way.

The real explanation, as others see it, must be found elsewhere. It lies in the fact that Jay is Wilson's secret weapon.

Wilson is a great student of Macmillan. And he is quite conscious that the break in Macmillan's career – when, instead of turning everything he touched to gold, he turned even gold into lead – came after his failure to get into the Common Market. After building up an irresistible momentum, Macmillan met the immovable obstacle – de Gaulle. The result was national disillusion.

Here, so this view runs, lies the real explanation for Jay's nine lives at the Board of Trade. Nothing suits Wilson better than to have Jay around pulling long faces at the prospect of entry into Europe (apart from anything else, Jay quite simply doesn't like going abroad – and tends to prefer sandwiches to foreign food). For the one impression that Wilson doesn't want to get around is that Britain has no alternative except to join up with the Six. At least, not until Wilson knows that he can actually get into Europe.

Perfect Fit

Hence the importance of Jay. He is there to apply the brakes to a band-wagon which Wilson doesn't want to run away with him. He is there (alongside such characters as Mr Fred Peart, the Minister of Agriculture) to make sure that Wilson doesn't face a united Cabinet all urging him to go into Europe. He is there, in the last resort, to keep the anti-Common Market door open for the Prime Minister.

It is a role which Jay fills to perfection. If, say, Mrs Castle or Mr Crossman were allowed to fill it (though the former is too busy playing trains, and the latter too busy reforming Parliament), there might be trouble if Britain did join the Six. Either of these would be an embarrassment as back-bench critic, giving the Left a leader which it now doesn't have.

But Jay, even assuming that he would ever carry opposition to the point of resignation, is dispensable. The man who wanted the Labour Party to change its name isn't likely to emerge as the leader of the Left, and most of his friends on the Right are ardent Marketeers.

Given this interpretation of Jay's role, as the licensed anti-Marketeer of the Cabinet, his eruption last Tuesday makes admirable sense. His timing was, of course, disastrously wrong (as his lack of political touch might suggest) but at least he was playing the part for which the Prime Minister had deliberately cast him.

For while there can now be little doubt that Wilson wants to get into Europe, there can be equally little doubt that he wants to avoid being rushed into a situation where he has no choice left. As he himself gaily pointed out in the House of Commons recently – breaking into verse – when asked to take a long-range view on some issue: –

> . . . *I do not ask to see*
> *The distant scene;*
> *one step enough for me.*

22

A Man for All Classes

THE OBSERVER
5 March 1967

Not since the days when Charles I used to dismiss contumacious Parliaments have MPs been dressed down in quite such brutal language. But Mr Wilson's threat to go to the country if his backbenchers don't behave themselves is only part of a strange new pattern of politics.

If anyone had prophesied three years ago that a Labour Prime Minister could tolerate 600,000 unemployed, slap down the trade unions and survive the abstention of some 50 of his MPs on a key issue, he would have been advised to see a psychiatrist. Yet all this, and more, has happened.

It is a very odd situation – though Mr Wilson's ability to turn defeat into apparent victory has hitherto concealed just how odd.

Of course, the Prime Minister's reputation as the man who can walk the waters could easily be dented by the coming by-elections or local elections. Of course, he is a superb political technician.

But there is more to it than that. In a way, Mr Wilson is a new political phenomenon. It is almost as though, without knowing it, we have entered the Gaullist phase of British politics.

It's not just that Mr Wilson has gone a long way to uphold the theory that Britain has moved into the era of presidential politics. He has, certainly, done that: he can afford to rough-ride over the opposition of the Parliamentary Labour Party because his appeal is direct to the electorate. Labour MPs may loathe him, distrust him or disagree with him – but they are not going to get rid of him while he tops the opinion polls.

Thus Mr Wilson has used television as a direct link to the voters, with great frequency and enormous skill, to by-pass Parliament. Equally important, he has used television in order to project himself in a particular way: as a kind of British de Gaulle, above the pettiness of party politics, who speaks for the national interest. His technique is to brand his critics as partisan and factious.

Take the example of Rhodesia. Poor Mr Heath did his best to maintain some elements of a bipartisan policy (admittedly at the cost of fudging some issues). Whereupon the Prime Minister turned on him, and accused the Conservatives of playing party politics. The standing of the Opposition Leader, whose stock-in-trade inevitably is criticism, has fallen. He has been branded a niggler.

The fact that Mr Wilson has been able to do this is a tribute to his skill in the illusionist's art. As my colleague Nora Beloff shows on another page, the Prime Minister is far more concerned with, and worried about, the intricacies of domestic Labour Party politics than his public stance would often suggest. Obviously the comparison with President de Gaulle should not be pushed too far.

But it is quite conceivable that Mr Wilson may even be able to turn the present Labour 'rebellion' on defence to his own advantage. Just as his toughness towards the trade unions has won him credit, so his toughness towards his own party may reinforce his image as the man prepared to subordinate narrow political considerations to wider, national needs.

For Mr Wilson's tactics seem, instinctively and intuitively rather than consciously, to reflect a new national mood. The age of the pragmatic voter has produced the pragmatic Prime Minister.

In the fifties psephologists like Mark Abrams showed us that, with rising prosperity, the working classes were abandoning their cloth caps. In the sixties it is now becoming apparent that our stereotypes of the middle classes are becoming equally out of date.

All classes, many sociologists now argue, are undergoing a seachange. An over-simple illustration: the old working-class community of London's East End, tightly knit and cohesive, is breaking up as people move into new housing estates. At the same time the traditional symbols of the middle classes, the rows of semi-detached houses, are being replaced by new-style housing estates where neighbours can't help knowing one another: the lace curtain is giving way to the picture window. The working classes are losing some of their feeling of being brothers in arms marching together, just as the middle classes are gaining some of this sense of community.

Again, what is the middle class? To listen to the Conservatives one might think that the typical member of the middle-class 'salariat' is the thrusting executive on his way to the top – interested chiefly in financial incentives. But the statistics issued by the Inland Revenue only last week suggest a very different picture. The great bulk of salary-earners, 3,200,000 of them, get less than £1,500 a year. Another 1,300,000 earn between £1,500 and £3,000. Only 250,000 earn more.

Mr Wilson has realised that the new middle classes may be more interested in stability (hence the wide public support for incomes policy) than in thrusting progress. He is aware that more middle-class voters are interested in having good comprehensive schools for their children than in preserving the public schools – to which most of them cannot aspire.

Above all, Mr Wilson's success suggests that today's electorate is far more atomised, far less committed to inherited political attitudes, than in the past. Precisely because people are less sure of their place in society – precisely because many working men earn more than some teachers and office workers – they are prepared to turn to a de Gaulle-type figure. All the more so when that figure is someone (like Mr Wilson) who doesn't fit easily into any class category – who, in a peculiar kind of way, manages to belong to all classes and to none of them.

If this interpretation of Mr Wilson's ability to maintain his authority in the face of hostile events is right, then it is clear that his advent marks a watershed in British politics. It does not necessarily follow that Labour has become the permanent part of power, or that Mr Wilson is personally invulnerable. But it does follow that the Conservatives will have to become a very different kind of party if they are to return to office.

23

Controlling THEM

THE OBSERVER
26 March 1967

When men with such different and opposed philosophies as Mr Enoch Powell and Mr Frank Cousins agree, as they do in condemning the Government's incomes policy, it is tempting to conclude that the man in the middle must be right: that their criticisms cancel each other out. But this is too easy. In an important sense Messrs Powell and Cousins are right.

The implications of the Government's attempts to introduce an incomes policy are far more revolutionary than Ministers have cared to admit either to the public or perhaps to themselves. They represent a basic shift in the balance of power between the individual and the State.

The extent of this change has hitherto been concealed by the Government's own rather confused tactics: it's been a revolution introduced on the instalment plan and diguised in the woolly language of White Papers. Last week we had a White Paper laying down the 'norms': soon we'll have another one telling us what power of compulsion the Government intends to introduce to stiffen the back-bone of its 'voluntary' incomes policy.

But although at times the Government gives the impression of having introduced its incomes policy in a fit of absent-mindedness, the drift of its actions is clear enough. For the first time the State is claiming the power – and, indeed, exercising it – to quash freely negotiated wage agreements.

State Power

The gradualness of the process by which we have reached this point shouldn't be allowed to conceal the enormous implications of what is happening. All the more so since this forms part of a consistent trend towards strengthening the power of the State during Mr Wilson's administration.

The Government disposes of a large and increasing share of the national income; it's now above the 40 per cent mark. It directly controls a large sector of the economy and will control even more when steel is added to the list of nationalised industries. It has introduced strict controls on office building. The emphasis on regional development has meant much more direct and selective Government interference with industry. The number of civil servants needed to administer these policies is shooting up: by 24,000 in the past 12 months.

It is all rather alarming and spine-chilling. And an incomes policy neatly fits into the pattern of a drift towards an all-powerful and all-embracing State paternally making decisions for the individual, whose freedom of choice is inevitably curtailed.

In such a situation the temptation, of course, is simply to attack the trend in an attempt to reverse it to argue that the only answer is deliberately to cut back the growing power of the State – to 'set the people free', as the Conservatives put it in their successful 1951 election campaign.

But, in fact, the dilemma is much more subtle and needs a more sophisticated answer. For the paradox of the present situation is that the growth in State power in some respects actually adds to the sum of freedom enjoyed by the people in this country even while curtailing some hitherto accepted individual rights.

Take town planning. Forbidding people to build houses or factories in a Green Belt obviously is a limit on their freedom. But it is a necessary limitation if the rest of the population is to have an opportunity to enjoy the countryside. Again, while a compulsory incomes policy (assuming that it could work) would limit the freedom of some people, in theory at least, it would give the community as a whole greater economic freedom of choice. Planning often is a way of safeguarding those freedoms which the individual himself cannot protect.

Frustration

The trouble is that this process inevitably means limiting the individual's freedom of choice. It may be a socially necessary limitation. But that doesn't necessarily make it psychologically acceptable.

To the extent that the Labour Government neglects this source of frustration, it may be digging a grave for its own policies. Obviously we have come to accept far more limitations on our individual freedom of action than our grandfathers would have thought tolerable. Obviously it

may be possible to condition people to accept even further encroach-
ments by the State.

But it would be a mistake for the Government to gamble on the
continued willingness of people to accept such a diminution in their
freedom. Its aim should rather be to anticipate the inevitable discontent
by preparing to offer an alternative.

The real alternative is not to dismantle the whole machinery of State
planning (which even Mr Powell doesn't want). It is to adopt a deliberate
policy of trying to widen the area of choice available to the individual
and of giving him a greater say in the evolution of those policies where
the decision must be taken by the community as a whole.

Partly this means a new approach to planning, with the Government
providing a framework within which individuals can then exercise their
freedom of choice. Incomes policy is a case in point. At present this is
based on the assumption that individual pay packets must be subject to
Government scrutiny. But it is equally possible to conceive a policy which
limits the total amount of wages paid out by firms while leaving it to
them and the unions to decide how to share it out.

But it also means a new approach to the whole process of administration. At one level it means accepting that parents are not just a nuisance,
but should have a say in the running of schools. At another level, it
means recognising that government should not be a mystery in which
only the elite are qualified to take part but a dialogue between the
governors and the governed – a dialogue which should take place in
public. Similarly, it means a readiness to try new social experiments, e.g.,
workers' participation in the management of industry.

It's not going to be easy. But unless we are prepared to give a new
meaning to democracy – to define individual freedom in terms of freedom
to influence and take part in the shaping of public policy (instead of just
voting every five years in a general election) – we may end up discrediting
the idea of a planned society. For what is wrong about present trends
(which are equally apparent in other Western countries, even America)
is not so much the growth in State power. It is that we have uncritically
accepted what's happening without recognising that we must make a
conscious attempt to balance it by increasing public participation in
decision making. The aim should be not so much to cut the Government
down to size but to ensure that the institutions of public control keep
up with the increase in its activities.

24

You Won't Read This ...

THE OBSERVER
9 April 1967

The great temptation in writing about the reform of local government is to abandon the attempt even before starting. Statistics suggest that only two out of every five readers of this article are likely to vote in this week's council elections. Intuition suggests that most of them are going to feel like stopping reading as soon as they know what the subject is about.

Which is, of course, precisely why reform of local government – now being brooded over by a Royal Commission – is so urgent. Here we have more than 8,000 elected authorities spending something like £4,500 million a year. And yet there is this ocean of bored indifference, on which the politicians have hardly been able to produce a ripple of interest in weeks of hard campaigning.

The fact that polls are low doesn't matter too much in itself. Far more disturbing is that most of the people who vote do so for reasons which have very little to do with their local council. All the available evidence suggests that most of those who turn out do so out of party loyalty: in effect, the party machines flatter the degree of public interest.

It's worth stressing this, if only because of the danger that the Royal Commission may interpret its brief too narrowly: that it may be too concerned with bringing about administrative efficiency (which is relatively easy) and too little concerned with making the system more democratic (which is fiendishly difficult).

Power Struggle

For if local government is to retain any kind of effective existence, it will have to reclaim some of the powers now exercised by the central government. And it will never do that if it cannot generate popular pressure for its claims.

The first need is for units big enough not to require child guidance from Whitehall. This means some form of regional government – whether a dozen or fewer big geographical regions or 40-odd pseudo-regions (the policy, alas, favoured by the Ministery of Housing). The present system of having 160 planning authorities, 1,190 housing authorities and 165 education authorities is obvious nonsense. It spreads skilled manpower too thinly; it neglects the economies of scale; it ignores the fact that the old frontiers between town and country are becoming increasingly blurred and meaningless.

Moreover, big authorities could do things which the present ones simply cannot do. They would be able to get rid of the straitjacket of the rates system – a cheap but inflexible system of raising money. They would be able to argue (as Roland Freeman does in a Conservative Political Centre pamphlet, 'Money for the Council,' published last week) for new sources of revenue: whether a local incomes tax or a local sales tax. Once again, they would be less dependent on the central government.

London Snags

So the case for some form of regional authorities – and the bigger, the better – is overwhelming. But this will throw up some entirely new snags. The Greater London Council is the nearest thing to a regional authority we have now got. And it is already clear that the creation of such a body creates almost as many problems as it solves.

Last year, Mass-Observation carried out a special survey on behalf of the GLC which provided some disquieting evidence of how local government reform can simply by-pass the people most concerned. While 58 per cent of those questioned could identify their MP, no more than 5 per cent could name their local borough councillor and only 2 per cent knew who their local GLC representative was. There was a great deal of confusion between what the GLC did and what the boroughs' role is. As the report sadly remarked: 'It is very difficult to see how Londoners can identify themselves with the Greater London Council when they are so very unaware of the amenities, functions and services provided by the GLC.'

The GLC's reaction to this – bitterly attacked by the Conservative opposition – was to increase spending on its information services. At best, this can be only a partial answer. Facts are dead things unless people feel that they matter to them personally. And it is this which is lacking.

Here it's worth remembering what happened when it was proposed to tidy the County of Rutland (population, 27,500) out of existence. Despite the fact that Rutland is an administrative absurdity, which ought to have been abolished, local feeling forced Ministers to retreat. It is impossible to imagine a similar uprising if, say, it was proposed to abolish my own local authority – the borough of Haringey (population, 255,000). This synthetic creation – the result of the reorganisation of London government – has no geographical, social or historical reality. It is an administrative unit, nothing else.

It's essential that the Royal Commission should avoid repeating the mistake of creating another lot of anonymous authorities. The second level of authorities, below the regions, should therefore be of a size to mean something to the people living in their areas. Of course the result could be to create councils too small to be of any use. But this depends on how their functions are defined. To the extent that the second-level authorities are expected to be the same kind of animal as the regions – exercising the same kind of power in a more limited sphere – we will condemn ourselves to a new form of giganticism.

New Model

But it's quite possible to conceive of a rather different kind of authority. For there is all the difference in the world between *strategic* decision making (which requires to be big in scale) and the *tactical* execution of policies (where small size can be an advantage).

So a new model of local government might see the big regional councils taking the planning decisions and carrying out major projects, while leaving it to the small authorities to administer them in the light of local needs. Indeed, it's quite possible to imagine an even more radically new pattern. This is that the elected second-level authorities should represent not so much geographical units but special needs: schools, housing estates and so on.

But the revolution – for it would be no less – should not stop there. At present councillors are hybrid creatures who make policy as well as taking part in its administration. As a result, they are not only swamped with paper work; they are also expected to handle their constituents' complaints against the bureaucratic machine of which they themselves are part.

Public Grumble

It would be far better if the majority of councillors, like back-bench MPs, dealt only with policy-making while leaving it to the officials and salaried committee-chairmen (the equivalent of Cabinet Ministers) to do the actual running of the regional authorities. This would help to reinforce the role of councillors as the people's representatives, and halt the present trends which are turning them into amateur bureaucrats.

Nor need democracy stop there. I remember my astonishment when, travelling in the United States, I came across Sioux City (population, nearly 100,000) where every town council meeting is thrown open to the public – where every citizen can personally voice his complaints and grievances. Obviously this would not work in the regional councils. But why not try it in towns the same size as Sioux City?

Of course, this would be an unprecedented experiment, in this country at least. But then this is what local government reform should be: an unprecedented exercise in social engineering designed to find out whether efficiency is compatible with participation. The Royal Commission's aim should not be to produce tablets of stone for all time, but a system flexible enough to allow trial and error – a system which can be adapted to local needs in response to local pressure.

25

Curbing Whitehall

THE OBSERVER
4 June 1967

Despite its deceptively innocuous and technical title, the Maud report is really about our entire conception of democracy. What do we really mean when we talk of Britain as a democratic country? What is the distribution of power most calculated to ensure the democratic control of decision-making? And how do we see such a democratic control working out in practice?

On the face of it, Sir John Maud and his committee on the Management of Local Government have recommended only that local councils should change the way they run their own affairs. But, in effect, the Maud Committee has challenged the basic assumptions underlying our present system of local government; about its relations with the central Government in Whitehall and about the role of the elected councillors.

These questions are all the more worth teasing out because they are implicit in the Maud Committee's recommendations without ever being quite fully spelled out. These recommendations rest on two basic arguments. First, that the dependence of local government on Whitehall finance ought to be lessened and that Ministers ought to exercise less detailed control. Second, that the councils themselves should behave more like the House of Commons: approving the broad lines of policy laid down by a Cabinet-type board of management but leaving day-to-day decision-making to officials.

School Plans

The implications of the Maud Committee's report are all the more important because Sir John is also chairman of the Royal Commission now considering the future geographical pattern of local government. Basically, the committee has come out in favour of a pluralistic system of government for Britain.

It's certainly feasible – particularly if the Royal Commission comes out in favour of larger units of local government which could then tap new sources of revenue, like local income or sales taxes, to supplement the rates. This, in any case, is the pattern in most of the other countries – Sweden, Germany and the United States – at which the committee looked.

But it implies also a deliberate attempt to reverse the trends of the past century which have seen the powers of Whitehall grow at the expense of those of the town hall. And this raises some very touchy questions. The degree of central supervision at present often verges on the ridiculous. But can the Government stop at laying down broad guide-lines – particularly about expenditure – without seeing that the rules are observed? Could it, to take an example now very much in the news, be content to lay down that schools should be comprehensive without examining in detail the schemes put up by local authorities?

Again, the Government is responsible for overall economic planning. By diffusing decision-making, it may lessen the chances that one central decision will lead to a whopping mistake. But, obviously, it also weakens the Government's control – and thus also that of the House of Commons.

Hence the importance of the other part of the Maud Committee's report: the recommendations intended to make local government both more efficient and more responsive to public feeling. Here, in effect, the committee suggests an entirely new concept of local democracy.

At present, we have got participating democracy in local government. The 43,000 elected councillors actually take part in shaping the day-to-day decisions of local government – from choosing an assistant caretaker to laying down a multi-million-pound housing programme.

The committee suggests instead what might be called ballot-box democracy: the idea that democracy consists in being able to turn out a Government (or a local council) at election time.

Part-time

The Maud report argues that councils should be run by boards of management – again drawing on the example of other countries. The members of these committees – drawing part-time salaries of up to £1,000 a year – would exercise political supervision over the council's affairs, leaving it to the officials to take the detailed decisions. The other councillors would be stripped of most of their existing powers.

Obviously, this would make for more efficient local government. The report amply documents the drawbacks of the present system, with its proliferation of committees and paper work: its investigations discovered councillors who sat on 20 committees (the average number was six) and got up to 1,000 sheets of paper to read each month. Also the surveys sponsored by the committee show that the average elected representative spends just over 52 hours a month on his job, of which only seven and a half hours are devoted to dealing with the problems of his constituents.

The system proposed by the Maud Committee would therefore allow councillors to spend more time looking after their electors. It might also attract a wider range of candidates. At present small tradesmen and employers are over-represented and workers are under-represented. Compared with MPs, too, councillors tend to be under-educated: of the former, 51 per cent have had some form of higher education as against 15 per cent of the latter.

But there are dangers. Assuming that we get better-educated councillors and assuming also that more of the work of local government will be done by officials: are we in danger of sacrificing the representative nature of the present system with all its disadvantages to the demands of efficiency?

The Maud Committee is aware of the difficulty. It stresses the need for encouraging interest in local government in the schools. It asks that the town halls should be more accessible to the ordinary citizen.

But, regrettably, the committee turns down the proposal for a system of Ombudsmen attached to at least the big local authorities. Again, it doesn't even discuss the alternative ways of involving the citizen in the process of decision-making: by allowing him to vote on specific issues (local referenda) or, to take another example, allowing him to elect school managers.

Radical

Perhaps Sir John Maud will consider some of these possibilities in his other role as chairman of the Royal Commission on Local Government. It is precisely because he has shown himself ready to be really radical – to rethink the basic assumptions of our institutions – that it's all the more important that he should be willing to experiment daringly.

The operative word here is 'experiment.' In the past, Royal Commissions delivered tablets of stone: solutions to last for all eternity. Of course, eternity always proved to be matter of decades, and then the whole process had to start all over again. It would surely be far better to regard the whole process as a process of trial and error – to allow for different ideas to be tried out in different places to see which works out best.

26

Saving Labour's First-born

THE OBSERVER
23 July 1967

Since the aim of any Cabinet discussion is not to find the right solution but the most acceptable one, the most likely outcome to the present agonised argument about cutting Government spending is some kind of patched-up compromise. Some of the social service plans will be cut; some charges may be introduced or raised; some degree of selectivity may even be tried out.

The trouble about such a compromise solution, which carefully skates over the very real difficulties of political principle involved, is that it makes another crisis inevitable. For there are two distinct aspects to the present Cabinet debate about cutting the Government's spending.

There is the immediate problem presented by the Government's failure to achieve its plans for economic growth. And there is the long-term problem presented by the insatiable appetite of the social services for more funds.

Spending

To deal with the immediate problem first. The Government's present plans for the social services are based on expectations about economic growth which have turned out to be over-optimistic. If the Government does not cut the welfare budget it will have to hold back *all* other spending, Government and private. Between 1964 and 1970, consumer spending could go up at the rate of only $1^1/_2$ per cent a year – compared to 3 per cent a year in the previous decade.

But, more serious still, there is the long-term problem. This is that welfare spending seems to have a disconcerting tendency to grow faster than the economy – as France and Germany, as well as this country, are now discovering. Partly this is because the proportion of young and old people in the population – who make the heaviest demand on these services – is increasing relative to the number of those at work. Partly, too, this is because every improvement paradoxically underlines how much more there is to be done: because by raising standards we are increasing expectations.

It is this built-in trend, rather than the Government's immediate difficulties, which poses the real challenge. Is there, in fact, some limit to what a country can 'afford' to spend on the social services and pay out in social benefits? And to what extent is that limit affected by the methods used to raise the funds required?

It should be quite clear that there is no magic formula for determining what a country can afford to spend on the social services. Britain spends less of her resources than most West European countries – but far more than would have seemed conceivable 30 years ago.

But equally it is becoming clear that the way in which the Welfare State is financed may affect its capacity to expand. For here considerations of political principle and expediency set a limit to what can be done.

Britain's Welfare State depends very heavily on being financed out of taxation. Which means, in present circumstances, that taxes will have to go up unless the existing plans are cut.

Again, there is no magic formula which allows us to decide whether a particular level of taxation is tolerable or not. Mr Anthony Crosland – who, of course, as Minister of Education has reasons of his own for arguing against cutting public expenditure – was quite right, in his speech last weekend, to point out that the picture of Britain as a grossly over-taxed country is something of a national myth.

The difficulty is that any increase in taxes – without changing the basis of the tax system – would almost inevitably mean a move towards egalitarianism (it's no accident that Mr Crosland, in his days as a right-wing heretic, re-defined socialism as being about equality). Which, of course, has enormous political and social implications.

Unequal

Britain is still a very unequal society: there has, contrary to the general assumption, been remarkably little re-distribution of wealth in the past 20 years. The trouble is that soaking the rich won't pay for the needs of the Welfare State. Higher taxes would also hit those with incomes just above the average – precisely those whom Labour cannot afford to alienate.

To argue in favour of financing the Welfare State by means which require Ministers to cut their own throats politically is to ask too much of idealism. Indeed it is to condemn the Welfare State to perpetual inadequacy: for the unwillingness of politicians to find sufficient funds out of taxation has already led to the growth of a kind of private enterprise Welfare State, with an increasing number of people making their own provisions for education, pensions and medical treatment. (So taking a considerable burden off the taxpayer: it's easy to imagine Mr Crosland's embarrassment at this moment if his commission on the independent schools were to recommend their abolition and he had to find out of taxation the money which parents now pay in fees.)

And it is here that one comes to the really difficult political choice for Labour. To the extent that it wants to preserve its own creation, the Welfare State, it may have to abandon some of its own most cherished beliefs. In particular, it may have to reconcile itself to selectivity (e.g., to directing help to the 150,000-odd families below the poverty line, instead of raising all family allowances – which inevitably means either that the cost of the increase would be prohibitive or that the scale of the rise would be inadequate). Similarly, it may have to accept charges for particular services – something which it resists in principle, while accepting in practice (it abolished prescription charges but did not touch the charges for dental treatment).

There are considerable difficulties involved in such an approach. As administered at present, charges often act as a deterrent to those most in need: school meals are a case in point. But this surely is an argument for trying to devise less humiliating means for determining need, rather than against the whole idea. Again, it is an argument for looking at each issue – charges for school meals, loans for students, charges for visiting doctors – on its own, rather than abandoning the attempt and so condemning the Welfare State to eternal penury.

Impoverished

For this kind of approach is not a way (as some Conservatives are inclined to see it) of cutting State spending. It is a way – arguably the only way – of extending the Government's capacity for financing the Welfare State. For the main remaining reservoir of finance is now the willingness of people to pay for services out of money which would otherwise go on personal consumption.

To the extent that Labour is prepared to harness this willingness to the Welfare State, so the social services can be expected to survive in their present form. But if it refuses to leap this particular ideological ditch, the result will be an impoverished Welfare State catering for the poor with the better-off making their own provisions – precisely what Labour wants to prevent.

27

The Message is McLuhan

THE OBSERVER
1 October 1967

Some have compared him to Freud and Marx; others have dismissed him as an intellectual clown, a fashionable prophet who disguises his poverty of thought in a torrent of words. But no one has ignored Marshall McLuhan.

The sometime Professor of English at Toronto University – a Canadian in his fifties – is already a well-established cult figure in the United States, broadcasting, lecturing and delivering opinions: one of the great oracles of the pop-soc – popular sociology – scene. And now, with the publication of his collected works here, he is making a bid to extend his beachhead in this country.

Is he worth taking seriously? The question is not all that easy to answer. For the mere fact that he has made such an impact – that a reference to McLuhan is an essential item in any do-it-yourself kit for being intellectually up to date and in the know – is important. If nothing else, his popularity tells us something about the world in which we live. For even if he turns out to be a phoney prophet, there is significance in the hunger for the kind of prophecy which he delivers.

His Slogan

For McLuhan *is* a prophet. He is not just analysing the world around him. He is telling his readers that he has discovered which way the world

---

'The Mechanical Bride,' 45s; 'The Gutenberg Galaxy' (paperback), 20s. Both published by Routledge and Kegan Paul. 'Understanding Media' (paperback), Sphere, 10s. 6d. 'The Medium is the Massage,' Allen Lane, 42s.

is going, and that they'd better climb on to the bandwagon of history before it leaves them behind.

For McLuhan's basic idea – though not his way of expressing it – is simple. It is that the way people communicate is more important than what they say: hence his famous slogan, the medium is the message. Or, in other words, the technology of communication shapes the way people see the world around them, the way they behave and the way they think.

Tribal man, before the invention of the phonetic alphabet, lived as part of his environment. He was totally involved in it, in his sense of sight, in his sense of touch and in his sense of hearing.

But then came the invention of the phonetic alphabet (all this is fully set out in the 'Gutenberg Galaxy' originally published in 1962, the most searching and best-worked-out of all McLuhan's books). There followed the expulsion from Paradise, the fall from innocence. Gradually man's sense of wholeness disintegrated – he lost his capacity to regard things in an 'audio-tactile' way – i.e., using his sense of hearing and touching. He became increasingly, and finally, exclusively visual.

The revolution was completed with the invention of printing in the fifteenth century. This not only made men irredeemably visual but created a new tradition of thought: like the movable type of the printing process, man came to think in terms of logical sequences. Man himself became a movable, replaceable part – an individual entity in himself, instead of part of the collective.

But now, as McLuhan expounds in 'Understanding Media' (1964), we are in the middle of yet a further revolution: the electronic revolution, of which television is the most important feature. And we are re-creating tribal society on a world scale: the globe, in McLuhan's phrase, has become a village.

Television is a 'cool' medium – another key word in McLuhan's terminology, very personal, sometimes rather weird. That is to say, it involves its viewers as participants – unlike 'hot' media, like newspapers, which simply deliver messages to them. It engages their emotions, it demands their attention and invites them to react.

To take a specific example. In an interview published in *Encounter,* McLuhan expatiated on this theme: 'TV news coverage of Vietnam has been a disaster as far as Washington is concerned because it has alienated people from that war. Newspaper coverage would never alienate people from the war because it's "hot"; it doesn't involve. TV does, and creates absolute nausea. It's like public hangings – if there were public hangings there would be no hangings: because public hanging would *involve* people.'

So we are moving into a new era – as McLuhan explains in 'The Medium is the Massage' (joke!), the latest, most prophetic of his books, which has now appeared in this country. Here, with a minimum of words and a maximum of pictures, he sums up his main themes. We are moving into the age of 'mass culture . . . a world of total involvement in which everybody is so profoundly involved with everybody else and in which nobody can really imagine what private guilt can be any more.' Man and his environment are at one once again. The split between man and society, between the individual and the crowd, between nation and nation, has been healed by the wonders of technology.

New Freud?

So much for the main outlines of McLuhanology. Where does this leave him – a new Freud or a false prophet?

McLuhan obviously has some valuable insights. He is a man of genuine perception. What he says may very often seem obvious, even platitudinous, once he has said it. But the important thing is that he said it. We didn't recognise his epigrams as platitudes until he had drawn our attention to them.

It's self-evident now (but it wasn't until McLuhan pointed it out) that television does affect our way of seeing things, that the screen isn't simply an extension of the book or the newspaper. Television, for example, is bad at presenting a logical argument. But it's marvellous at bombarding us with images which set up a great many reactions.

Take political broadcasts. In the age of radio, a Prime Minister would address the nation – and that would be that. Now he is interviewed. There are films of interviews with people. There is an attempt to persuade the viewer to identify himself with what he sees on the screen – whether with an unemployed man on the dole or Mr Wilson dealing with the verbal darts of the interviewer.

Again, McLuhan seems to have correctly diagnosed a new desire, particularly among the young, to participate: whether simply by jiving to records instead of sitting still or by listening to public readings of poetry.

But though it may be absurd to compare McLuhan with figures such as Marx and Freud, he does resemble these prophets in one important respect. It is that he attempts to give one explanation to make sense of all the many, perplexing changes through which we are living. He has tried to produce one all-enveloping system of thought to produce a master-key to our time – with electronic technology taking the place of the class struggle. It is this which explains both his popularity – for all of us, after all, would like to make sense of the chaos around us – and his failure.

For the great mistake – fostered by McLuhan himself – is to see him as a neutral observer, emotionally detached and eager only to analyse without involvement. He is none of that, even though he goes out of his way to explain that he personally is rather distressed by many of the phenomena of the electronic age.

The key to McLuhan lies in his first book, 'The Mechanical Bride,' published in 1951, which he now tends to dismiss as having been written before the age of television had revealed the truth to him. In this he takes a series of newspaper advertisements and strip cartoons as slipways from which to launch essays on the state of American society. And what emerges is a picture of a man in revolt against his environment. A man, moreover, who far from refusing to judge what he sees – his position now – not only judges but condemns.

He condemns the American cult of individual competitiveness. He condemns the American system of co-education as designed 'to prepare boys and girls alike for the neuter and impersonal routines of production and distribution.' He condemns 'the view of the human body as a sort of love machine capable of merely specific thrills.' And so on.

Dangerous

No wonder, given this disenchantment, that McLuhan sees the new electronic age as a release: the new era which, like the classless society for Marx, will solve all our problems. No wonder, then, that television and all the rest of the wonder equipment assumes magic properties for him, explaining everything and reconciling everybody.

And it is this which makes McLuhan not so much a false prophet (much of what he says may be true or become so – no one, and certainly not the prophet himself, can tell) as a dangerous one. For, unlike Marx and Freud, he relieves us of personal responsibility. His is no programme of action. Relax, and welcome the inevitable is his message. No wonder he is the centre of a new cult – which demands no effort and apportions no responsibility.

Equally dangerous, however, is his way of presenting his message (and since he stresses the importance of the medium, it's only fair to analyse his medium). He doesn't argue. He asserts. He doesn't prove. He ransacks the books of anthropologists, historians and scientists – so giving his books a formidable if slightly spurious air of scholarship – for examples and quotations which will support his views.

Moreover, he has a short way with critics. The critics, he replies, simply don't understand that he is doing something entirely new which demands new methods. So, clearly, their objections simply reflect their out-of-date prejudices.

While the early McLuhan of 'The Mechanical Bride' called for 'rational self-awareness' to counteract 'the behaviour mechanisms of the machines that frighten and overpower us' the later McLuhan tends to dismiss any criticism of current trends as an exercise in spitting in the wind. Like Marx, he claims to have devised a new method of inquiry. Unlike Marx, though, his method denies rational refutation: those who differ from him, by definition, haven't understood him. To aim at 'rational self-awareness has become the inability of the old-fashioned 'visual' man, brought up on the print culture, to understand what's happening.

McLuhan is the master of the brilliant half-truth and the dogmatic overstatement. Everything is explained exclusively in terms of his dominating theme. The Roman Empire crumbled because supplies of papyrus from Egypt were cut off; Hitler rose to power because television had not yet been invented. And so on – a great cataract of statements which may contain a germ of truth but which are far short of the whole, complex truth.

Insights

McLuhan himself tends to dismiss those who object on these grounds as lacking in a sense of humour: to argue that he is dealing in poetic, not literal, truths. But if so, he is pulling the carpet not only from under his readers' feet but from under his own.

Considered as a prophet, McLuhan must therefore be considered as a false one. Considered as a cult figure, he must be regarded with cautious scepticism – as encouraging the belief that there are simple solutions to complex problems. Only considered as a man with brilliant insights – no more and no less – he should command our attention.

Some McLuhanisms

- 'Our new electric technology that extends our senses and nerves in a global embrace has large implications for the future of the language. Electric technology does not need words any more than the digital computer needs numbers. Electricity points the way to an extension of the process of consciousness itself, on a world scale and without any verbalisation whatever. Such a state of collective awareness may have been the preverbal condition of men.'

- 'Television demands participation and involvement in depth of the whole being. It will not work as a background. It engages you. Perhaps this is why so many people feel that their identity has been threatened.'
- 'In both new attire and new dwellings, our unified sensibility cavorts amidst a wide range of awareness of materials and colours which makes ours one of the greatest ages of music, poetry, painting and architecture alike.'
- 'Any expensive ad represents the toil, attention, testing, wit, art, and skill of many people. Far more thought and care go into the composition of any prominent ad in a newspaper or magazine than go into the writing of their features and editorials . . . it is obvious that any acceptable ad is a vigorous dramatisation of communal experience.'
- 'Just as we now try to control atom-bomb fallout, so we will one day try to control media fallout. Education will become recognised as civil defence against media fallout. The only medium for which our education now offers some civil defence is the print medium. The educational establishment, founded on print, does not yet admit any other responsibilities.'

28

The Doers and the Done-to

THE OBSERVER
29 September 1968

A public opinion poll taken recently in the United States showed a majority of Americans to be agreed on one issue: in their dislike of all three presidential contenders. More than half of the electorate would prefer not to have any of the candidates – Nixon, Humphrey or Wallace – as their country's leader. It is a result worth pondering by both Mr Wilson and Mr Heath as they prepare for their party conferences. For it would be surprising if a similar poll taken in this country were not to show a similar rejection of the leadership.

It's a mistake to over-interpret the result of polls. People had high temperatures long before the thermometer was invented. Voters distrusted politicians as self-seeking careerists long before they were asked to record their distrust by the pollsters.

But this said, it is possible to detect a new mood, a new intellectual atmosphere. For the past 10 years political discussion has centred very largely round the techniques of managing the nation's affairs: the politics of planning. For the next 10 years political discussion looks like centring round the question of who should be managing whom: the politics of participation.

There is a growing feeling – expressed in innumerable articles, pamphlets and speeches – that it is not enough to discuss ways of promoting economic growth. The question now is: growth for what? Does it make sense to define the 'quality of life' – a much-favoured phrase – in terms of refrigerators and hospitals, cars and schools? Or should it take into account man's relationship with his fellow citizens and society?

Allies Against Bureaucracy

The question has been put most stridently and aggressively by the students of the revolutionary Left. It is increasingly echoed by the intellectuals of Labour's centre. And it is also being asked by a growing number of Conservatives. For Left and Right are linked in their shared dislike of bureaucracy, in their suspicion that the growth of State power has brought about not an increase but a diminution of democratic control.

For a great deal of the emotional steam behind the Conservative demand – sure to be voiced at Blackpool when the Tories meet there next month – for cuts in State spending, for sacking civil servants, spring from a vague, confused and hardly articulated feeling that the ordinary citizen is losing his freedom. There is, of course, also the more primitive and old-fashioned dislike of having to pay taxes.

But certainly the more sophisticated advocates of a market economy, particularly those associated with the Institute of Economic Affairs, have developed a coherent philosophical base for their theories. They argue that the most effective way for the ordinary citizen to participate in decision-making is to allow him to make his own decisions. Why, they ask, should the State paternalistically decide who should go to what schools? Why not give all families vouchers which will allow them to buy whatever education they prefer for their children? The middle classes do so already. Similarly with other social services: why patronise the working classes by assuming that they cannot exercise freedom of choice?

It is an attractive approach. But it does raise some very prickly problems. There are some decisions, e.g., town planning, which cannot be left to the individual. So, whatever the arguments in favour of increasing the area of choice, it is not a complete answer.

Obsolescent Rituals

At the other extreme are the latter-day Marxists working for the day when students will be running the universities, when workers will take over the factories and when the State will wither away. Their agitation is significant chiefly for the mood that it reveals. For this kind of approach is rapidly by-passing the thinking of Labour's traditional Left. It underlines the belief that nationalisation doesn't make much difference either to workers or to the public.

The Labour Party conference this week may be too busy with its ritualistic self-laceration to spend much time on this subject. But it is simmering away, and could soon boil over. There was Mr Anthony Wedgwood Benn's speech calling for greater participation – a demand now reflected in the Labour Party's mid-term manifesto, with its emphasis on involving the ordinary citizen and on creating an industrial democracy.

But to call for more participation and to argue for industrial democracy is all very well: it's the kind of political sermonising which instantly has the whole audience nodding in agreement. Indeed there is a danger that 'participation' will come to be regarded as the cure to all the ills of a technological society, that it will develop into the slogan of a new kind of secular religion which gives comfort to its adherents without imposing any great burden of thought on them.

The reasons for this longing to find a new theology of democracy are not difficult to analyse. Traditionally society has been divided into the middle classes and the working classes. But a more accurate division would now be into the doers and the done-to. There are those who take decisions – whether managers or civil servants – and there are those who have decisions imposed on them – whether workers or clerks.

In one sense there is nothing new about this. The real difference is that an increasing number of people are no longer prepared to accept this state of affairs: the expectations aroused by the democratic myth have come home to roost.

The number is bound to increase with education. For the remarkable thing about those who have taken to the streets in protest – as a study by Frank Parkin of the CND movement showed – is not that they are alienated from society. They are predominantly young people with a good education who believe that they *ought* to have a say in how things are run. In short, the expectations of the traditionally small ruling élite are now shared by a growing number of people.

Granting all this, what does 'participation' mean? What does 'industrial democracy' imply? As soon as one starts trying to answer these questions, it immediately becomes apparent that there are two different approaches to the whole problem.

The first approach is to accept, the concentration of power in an advanced industrial society. It is to acknowledge that the decisions which Ministers and managers have to take require a great deal of technical expertise which cannot be reconciled with the demands of head-counting.

Proponents of this view, like Professor Bernard Crick, believe that, while it is impossible to involve people in the actual decision-making process, it is therefore all the more important to keep them in touch with what is happening. The emphasis is on communication: on letting students know what is happening in their universities, on letting workers know what is happening in their factories, on letting the public know what is happening in Whitehall. Let us have less secrecy about decision-making, let us have more inquiries into Government, let us use opinion polls to find out what the public wants, but don't let us pretend that there is some magic formula for participation – so runs this line of argument.

Skyscraper Nonsense

Obviously there is a great deal to be said for this approach. If anyone had seriously tried to establish people's preferences about where to live, it's very unlikely that the nonsense of building skyscraper blocks of flats would have been perpetrated. If more were done – on the model of Coventry – to consult people's views about replanning their cities, there would be less of a feeling that town planning is something inflicted on the ordinary citizen.

But is communication really enough? A recent study of the John Lewis Partnership by three distinguished sociologists, Allan Flanders, Ruth Pomeranz and Joan Woodward, suggests that it is not.

The John Lewis Partnership is not only a profit-sharing concern. It also has a most elaborate machinery for consulting and informing the 'partners,' i.e., the workers. But the powers of decision remain with the managers. And, the three sociologists found, the attitude of the partners is much the same as the attitude of the workers to their employers in other firms: they do not, in any real sense, feel a sense of belonging. Information and communication are a means of improving management efficiency, not for creating an 'industrial democracy.'

Hence the emphasis of the other kind of approach: which is to stress the need to allow more people to share in the exercise of power. This line of argument can be applied to a variety of institutions. For example, creating new regional authorities in place of some of the existing councils does not necessarily increase participation. But allowing more direct elections to, say, school boards of management might be a way of promoting direct participation.

Again, in industry, workers often participate in the decision-making process only when they go on strike. This may be their most effective way of making sure that their views are heard by the management. Hence the argument, put forward by Professor Elliott Jaques, that it is much better to give workers the right to be involved in all strategic decision-making from the first – rather than waiting for strikes to force managements into a position where they have to concede this right. At the Glacier Metal Company, from whose experience Professor Jaques draws this conclusion, no major decision can be taken without the unanimous agreement of both workers and managers.

Conflict of Loyalties?

Hence the Liberal Party's proposal that there should be a works council in every plant with the right to be consulted. Hence the slightly weaker proposals of the Labour Party that workers should have the right to information about their firm's activities.

But should such rights be backed by workers' directors on the boards of their companies, as recommended by a minority of the Royal Commission on Trade Unions? It's a proposition which is rejected by a great many trade unionists, who see it as a means of blurring the lines between unions and managements.

The difficulties are not, however, insuperable. The problems thrown up by involving workers' directors in day-to-day decisions of management – where a conflict of loyalties could easily arise – can be partly resolved by having, as in Germany, Supervisory Boards. These do not interfere in day-to-day management but (rather like the part-time outside directors on British company boards) represent other interests, including those of the workers.

There are plenty of obstacles in the path leading to the promised land of participatory democracy. Indeed, the promised land may turn out to be a mirage. But it is only by advancing towards it – by trying out, on a cautious experimental basis, new methods of involving people in the management of government, of universities and industry – that we shall be able to find out.

29

Masters Into Managers

THE OBSERVER
30 June 1968

Tarting up old buildings is a dangerous business: an old beam comes out and down falls the ceiling, a bit of panelling is removed to reveal dry rot, and soon everybody starts asking whether it wouldn't be more sensible to pull the whole thing down and start afresh. And this, of course, is precisely the question provoked by the Fulton report on the Civil Service.

Its members were in effect told to provide the design for converting a Victorian mansion into a modern office block. And, admirable though most of their ideas are, the main impression left by their report is that it would have been better to start on the building: that before deciding on what kind of civil servants are needed, it would have been best first to determine what kind of machinery of government they are going to run.

Taking Risks

As it is, one's got to start the other way around. The Fulton Committee's basic assumptions were that the needs of government today require a greater emphasis on management rather than administration, on taking rather than avoiding risks, on personal responsibility rather than a collegiate system which gradually evolves decisions, on research and figuring rather than on educated hunches. Given all this, what follows?

For example, the Fulton report condemns the system of switching civil servants from Ministry to Ministry. But if civil servants are to stay longer – and if, at the same time, they become more 'expert,' as the report recommends – doesn't this make it all the more necessary that Ministers also should stay longer in their jobs? Otherwise they will be far more at the mercy of their civil servants than they are now; the reason why Ministers now can so often resist domination by the bureaucracy is that the civil servants may be almost as ignorant as the political heads.

One Minister recently suggested in private that nothing less than a three-year term in office makes sense (though obviously three months is too long for an incompetent incumbent). So one conclusion to be drawn from Fulton is that, if there is to be efficient government, there will have to be far fewer Ministerial changes: in particular changes (like those at the Department of Education) which have been prompted not by any desire to improve the Ministry but by the political desire to shuffle the pack.

Indeed, to the extent that the civil servants become more professional and expert, so it's going to be increasingly important that the politicians should become more efficient in carrying out their task. At present civil servants are to some extent political animals: not in the sense of owing allegiance to any one party but in that they take account of political arguments in shaping their decision. If they are going to become more managerial in their approach, then it is all the more essential that Ministers should be better equipped than they are now to frame the terms of references within which the bureaucrats act.

The Fulton Committee's proposal for a special policy planning department within each department, responsible directly to the Minister, should help (something along these lines was recommended by the Haldane Committee on the Machinery of Government 50 years ago: this said: 'In the sphere of civil government the duty of investigation and thought, as a preliminary to action, might with great advantage be more definitely recognised').

But even more important, surely, is the overall planning of government policy. For as the report of the Management Consultancy Group, which advised the Fulton Committee, put it: 'In big firms the evaluation of different courses of action based on research is a major concern to top management. In the Civil Service, top management is largely preoccupied with reaction to such immediate pressures as Ministers' cases, Parliamentary debates and questions, reports of Parliamentary Committees and deputations.' And what goes for the Civil Service applies even more strongly to Ministers, in particular to the Cabinet.

In making the case for Civil Service reforms to remedy this weakness, the Fulton Committee was by implication making out a similar case for Cabinet reform. The argument points in the direction of a smaller Cabinet (along the lines of the Parliamentary Committee which Mr Wilson has already introduced) which concentrates on taking the essential decisions, isn't cluttered up by trivia and is fully equipped with facts and figures.

But there's an obvious danger if the machinery of government – political as well as administrative – were to become too managerial in its approach. For there is all the difference in the world between running a business and running a Government (however much the latter may usefully learn from the former's methods). In business the aims of the enterprise – crudely speaking, to make money – are clearly defined and are not the subject of debate. The whole process of government, by contrast, is a way of defining and adapting those aims – to take account of conflicting interests, changing circumstances and political ideas.

Obviously once those aims have been defined, then there is every reason for letting the civil servants get on with the job in a managerial way (one of the main themes of the Fulton report). Hence the case – touched on by the committee – for hiving off some government functions to administrative agencies on the Swedish pattern. Hence, too, the case for devolving power to the bigger authorities which are likely to be recommended by the Maud Commission on local government.

MPs' Powers

But if Whitehall sloughs off some of its existing responsibilities what happens to Parliamentary control? How can MPs exercise a check on the activities of such agencies without intolerably meddling in detail?

This problem has already arisen in the case of the State-owned industries. And the rough outlines of a solution are already clear. In return for renouncing some of their power to inquire into the details of policy execution, MPs should be given greater power to help shape the framework of those policies.

What this means in practical terms is an extension of the system of committees which look into the work of Government departments (also recommended by Haldane 50 years ago). MPs could then concentrate on arguing about what the aims of policy should be – rather than spending time on niggling details.

But niggling details do, of course, matter – for they are those which usually affect the public most directly. And to the extent that civil servants are encouraged to act in a more entrepreneurial way, so the protection for the citizen will have to be strengthened. It may be no accident that in countries like France, where civil servants are encouraged to use their personal initiative, there is also a system of administrative law which lays down rules of conduct and gives the citizen a right of redress.

But, of course, there is a further protection for the citizen: publicity. The most effective restraint on the Civil Service (as Fulton recognises) is the ability of the public and the Press to find out what is happening. Managerial government should mean the abandonment of the present, introspective habits of secrecy.

Saving Time

These are all very large questions. And the time has surely come for Mr Wilson to set up a committee (however reluctant one is to suggest yet a further inquiry) to look into all these matters. Here the Haldane committee once again provides a precedent: this did its work within 18 months. And, to save the Prime Minister time, here's a list of possible members – chairman, Mr Douglas Houghton, Labour's most distinguished backbencher and chairman of the Parliamentary Party, backed by Mr John Mackintosh (a Labour MP and former academic specialising in constitutional matters), Mr Jo Grimond, Sir Keith Joseph (who as well as being an ex-Tory Minister has business experience), Mr David Howell (a young Conservative who has done much work on this whole subject) and Sir William Armstrong (the new head of the Civil Service).

If such a committee were appointed now, it could report before the end of next year. And Britain might go into the seventies with a machinery of government, as well as a Civil Service, adapted to contemporary needs.

30

Participation v. Efficiency

THE OBSERVER
29 December 1968

It was the year that discontent infected the student body with all the virulence of an influenza epidemic. It was the year that theatre censorship was abolished. It was the year that 'Look Back In Anger' was revived. It was the year that John Lennon was fined for possessing cannabis. It was also the year in which the Labour Government seemed to be continually teetering on the edge of political disaster, while all the attempts to exorcise the ghost of economic crisis failed conspicuously.

Indeed, a cartoonist trying to sum up the year might well picture Britannia as a raddled old hag in a miniskirt on her way to the bankruptcy court with an armful of parcels collected in a last, defiant shopping spree. In the background is the iconography of 1968: dockers marching in support of Enoch Powell, a theatre poster advertising 'Hair,' a policeman being kicked, a demonstrator with blood streaming down his face, the weary, no-comment visages of Ministers disembarking from official cars outside No. 10.

No doubt this is a gross, outrageous and inaccurate caricature. But in one respect it does catch a characteristic of 1968. Unlike other years of disillusionment and doubt (and when was there last a year when one was not tempted to use these twin adjectives in writing its obituary?) 1968 had a special flavour about it. It was the year in which disenchantment sprang not from a revolt against oppressive symbols of the past but from disappointment with the achievements of yesterday's iconoclasts and reformers.

Looking back over the past 12 months, the remarkable thing is the rapid rate of change: like the crew of a leaking old ship, Ministers have been jettisoning old ideas, old policies and old ideals.

The military withdrawal from East of Suez was hastened in the wake of devaluation. Prescription charges were introduced. The plan for raising the school-leaving age was abandoned, precipitating the resignation of Lord Longford. At times the slaughter of sacred cows proceeded at such a pace that the gutters of Westminster seemed to be running with political blood.

Indeed, as the year went by, the process seemed to gain momentum. The Seebohm Committee drew up a new blueprint for the country's welfare services. The Fulton Committee denounced the cult of the generalist in the Civil Service and proposed a much more managerial body to run Whitehall. The Donovan Commission called for trade union reform though, inhibited by the presence of Mr George Woodcock among its members, it seemed to think that this could be brought about by pious exhortations. The Labour and Tory leaderships agreed on a plan to eliminate the hereditary element in the Lords.

Found Wanting

It was as though the previous autumn's devaluation had broken the dam of inherited inhibitions. Radical reform was the year's orthodoxy.

For 1968 marks the point where the reforms advocated over the past 20 or more years were largely carried out – and found wanting. After decades of trying to clear up the problems of the past, Britain found herself facing the problems of the future.

The 12 years which went by between the premiere of 'Look Back in Anger' and its revival in 1968 has made what once appeared as a challenge to society something closer to a theatrical requiem for a society that is passing away. Anger has given way to frustration with a society which assimilates its critics (including John Osborne himself) and which is too unsure of itself to provide the simple, self-evident and indefensible targets which were still available in the immediate post-Suez era. Even the theatre censor has gone. How can one commit sacrilege in a church whose priests nod benignly at four-letter words?

It is a situation which produces its own ironies. A decade ago, demonstrators paraded their indignation at Britain's shoddy pretence to be the world's policeman. In 1968 the young were indignant because Britain lacked the power or the will to try to influence events in Vietnam, Biafra and Greece.

It is also a situation which creates its own stresses. For tolerance is a two-edged weapon. It is an effective (and humane) way of dealing with would-be revolutionaries. Nothing, after all, is better calculated to neutralise the self-styled enemies of society than turning them into the equivalent of showbiz personalities on television.

The Conflict

But tolerance can also tempt society's critics to raise the temperature of controversy: to try to attract attention by breaking windows or heads when hard words fail. Moreover, militant tactics can sometimes work: a year starting with the sit-in at the Hornsey College of Art and ending with students at Birmingham rifling through the Vice-Chancellor's files has brought large gains to the undergraduate population.

But the gains – and one wonders just how many students will want to sit on all those boring university committees once these have lost the charm of the unattainable – have been bought at a price. For 1968, while showing the extent of British society's tolerance of dissent, has also demonstrated that this particular piece of social elastic has its breaking-point.

It has spelled out what previous years have only hinted at: Britain, like other advanced industrial societies, is now facing a conflict of two distinct political and social cultures, partly – but only partly – embodied in the traditional conflict of generations.

There are those whose tribal memories encompass the past: who see in the political system a method of apportioning scarce resources by means of a peaceful, if not entirely rational, method of bargaining and compromise. Their tradition rests (at its best) on self-discipline and (at its worst) on authoritarian paternalism. They tend to believe in collective action, through trade unions or professional bodies.

As against all this, a new culture is developing: one which isn't haunted by the ghosts of the past and which takes the achievements of the post-war period for granted. It is both generous and naïve. Generous because it takes the abolition of things like poverty for granted (and is therefore appalled to learn that homelessness is still a problem.) Naïve because it assumes that all would be well if only society were not run by a reactionary bureaucracy, if only students were allowed to run universities and workers were permitted to run factories.

In a sense, it was absolutely logical that British students should be infected by the wave of unrest that swept the universities of the world in 1968. Not in spite of the fact that they are better off than most of their contemporaries elsewhere but because of it: because their eyes are on the problems of the twenty-first century, the problems of affluence and leisure, rather than the problems of removing the debris of the nineteenth century.

There is another strand in this development. The new movements in the arts proclaim the value of individual and spontaneous experience and reject the framework of social and historical tradition.

At one end of the scale this new form of individualism takes the form of arguing for legitimising the use of 'pot' and other means of 'stretching the mind.' At the other end of the scale it takes the form of composing music in which the fidgetings of the orchestra play as integral a part as the notes on the composer's score.

But this form of individualism is a luxury: the luxury of those who, whether as pop stars or actors, whether as subsidised students or affluent teenagers, can afford to opt out. Hence much of the resentment that became evident in 1968: the resentment of those who perhaps envy the freedom enjoyed by the younger generation – but are also conscious of the precariousness of that freedom and of the struggle needed to make it possible.

This, as public opinion polls during the year confirmed, was the reaction of a majority which was all for cutting the students down to size and for emphasising the traditional values of 'law and order.'

Once again this is hardly surprising. In a period of change people inevitably seek to cling to those parts of the established order which have escaped shipwreck.

Certainly this fear of change underlies much else that happened in 1968. It was one ingredient (though perhaps not the main one) in the nearest thing to a popular movement: the response to Enoch Powell's 'rivers of blood' speech. For this, while it was certainly fuelled by feelings of racialism, also touched society on a raw nerve. It raised the fear that a society in which a great many men and women were already worried that their traditional skills and social habits were becoming obsolescent would change its nature in a still more fundamental way, with the injection of a large, permanent coloured minority.

Some of the fears are rational enough – though their projection on to the immigrant population was not. Ministers have for so long been proclaiming their aim of 'restructuring' British industry, to use the official jargon, that it was difficult to realise that this was actually happening in 1968.

But happen it did, as the continued closure of pits and the accelerated tempos of mergers showed. And industrial and technolgical change inevitably means social dislocation: not only the miners but workers hit by mergers demonstrated their discontent during the year.

These demonstrations underlined another theme to emerge in 1968. The demands of economic efficiency and the demands of social tranquillity often point in opposite directions.

A great many people in Britain want to preserve the amenities of peace and quiet: the year began with a famous victory when the Government was forced to abandon its plans for Stansted airport. But how many are prepared to pay the cost of doing so?

Again, a great many people in Britain want to preserve their traditional way of life. But what, as in the case of mining villages, if this conflicts with the dictates of economic efficiency?

The question was asked in a wider context still in 1968 when participation became the vogue word. The world of parish councils – where people meet to decide what affects their own immediate environment – is as much part of the native mythology as the belief that every Englishman is potentially a country gentleman.

But just as the mythology of an-acre-and-a-cow comes up against the facts of life in a small island with a large population, so the mythology of participation comes up against the fact that a great many services may be run more efficiently on a national rather than local scale. Moreover ideals can easily come into conflict with one another, as 1968 also showed. Against Labour's ideal of a comprehensive education was opposed the ideal of each local community being able to decide on its own form of education.

While nationalistic feeling continued to run high in Scotland – as signalled by the local election results – Northern Ireland came as a warning that conceding freedom also meant renouncing the ability to influence events. Again, while Mr Wedgwood Benn and others talked about participation, many voices were calling for the safe paternalism of a coalition government.

The year ends, therefore, bequeathing a whole horde of questions to its successor. Labour, having during the course of 1968 plotted a manic-depressive course of alternating despair and hope, seems destined to go down to defeat. Or is it? The country as a whole has seen its expectations of economic recovery frustrated by international crises. Can it now ride the underlying groundswell of prosperity created by devaluation or will the ship strike yet another hidden rock?

A sustained period of political stability and economic prosperity could well dispel 1968's sour smell of national frustration, just as further setbacks could increase the sense of introspective self-pity to dangerous proportions. No one can be sure. But this much is certain: the nation's basic dilemmas will remain. It will still be faced with the choice between managerial efficiency and participation, between the conflicting requirements of growth and the desire to maintain social cohesion.

.

31

Barbara's Strike Cure

THE OBSERVER
5 January 1969

When the unions denounce Mrs Barbara Castle for going too far and employers attack her for being too timid, it is tempting to conclude that her plans for reforming industrial relations represent a sensible half-way house. But this would be a mistake. For this is not a problem which can be solved by compromising, any more than the question of abolishing the death penalty could have been settled by deciding to half-hang murderers.

Indeed, Mrs Castle deserves sympathy in her present dilemma. Not only does she face the prospect of a political row within the Labour Party. But the problem she is trying to tackle is one of those complicated issues which defy simple diagnoses or easy remedies. For strikes are not a virus which can be cured simply by finding the appropriate social, legal or financial vaccine.

In the decade between 1955 and 1964, the latest year for which comparative international figures are available, Britain had a *better* record than, for example, the United States and Japan in terms of days lost through strikes (though a far worse one than Sweden or West Germany). But nearly 95 per cent of British strikes were unofficial: the British speciality is frequent, small-scale strikes whose effects may be quite disproportionate to the numbers actually engaged – as the recent disputes in the motor industry showed. Hence their peculiarly disruptive effect.

If one were starting from scratch in designing an industrial relations system, it would not be difficult to cure this condition. Obviously, better management is needed. Equally, it would help if there were always one union to represent the men in any one workshop. Again, as the Royal

153

Commission on Trade Unions stressed, it is essential to have clearly defined agreements for settling disputes quickly.

Beyond this one enters more controversial territory. Strikes often reflect a breakdown in communications. But how is efficient communication to be guaranteed? It may be that the answer is worker representation on the board of directors – a solution Mrs Castle seems to be flirting with tentatively. Or it may be more effective to have works councils in each factory with the right to be consulted before the management takes decisions.

But it is one thing to propound the solutions that are required. It is quite a different matter to put them into effect. And here the real perplexities begin. The majority of the Royal Commission persuaded themselves that very little could be done beyond exhortation.

Mrs Castle – judging by the details of her proposals that have leaked out – has rejected this approach. Instead, she has reconciled herself, somewhat gingerly, to stealing some of the Tory clothes and altering them to suit her own political style.

There is to be no question of making agreements between employers and unions legally binding. Instead, there is to be the power to impose a two-month 'cooling-off' period on unofficial strikers (with fines to be collected subsequently from their wage packets – so avoiding the danger of having to send hundreds of men to prison for refusing to pay). Also the Government would have the power to make the findings of the proposed new Commission for Industrial Relations legally binding in certain circumstances and to compel unions to hold a ballot before deciding to go out on strike.

In principle, one ought to be suspicious of any extension of the law into a new sphere of social activity. Indeed one of the ironies of the present situation is the confusion in which the parties find themselves. The Tories, who resisted race and incomes legislation, are in favour of industrial legislation. Many Labour MPs, who favoured race and incomes legislation, are suspicious of this incursion into a new territory.

But the case for legislating about industrial action is that strikes can, in certain circumstances, damage society as a whole. Hence the oddity of the unions presenting themselves as the champions of a new kind of *laissez-faire* – as though they were suddenly to argue that the State should have nothing to do with the siting of factories or with the emission of noxious fumes, however damaging such activities were to the health of the community.

The real objection to Mrs Castle's proposals is rather different. It is that they propose to regulate industrial relations by administrative action rather than the impartial workings of the law.

Under the Conservative proposals, all breaches of agreements – whether by employers, union officials or wildcat strikers – would be legally actionable (though, if one reads the fine print in the Conservative Party document, the parties to an agreement could agree *not* to make it legally binding – a loophole which, it might be thought, gives the unions plenty of protection). But under Mrs Castle's draft plan, it would be left to the Minister's discretion to decide when and where to apply the new legal powers.

This, as the history of the Prices and Incomes legislation has demonstrated, could be catastrophic. Thus the incomes policy is being applied to stop the farm labourers (who are in no position to strike) from getting a rise, but not to stop the tally clerks in London's docks from getting one. Thus, too, the university teachers immediately got the Prime Minister to repudiate Mr Aubrey Jones's strictures on their work habits, but no one imagines that he would have intervened if similar unpalatable things had been said about the rat-catchers' and mole-trappers' union. It is as though the law against robbery were to be enforced only against the small fry but not against the Train Robbers.

Yet unless the law is applied impartially, it will sooner or later fall into disrepute. At the moment there is widespread support for the idea that unofficial strikes should be made illegal: in a National Opinion Poll survey last year, 61 per cent favoured such a step; moreover, 56 per cent of Labour supporters and 57 per cent of union members agreed. This support could easily be dissipated if, like incomes policy, measures to regulate industrial relations were to be regarded as yet another short-term political expedient.

This would be a tragedy. There is much that is good in Mrs Castle's package. The idea of giving unions, like firms, public money to encourage rationalisation and mergers is excellent (though here I must admit to being prejudiced, having fathered this idea some years ago). So are the proposals for giving dismissed workers the right to appeal to an impartial tribunal and for giving unions the right to recognition in certain circumstances.

But the effect of all this can only be gradual. Hence the need to frame any legislation with the awareness that the prime aim is not to obtain any immediate short-term results but to change attitudes, to apply leverage to the conservatives on both sides of industry to change their traditional habits.

For the aim should not be to stop strikes. In a free society, strikes are inevitable. There will always be circumstances where there is a direct clash of interests between employed and employers.

The real aim, in which a change in the law has an important but subsidiary role to play, is to avoid the kind of pin-prick strike which results from misunderstandings or sheer bloodymindedness. It is to exert pressure on both sides of industry to create a situation where the inevitable friction can be resolved without strike action.

Other countries, notably Sweden, also have legal provisions for fining strikers who break agreements. But these work, one suspects, because Sweden also has a more efficient system of industrial relations. And the case for introducing legal penalties in Britain is that they would be a direct incentive to both sides in industry to improve the whole machinery of negotiation. If anyone has yet thought of an equally effective incentive to persuade them to do so, they have still to come up with the answer.

32

How to Live with Cannabis

THE OBSERVER
12 January 1969

Ego: What a pity that Lady Wootton and her colleagues didn't have the courage of their own arguments and recommend the legalisation of cannabis. It really is rather hypocritical to point out that 'the long-term consumption of cannabis in *moderate* doses has no harmful effect,' and then to come out in favour of tinkering with the penalties for smoking it rather than abolishing them.

Of course, I know why they have done this. There they all are, card-carrying middle-aged liberals, who no doubt smoked cigarettes and drank whisky while they brooded over their report. They just don't understand that the young may prefer to get their 'sense of excitement . . . followed as a rule by a sense of heightened awareness' by smoking pot rather than by consuming alcohol or nicotine.

Super-Ego: You obviously haven't read their report carefully enough. If you had only bothered to go through Professor Aubrey Lewis's appendix, reviewing all the medical literature, you would have seen that there is a vast mass of contradictory evidence. Everyone is agreed that more research is needed.

I know that the medical case against cannabis can't be proved. But the evidence doesn't justify saying that there is *no* risk. After all, we spent 350 years laughing at King James I for writing an anti-smoking diatribe before the doctors discovered the link with cancer. The joke isn't quite so funny now, is it?

Ego: Heaven knows what the long-term effects of injecting cattle with hormones or feeding battery hens with antibiotics may be. But I haven't noticed anyone demanding that farmers who do this should be fined or imprisoned. But perhaps that is because puritans like you only believe in stopping things that give pleasure and not those which increase profits.

Alcohol

In any case, since you have been quoting the report at me, can I refer you to the committee's conclusion. This is that 'in terms of *physical* harmfulness, cannabis is very much less dangerous than the opiates, amphetamines and barbiturates, and also less dangerous than alcohol.' And don't start telling me that cannabis is the first step to the hard drugs. The report says: 'It is the personality of the user, rather than the properties of the drug, that is likely to cause progression to other drugs.'

Super-Ego: There you go again, pillaging the committee's report to suit your own argument. Just after the sentence you quote comes another one which doesn't support your case. It is particularly difficult, the committee point out, 'to assess what changes even a moderate and seemingly responsible habit might bring in the smoker's relationships with family and friends, study or work.'

In other words, we just don't know about the long-term social effect. Again, I would advise you to read the report. 'It was significant,' it says, 'that even those of our witnesses who saw least danger in the drug were concerned to discourage juveniles from using it.' How would you stop young people from using pot if you legalised its use?

Ego: The fact that the sale of liquor to those under 18 is prohibited doesn't stop young people from experimenting with drink. The fact that you may land in jug if you smoke cannabis hasn't stopped the habit from spreading.

Indeed, I think it is the illegality which may be part of its appeal. Earlier, you quoted Professor Lewis against me. I now want to quote his findings against you. 'Those who have studied American college students who smoke marihuana,' he writes, 'conclude that they do so because they are alienated from the values of adult society; through this habit they can mortify their parents and flout authority.' By legalising pot, you would destroy it as a symbol of revolt.

Super-Ego: But at the end of the sentence you have just quoted Professor Lewis adds: 'This is a speculative interpretation of their motives.' And I think that's something of an understatement. We don't really know why people smoke cannabis. But we do have a pretty fair idea that – judging by some research carried out in America – the habit is acquired very early on: at adolescence, or even before.

Surely when you are dealing with what are little more than children you have got to protect them against themselves. It's better to take the risk of giving them something to rebel against than allow them to live in a permissive society where nothing is barred. If you make any rules, someone is bound to break them. But that is not a good argument against having rules.

Ego: But it is a good argument against making rules which are widely regarded as unfair. I think much of the bitterness about the penalising of pot smoking springs from the fact that those concerned feel that they are being punished for being young and different.

In 1967, there were 2,393 convictions for cannabis offences. Not only were 17 per cent of *first offenders* sent to prison. But, the report points out, 'there was notably greater emphasis on fines and imprisonment for possession of cannabis than of other dangerous drugs.' Doesn't this suggest a rather vindictive attitude on the part of the authorities?

Super-Ego: Well, I agree that everything isn't right in the existing state of affairs. And that is why I am on the side of Lady Wootton and her colleagues in trying to steer a middle course between permissiveness and repression. I think their emphasis on trying to distinguish between the use of soft drugs and hard drugs, between the ordinary consumer of cannabis and the professional pusher, is dead right.

It seems to me that their proposal is a very reasonable compromise: the ordinary offender would face a maximum penalty of a £100 fine and/or four months in jail (which would usually be suspended) while the trafficker would face an unlimited fine and two years in prison. But I am inclined to sympathise with the reservation of Mr P.E. Brodie, the Assistant Commissioner of Police, that the maximum penalty may be too low to discourage the professional criminal.

Ego: Well, my sympathies are on the side of the other member of the committee who has signed a note of reservation, Mr Michael Schofield. He points out that, under the committee's recommendations, it would be left to the prosecuting authorities and the courts to decide whether the major or the minor punishment should be invoked. Surely the distinction between possession for private use and possession for trading should be written into the law.

There's another thing that worries me. The police have virtually blanket powers to arrest or search 'on suspicion' anyone whom they think might have drugs, whether hard or soft. This is probably fair enough as far as hard drugs are concerned. But it seems monstrous in the case of soft drugs. I see that another committee are going to consider this. I very much hope they come out on the libertarian side.

Super-Ego: I think your last remark touches on the real, fundamental and irreconcilable nature of our disagreement. You put all the emphasis on liberty for the individual. I would put the emphasis on the right of society to protect itself, even at some cost to individual liberty.

The report quotes J. S. Mill's famous remark that 'the only purpose for which power can rightly be exercised over any member of a civilised community against his will is to prevent harm to others. His own good, either physical or moral, is not sufficient warrant.' But the committee quite rightly rejects this argument in the case of cannabis. In any case, it doesn't stand up to examination. It is very difficult to think of any action which doesn't affect society. If a man destroys himself by smoking cannabis this will affect both his family and society as a whole – which may be faced with a considerable medical bill.

Ego: The trouble about you is that you are not prepared to accept the logic of your own argument. If you are prepared to use the law to prevent a man from damaging his health by smoking pot, why aren't you prepared to use the law to prevent a man from drinking himself into alcoholism or smoking himself into the cancer ward?

The Risks

A footnote in the report records that 'In 1966 over half the number of riders of motor-cycles who were killed, or seriously injured, were in the age group of 15 to 19, i.e., 12,159 out of a total of 22,716.' So if you were seriously concerned to protect people against themselves, the single most effective step you could take would be to prohibit anyone under 19 from riding a motor-cycle.

Super-Ego: I agree; logically, I should. But I think when it comes to social action, you have got to strike a balance between a number of factors. You have to take into account the prevailing mood of public opinion, for it's no use legislating against the grain of the consensus. Even the modest recommendations of the Wootton Report are probably ahead of public opinion.

Also you have got to strike a balance between the risks involved. The tobacco habit is probably too ingrained by now to try to eradicate it by making smoking illegal. But that is all the more reason for doing nothing precipitate about cannabis. Once it's made legal, there would be no going back even if you did discover that it was noxious. Are you really prepared to leap into the unknown in such a reckless manner?

Ego: Yes, I am. I agree that there is a risk. But any extension of individual liberty – whether homosexual law reform or the abolition of theatre censorship – involves some kind of risk. As for your argument about public opinion, this surely isn't worthy of you. If that is to be the clinching factor, we would still be hanging our murderers.

However, I am prepared to concede that in this kind of problem you always have to strike a balance between a number of factors, as you put it. The trouble is that we put different weights on the factors involved, just as we have different ways of looking at society. You are a paternalist; I am a libertarian. And we will never agree.

Super-Ego: I would use rather different words to describe our positions. You represent permissiveness. I represent responsibility.

33

Who Should Run Our Schools?

THE OBSERVER
8 February 1970

'... the Government believe unequivocally in greater freedom for local authorities within the framework of national policies laid down by Parliament. The reorganisation of local government creates an opportunity, which the Government intends to seize, for achieving this aim.'

'Clause 2 enables the Secretary of State to require a local education authority to prepare and submit for his approval one or more plans showing the measures which the authority propose should be taken for the purpose of securing that secondary education in their area is provided in nonselective schools.'

The first quote comes from Mr Anthony Crosland's White Paper on the reform of local government, published last week. The second comes from Mr Edward Short's Bill, also published last week, which gives him power to compel local authorities to introduce comprehensive schools.

There is a nice irony in their juxtaposition. For here is a Government proposing, with one hand, to give greater freedom to local authorities and, with the other, planning to tighten Whitehall's grip on their policies.

It may be argued that the contradiction between Mr Crosland's aspiration and Mr Short's policy is more apparent than real. It has always been the function of central government to establish the main framework of national policy – to decide, for example, that the school-leaving age should be raised or that local authorities should be responsible for re-housing people made homeless by slum clearance schemes. The real question, it may be said, is how much discretion should be left to local authorities to work out the implications of national policies in the light of local needs.

Thus in the case of the comprehensives, a decision to abolish selection could still leave a wide area of discretion for local councils. There are many different patterns of organising comprehensive schools, and different areas may decide to adopt different methods.

But this argument only skims the surface of the problem which is going to face any government, whether it is Tory or Labour. For it implicitly accepts the traditional view of the relationship between local and central authority as a child-parent one. Some parents may be more indulgent than others, and actually allow their children to decide how to spend their pocket money (which is the drift of Mr Crosland's White Paper). There can be no question, however, of who is the ultimate authority.

It is particularly odd that the Government should adopt a paternalistic attitude on the issue of comprehensive schools. For, in effect, Mr Short is trying to introduce a more democratic system of education by limiting local democracy.

Local democracy, of course, often doesn't work very efficiently. Looking back over the past 100 years, the central government has probably done far more to instigate improvements in local services than the authorities themselves. There are enormous differences in the standards of the services provided by the best and the worst local authorities: in the number of home helps available, for example.

This, indeed, is why Mr Crosland has now committed the Government to a radical reform of local government. This will involve the creation of 51 authorities in England which, between them, will provide most of the main services – including education. The hope is that this will improve standards by attracting councillors and officials of a higher calibre.

But improving standards means more than imposing policies from Whitehall. Abolishing selection in education will end what is now generally acknowledged to be a social debit; stigmatising certain children as failures at the age of 11. This is undesirable not so much because the method of selection is fallible but because it tends to be self-fulfilling: those marked out as failures by being sent to secondary modern schools tend to live up to the label which society has pinned on them.

Going comprehensive is, however, only the beginning of a long process. A bad local education authority is going to run bad comprehensive schools; grouping together several indifferent secondary moderns isn't going to produce a good comprehensive. A comprehensive school which seeks to impose the same elitist philosophy as a grammar school, is going to reproduce the same tensions and strains within its walls that are now apparent in the education system as a whole.

There are further difficulties. Comprehensive schools drawing their children from a working-class neighbourhood are not going to make a contribution to breaking down class barriers – unlike the grammar schools which, whatever their faults, do act as a kind of social mixing bowl. Again the grammar school system is an effective rationing device: at a time when there is a shortage of certain specialist teachers, e.g., in mathematics and physics, they concentrate the available resources. The impact of this rationing may be harsh and discriminatory; the implication of abolishing it is that either the existing man-power will be spread too thinly or a great deal of money will have to be spent on increasing the resources.

It will therefore be crucial *how* local authorities set about running comprehensives. If they simply see reorganisation as a matter of re-arranging the educational bricks, without being willing to re-think the philosophy behind their school systems and without making extra money available, Mr Short's great exercise may turn out to be a disappointing failure.

This is why coercion may prove counter-productive. As it is, only 22 out of 163 authorities have refused to submit plans for abolishing selection – though there is also the fear that other Conservative-controlled ones may backslide if they are not prodded. To force councils to adopt policies in which they themselves do not believe is calculated to ensure that those policies will be pursued in a half-hearted and niggardly way.

Against this, there is the argument that a relatively small country that hopes to achieve a high degree of mobility cannot afford to have different schools systems in different parts of the country. But this is not wholly convincing. As the example of Switzerland shows, wide local variations are perfectly compatible with high general standards.

In Switzerland the cantons (some of which have a population which would scarcely qualify them for the status of a rural district council in this country) run the universities. And the schools are run by 3,000 *communes* or *Gemeinden*, only 65 of which have a population of more than 10,000 and many of which have fewer than 200 inhabitants. Greater Zurich, for instance, has 40 communes – in some of which the local school-master is appointed by the communal assembly (or parish meeting). This system produces its eccentricities: in remote rural areas holidays tend to be long – to allow the children to help with the harvesting. But overall the standard of education does not seem to have suffered.

It is always dangerous to translate a foreign example into a very different context. The Swiss (as the article in *Public Administration*, from which I have drawn these facts, makes clear) have a tradition of civic participation lacking in Britain.

But it is at least possible that this tradition has been maintained precisely because the cantons and communes, unlike their counterparts in this country, have real power: in government nothing corrupts as much as lack of power – and absolute lack of power corrupts absolutely.

If Mr Crosland wants to make his reorganisation of local government more than an attempt to increase bureaucratic efficiency, he may have to take a gamble on giving real freedom to councils – and to accept the price in diversity and occasional inefficiency. To impose uniformity and efficiency – Mr Short, please note – may in the long term lead only to bloodymindedness and resentment.

34

What is the Difference?

THE OBSERVER
19 June 1970

The face of it, there is one clear-cut difference between the parties. Labour believes in equality; the Conservatives believe in competition. This reflects a basic divergence of view about the nature of society, and illuminates their prospective attitudes towards education, taxation, the Welfare State, housing and, indeed, the social policies.

Traditionally, Labour has seen taxation as an instrument of social justice, a positive weapon which can be used to influence the structure of society by evening out some of the inequalities of wealth. The Tories tend to regard taxation as a necessary evil and talk less about justice and more about incentives.

Other things being equal, one can therefore expect a Conservative Government to put more emphasis on reducing taxation than a Labour one.

But other things are not equal. A Conservative Government would operate within tight constraints: much the same constraints as a Labour Government, in fact. They are imposed by the inexorable growth of State spending – a growth which reflects changing circumstances (more old people in the population, more students at the universities, doctors and other public servants demanding more money) as much as deliberate policy.

One can therefore be sceptical about the ability of the Tories to make any major tax cuts (as distinct from re-arranging the tax burden) while accepting that a Conservative Government would, in any given situation, give greater priority than a Labour one to this objective. The one near-certainty is that the Tories would make considerable changes in the tax system, that they would put more emphasis on taxes on consumption (like the Value Added Tax) and less on taxes on income.

In a neat and tidy world this ought to distinguish the Tories very clearly from the Labour Party. Historically, Labour has always favoured taxes on income – which means that you pay according to your ability to pay (the tax on a television set obviously hits an old-age pensioner much harder than a £5,000-a-year man). Indeed Labour has made much during the campaign of Conservative proposals to switch the tax burden onto the less well-to-do sections of the community.

But a Labour Government also has to operate within tight constraints. Taxes on income are all very well, but what happens when the great majority of average wage-earners have to carry the burden? Soaking the rich may be a good slogan, but it happens to be poor economics: even if they were to be squeezed dry, only a few drops would be produced in terms of the oceans of money that a modern State requires. One of the notable omissions from Labour's manifesto was any commitment to a wealth tax.

There remains the question of which party would do most to redistribute income in favour of the poor. In terms of party attitudes and sympathies, the answer ought again to be self-evident: Labour. But the past six years have seen very little, if any, redistribution in favour of the poor (though it is misleading to argue that the poor have got poorer: in fact their standards have improved, if perhaps at a slightly slower rate than the rest of the population). In practice both parties would face the same political dilemma: how, in a modern society, do you redistribute wealth – when in fact it is the great majority, and not just a small handful of the rich, who would have to meet the bill?

Spending

One of the most emotive phrases in the current political vocabulary is 'Government spending.' Mention it to a Tory, and he is likely to bristle and associate it with 'waste.' Mention it to a Labour supporter, and he is likely to associate it approvingly with better schools and hospitals.

Here again, there appears to be a well-defined division between the parties. On the one side there is the Labour Party which sees the State as defending the community against selfish private interest. On the other side there is the Conservative Party which sees the State limiting the individual's freedom by taking decisions (and spending money) on his behalf.

On the face of it, the record of the Labour Government would appear to support this model of the political parties. Government spending *has* increased at a fast rate under Labour: there has been a marked switch from private expenditure by individual citizens (which has crept up slowly) to State expenditure (which has moved up smartly).

But the political significance of this development is largely illusory. To an extent, the switch of resources under Labour from the individual to the State has been an accidental stumble. When Labour came into office, it made its plans for public spending on the assumption of a fast rate of growth. The growth didn't happen – but by then the Government couldn't reverse its plans for spending.

There is a further irony in the situation. Much of the impetus for the expansion of State spending under Labour came from commitments inherited from the Conservative Government. Public expenditure is an escalator: once on it, once committed to a road or hospital building programme, it is just possible to slow it down but virtually impossible to stop it altogether.

Indeed, the traditional situation of Labour planning to spend more and the Tories promising to retrench has, to some extent, been reversed. In its recently published five-year plan for public expenditure Labour has sharply applied the brakes – so sharply that the Tories have denounced the inadequacy of the provision made for education, to take only one example.

There is only one safe prediction to be made. Government spending will go on increasing, whichever party is returned to power on Thursday. Significantly, some Labour Ministers have used the election campaign to put in new bids for more money: Mr Edward Short jumped in with a promise to raise the school-leaving age to 17 (an expensive commitment) and Mr Richard Crossman asked for an extra £350 million for the National Health Service.

The main difference between the parties is likely to hinge not so much on the total spent but on the methods used to raise the money required. A Labour Government will tend to accept that the best way of financing State spending is through taxation; a Conservative Government to look for alternative methods of raising the cash.

For instance, the parties have rival methods of financing the Welfare State. The case needs of the Welfare State are expanding faster than the willingness of the taxpayer to meet the bill: hence the schools with out-door lavatories, the 19th century hospitals and the pockets of poverty in our society.

Labour's emotional bias is to maintain and extend the existing ways of raising cash to finance the State services: to disguise taxation (as in the case of Mr Crossman's plans for old-age pensioners) as insurance. The Tory bias is to encourage the individual to make his own provision (by taking out a private health insurance policy or joining an occupational pension scheme) and so relieve the burden on the State.

The difference, in practice, is largely one of emphasis. Emotionally, Labour may disapprove of private health insurance: but it can't afford to get rid of it in the only legitimate way – by raising standards in the NHS to the point where no one wants favoured treatment. Emotionally, the Tories would like to make provision for old age an individual responsibility, but they may not be able to solve the problem of protecting pension rights and values without a considerable degree of State intervention.

The real puzzle is to know how far Labour can reconcile its instinctive bias towards providing universal, non-discriminating and non-selective services (in the name of equality) with the hard economic facts: can enough cash be raised to avoid making universality synonymous with inadequacy?

In turn, while the Tory approach carries the promise of raising extra cash by tapping people's willingness to pay for direct personal benefits, it also creates the danger that the State provisions may come to be regarded as second-class services for the socially under-privileged.

One's best guess is that both parties would qualify the principle of universality by a large degree of selectivity – Labour out of necessity, the Tories out of conviction. Indeed, the chances are that both parties would move towards the idea of 'universal selectivity,' so neatly squaring the doctrinal circle: Labour would produce a national standard means test (in place of the many different ones now used), applying to all applicants for the various forms of fringe social benefits, and the Tories would move towards a form of negative income tax, i.e., a guaranteed minimum cash income.

In fact, the party attitudes summed up in the phrase 'private v. public spending' (or, more emotively, 'private affluence v. public squalor') are becoming increasingly unreliable as guides to action.

Pollution, for example, whether of rivers by factories or of towns by car exhausts, can be dealt with either by regulation (fining those who emit noxious fumes or waste) or, as some American economists are now arguing, by levying pollution charges (and leaving it to individuals to decide whether it's more economic to pay up or to reduce the pollution).

Technically, this could be done almost overnight by either party, and there is nothing in either's ideological kit to prevent it. The real difficulty is that to tackle pollution is to pre-empt scarce resources. Eventually, the cost would have to be paid by the community as a whole, even if in the first place it were to fall on factory owners or car drivers. For creating a better environment is expensive – and has to be paid for in terms of a slower growth either in personal consumption or in public spending. As yet, neither party has given any indication of the priority it would attach to this issue.

Paternalism

A tempting parlour game is to divide all politicians into paternalists or individualists, into Roundheads and Cavaliers, into those who believe that the State's function is to improve people and those who think that the people themselves know best. It is a categorisation which also throws up some significant contrasts between the parties.

The difference comes out most clearly in the BBC v. ITV syndrome. Labour sees broadcasting as a public service embodying certain values: its function is to improve the moral tone of the nation. Hence Labour's decision to put local broadcasting under the umbrella of the BBC. The Tories see broadcasting as the provision of a service like any other, not essentially different from laundries or petrol stations. Hence the Conservative commitment to the commercial principle in local broadcasting.

The difference runs deeper still to reveal an emotional divide between the parties. Labour tends to be suspicious of much of the paraphernalia of the consumer society, notably advertising. Tories tend to become emotional about the free play of the market, forgetting that the market can destroy as well as create freedom of choice – as when the supermarket displaces the local delicatessen.

This faith in market forces is not, of course, shared by all Conservatives. Tory attitudes range across a wide spectrum, with Mr Reginald Maudling (representing a traditional Toryism, which accepts the need for State intervention) at one end, and Mr Enoch Powell (who has an almost mystical belief in the play of the market) at the other. Mr Heath's Conservative Party has become heir to two formerly antagonistic currents in British political history: the traditional squirearchical Toryism, protectionist and interventionist, and nineteenth-century classical Liberalism which was centred on the individual, *laissez-faire* in its approach to the economy and suspicious of State power.

So the Conservative Party cuts across the paternalistic v. individualist classification, making it difficult to predict how it will react when this particular ideological issue arises. For example, the pure market doctrine would mean that when a shipyard goes bankrupt, the State should not come to the rescue. In practice, however, the paternalistic tradition (let alone the fear of losing votes) suggests that the State doesn't let the workers go on the dole – or companies out of business.

The Labour Party, too, has its paternalists and individualists. But the historical currents which have shaped their attitudes are rather different. Much Labour paternalism stems from the bureaucratic élitism injected into the party by the Webbs: the feeling that the more power is concentrated in Whitehall, the greater scope there will be for the Socialist elect to do good. But another, older, more deeply-rooted tradition puts the emphasis on the sharing of power and sees Socialism as a way of life rather than as a series of decisions imposed from the centre.

Much of the disillusion within the Labour Party about nationalisation springs from the collision between these two historical attitudes. Taking industries into State ownership may have strengthened the power of Whitehall; it did nothing to change the position of those working in them. Hence, perhaps, the present, still rather fuzzy pre-occupation with giving workers a greater voice.

Again, the two attitudes can be seen in Labour's approach to the reform of the system of government. There have been attempts to apply the logic of more efficient bureaucratic control by producing a neater, tidier system of local government and strengthening central control over the Health Service. But there have also been attempts to balance this trend by introducing the Ombudsman to defend the individual citizen. It's unlikely that Labour would move dramatically in either direction; more probably it would continue to balance the bureaucratic paternalists against the individualist participators.

Much the same trend is likely under the Conservatives. The individualists are in favour of 'cutting the State down to size.' They can buttress their case by arguing that if government departments were less cluttered up by having to take detailed decisions on petty issues, they would be more efficient. But the paternalists would not want to give up too easily the powers of the State. Again, the most likely outcome is a compromise – with no basic change in the power structure, but more measures to protect the individual along the lines of the Bill of Rights advocated by Mr Quintin Hogg.

Hence the dangers of prediction: both parties are not only coalitions of interests but, as this analysis has tried to show, rather untidy rag-bags of sometimes conflicting attitudes, ideologies and emotions. This is why, in the last resort, the future policies of any Government, Tory or Labour, are likely to be shaped by the ability of their leaderships to create enough freedom of manoeuvre for themselves – by avoiding financial crises, by securing faster economic growth – to impose their own pattern and priorities on their parties.

35

The Wilson Era

THE OBSERVER
19 June 1970

The perspective of defeat is cruel and diminishing. Looking back over the five years and eight months of Labour Government immediately after Mr Wilson's spectacular – because unexpected – rejection by the voters, it is tempting to remember the failures rather than the successes of his Administration.

The real difficulty in trying to assess the record of Mr Wilson is to know what yardstick to use. Depending on one's starting point, very different conclusions are likely to emerge – conclusions which are going to be highly relevant to the internal dialogue within the Labour party that will erupt as soon as the initial shock of defeat has worn off. For then the inevitable questions will be: what lessons from the past should we be applying to the future?

If the record of Mr Wilson's Government is to be judged by its own promises in 1964, the verdict must be a severe one. For the vision then held out was one of euphoria based on the promise of economic expansion: the economy would be put right, there would be steady growth and everything would be possible – bread for the people and butter for the Welfare State.

Nothing of the sort happened, as we know only too well. The bread turned out to be stale; the butter turned out to be rancid. Living standards crept up; social expenditure shot up – but neither increase satisfied expectations. Mr Wilson fought a stubborn rear-guard action in defence of the pound, and the Labour Government never recovered from the economic blood-letting that it suffered during this battle. Unrealistic expectations, created by Mr Wilson and his colleagues, exacted their vengeance by creating cynicism and disillusion.

If Mr Wilson's record is to be judged against traditional Labour aims and ideology, the verdict is only slightly less harsh. There has been virtually no redistribution of income. The best that can be said – and it is quite a lot – is that even in the period of economic panic, Labour Ministers used a blunt and reluctant axe on the social services. Given the constraints imposed by their failures in the economic field, Labour Ministers stuck to the traditional priorities but lacked the resources to make their intentions effective.

It is when one tries to look at the Wilson Government in a rather different perspective that its real achievements stand out. The party that took office in 1964 had only barely recovered from an era of dissension and theological in-fighting. And it is one of Mr Wilson's major achievements that the notorious in-growing toe-nail of the Labour Party – nationalisation – is now only a dim memory. He de-mythologised Labour (though no doubt there are some in the movement who would argue that, in so doing, he also de-natured it).

Here it's important to stress that what was remarkable about Thursday's result is that it was unexpected. Given the economic record, it is surely astonishing that Mr Wilson should ever have been able to reach a position where everyone thought he would win. That, and not the final result, is the most significant aspect of the election – and it can only be explained by Mr Wilson's success in making Labour a party of government rather than a party of the faithful few.

Achievements

When one tries to find a thread linking the various indisputable achievements of the Labour Administration, it is provided not by tradition, not by ideology, but by the presence in the Wilson Government of some men of outstanding competence who used the opportunities of office with imagination and humanity. The Wilson Government may not have transformed the country, as it promised to do, but it provided a platform for the reformers. There was Mr Richard Crossman who, in the various offices he held, left a trail of both political indiscretion and innovation: protection for tenants, a Royal Commission on local government, and parliamentary committees to investigate Government policy. There was Mr Roy Jenkins, who, although condemned to the ungrateful role of the Iron Chancellor, had earlier brought a new tone to the Home Office: who showed that it was necessary to be tough-minded in defence of tolerance.

A paradox of the Labour Ministry was that it appeared at its best when it was tough-minded: when it showed that liberalism does not mean a sloppy pursuit of vague objectives, but a hard-headed examination of various policy objectives. Mr Denis Healey at the Defence Department has been an outstanding example of this approach. So has the emphasis (for which Mr Wilson probably deserves credit) on improving the quality of Government statistics – an unglamorous aspect of his Administration, but one from which the Conservatives will greatly benefit.

The catalogue of successes could be extended. There has been the generous treatment of the arts. There has been the programme of law reform. There has been the abolition of hanging, the introduction of abortion and divorce law reform (encouraged, though not introduced, by the Labour Government). There has been a series of Commissions dealing with various fundamental aspects of the nation's life: the Civil Service, the Constitution, and trade unions. There has been the 'green paper' experiment – offering the Government's proposals for public debate.

This is not a negligible record. And indeed some of Labour's achievements may still belong to the future. Industry has been forced to rationalise itself (though sometimes rescued from the consequences of its own mistakes). More men are being retrained in new skills. There has been the acceptance, helped by higher unemployment benefits, of the need for greater mobility. These are changes which can show results only over a period of years.

Yet a sense of disappointment is perhaps the most important legacy left by Mr Wilson's Government – and not just because of its economic failures. Part of the explanation may lie in the fact that, starting out against the background of the 1964 balance of payments situation, it never quite recovered its equilibrium: it always gave the impression – reinforced by the Prime Minister's personal style – of living from day to day. Again, the Wilson Administration found itself caught up in what can only be called an international crisis of government: with all the institutions of authority becoming increasingly questioned in the United States and France, as well as in Britain.

Against all this, Britain is still a placid country, a country where the stresses of social adjustment at home and the change in Britain's status abroad have, as yet, not exploded into conflict: here, in a sense, Mr Wilson's basic conservatism may have paid dividends. But whether this placidity is illusory and temporary, whether the stability will turn into a narrow-minded parochialism or even into a destructive reaction against tolerance and liberalism, isn't clear yet. But it's probably by this touch-stone – rather than by an examination of the accounts – that history will judge the Wilson Government's success or failure.

Part 3

From Public to Social Policy

Rudolf claims that his conversion from public to social policy work was based largely on happenstance. His story is that a series of accidents plunged him into social and health policy when he started work in various academic establishments. Particularly at the time he joined the London School of Hygiene, no-one was looking at the politics of health policy and he saw that there was a vacuum to be filled. However, the problem with Rudolf's own simplified account of his changing work focus in the mid-to-late 1970s is that it does not explain why the academic world into which he leapt was full of these vacuums waiting to be filled by an outsider.

The papers in this section are about the politics of policy-making and cover twenty-two years of Rudolf's contribution to the idea that there is actually a politics of policy-making. This is not to say that he made the whole of his conceptual contribution take place within this twenty-two-year period but rather that my selection of papers happens to fall into this time span.

But while this collection marks a conversion from one field of interest to another, it also demonstrates just how skilfully Rudolf made the transition from one trade to another. He plunged into academic research out of journalism without a gear change. The articles about football and the opera have gone but the sharp observations and the keen analytical style are evident still in these academic papers. Nor has he ever conceded that dullness is a necessary requisite for seriousness.

36

The Management of Britain

MANAGEMENT TODAY
March 1971

In politics, as in the rag trade, fashions change rapidly. And as the fashions change, so do the vogue words linked to them. Once the magic word was growth, but its attractions have diminished as the prospects of achieving it have receded. Then it was planning; later still, participation was given an outing. Now the political hemline has changed once again, and the key word is efficiency. Mr Heath has produced a White Paper outlining his plans for improving 'the efficiency of government'. The Whitehall kit of departmental building bricks has been given a shake-up to produce new super-Ministries. Businessmen have been brought into the Treasury. Lord Rothschild has been hired to head 'a small multi-disciplinary policy review staff' attached to No. 10. The language of the business schools has become the language of Whitehall, as civil servants discuss 'output budgeting' and 'accountable units of management'.

To raise doubts about this efficiency drive would, perhaps, be as offensive to Mr Heath as raising doubts about the existence of God would have been to Mr Gladstone a century ago. Who, after all, can be against efficiency? Who can oppose more businesslike government and better managerial techniques in Whitehall? The answer, of course, is no one. The real difficulties begin when one tries to analyse what efficiency in government means. How is it to be measured? What are the criteria for success? What indices of performance are to be applied to the Whitehall managers?

In a business, it is relatively easy to measure efficiency – though even here accountants do run into difficulties. There are clearly defined inputs: labour, capital and raw material. There are clearly defined outputs: drawing pins, transformers or whatever else is being produced. There is a generally accepted measuring rod: money. And there are various indices man employed, and so on. Trying to assess efficiency in government is far more complex. It is, of course, perfectly possible to talk of inputs and outputs; respectively, taxes raised and services provided. Equally, it is just possible to devise indices of performance: if the same number of civil servants manage to write more letters, then productivity has gone up. But any attempt to push the comparison with business management much further comes up against three basic difficulties.

First, if companies are profit-maximizing organizations, governments are vote-maximizing machines. As important as the input and output of real resources is the input and output of political resources. A government needs an input of votes if it is to take office in the first place, and an output of voter satisfaction if it is to continue in office. And economic efficiency – i.e., making the best use of real resources – is not necessarily the same as political efficiency.

Thus, political efficiency means the ability to attract more voters than the rival company, just as economic efficiency means attracting more customers, among other things. But while a supermarket which pulled in customers by giving away its goods would end up bankrupt, a government which follows the same tactics stands a high chance of being re-elected. The political equivalent of giving away goods is, in this case, staging a pre-election boom: a promotion ploy which succeeded for Harold Macmillan in 1959, and for Harold Wilson in 1966, and which only narrowly failed in 1970.

The second difficulty about measuring the efficiency of government is that the most important output of government is not services, but decisions – and, what is more, decisions of a very special kind. While business decisions are inner-directed (i.e. they are decisions about what people inside the organization should do), the crucial government those outside the machine – individuals, firms or local authorities). Perhaps the most crucial index of a Government's performance is its management of the economy. But this does not only mean regulating or manipulating the behaviour of others. It also involves trying to strike a balance between often conflicting interests and considerations. For the other unique characteristic of government decisions is that they involve subjective judgments which cannot be translated into a balance sheet. For example, what is the right 'mix' between unemployment and inflation, or between growth and balance of payments considerations?

In short, government is largely a continuous process of determining the criteria of success – while in business these criteria (profits, return on capital, etc.) are the accepted tools of management. To return to the first example: if the Government decides that civil servants should step up their letter-writing rate, even if this means shorter replies to the public, what is the test of success to be? How can a balance be struck between greater efficiency (good) and more complaints from the public (bad)?

The third and last difficulty, stems from the problem of built-in political obsolescence. In business, the customer rejects the product when it stops satisfying him; in government, he rejects the managers. Equally, the political equivalent of changing the packaging or brand-image of a product is to change the Minister responsible for it. Thus Britain has had 12 finance directors, or Chancellors, in the 25 years since the war: a record equalled by few other countries and by few companies.

The converse of this exceptional mobility among those responsible for making policy is the exceptional immobility of those responsible for executing it: the civil servants who enjoy a life-tenancy of their jobs. In turn, this points to a basic characteristic of the government machine which distinguishes it from other organizations. In the last resort it is more important that government should go on than that it should be efficient. After the crash of Rolls-Royce, aero-engines went on being made. If the Government were to go out of business, there would be a vacuum. Hence the crucial importance of the principle of continuity and of 'the high priests of the machine', as one Minister has described the civil servants.

There is a further constraint on efficiency in government. This is not the obvious one of its size and complexity: the public sector now employs about 6.25 million, of whom 720,000 are civil servants working directly under Ministerial direction. The constraint is the doctrine of Ministerial responsibility, which says that a Minister is accountable to Parliament for whatever is done in his department. This doctrine prevents the delegation of responsibility which alone would make it tolerable to direct a machine of this size. For how can you delegate effectively if you are liable to be hauled over the coals by MPs if a minor official of your Ministry in Darlington steps out of line?

A flick through any random collection of *Hansards* shows the drain of top management time imposed by the doctrine of Parliamentary responsibility. One MP asks about the rule governing the flying of flags from Government House, Hillsborough, Northern Ireland. Another asks for a statement about a recent fire at Gordon Barracks, Gillingham. A third wants details about restoration work going on at St Catherine's Chapel, Abbotsbury. A fourth asks how many British passport holders are resident in Zanzibar. A fifth wants to know what the Minister proposes to do about increased charges imposed by the Stoke City Football Club. And all this is on top of the thousands of letters sent annually by MPs direct to Ministers, with the implicit threat of a question in Parliament if a satisfactory answer does not come through.

There are perfectly respectable arguments in favour of this system: for if the Minister were not answerable, who would be? But it does mean that both Ministers and civil servants are liable to be sucked into a morass of detail. 'I used to get so many briefs,' recalls one Labour ex-Minister, 'that it made more sense to toss a coin rather than to try to read them all before reaching a decision.' In practice, the good Minister doesn't try to read all the papers thrust before him: he selects the important issues. Even so, the tension between the demands of politics and management efficiency remains.

Two sets of figures illustrate this point. A survey of Cabinet Ministers in the last Government showed that they worked an average of 61 hours. Of this time, 25 hours were devoted to Cabinet discussions, Parliamentary and party business; 19 hours were spent seeing people, meeting delegations, attending receptions and making formal tours of inspection; two hours were given up to constituency matters – and 15 hours, less than a quarter of the total working time, went on the paper work and office meetings of their departments.

A survey of how administrative-rank civil servants spend their time mirrors this picture. More than a fifth of their time, 21%, was given up to helping Ministers in their political role: preparing answers to Parliamentary questions, drafting speeches and so on. Slightly less time, 20%, was given up to the 'consideration of projects in the light of financial and policy control', to use the stiff phraseology of the questionnaire prepared for the Fulton Committee on the Civil Service.

The result, often, is mutual frustration. There has long been an academic debate about who really runs the country; the politicians or the civil servants. But the more important question is whether anyone runs the country, in the sense of taking long-term strategic decisions as distinct from keeping the machine running and reacting to events. Here the result of an American laboratory experiment is relevant. In this the subjects were made responsible for managing an inventory control system. They were told to pass on routine information to clerks, to allocate clerks so as to maintain an even work-load and, thirdly, to suggest changes in procedure. All three tasks were to be given equal importance. In practice all the subjects spent more than a third of their time on the routine part of their job, and as the amount of information increased so the amount of time spent on planning decreased – until eventually, at peak load, no planning at all was done. This is what a former civil servant turned academic, R. G. S. Brown, has christened the Gresham's Law of Planning – that daily routine drives out planning. And nowhere is there more daily routine than in government.

Talking to almost any Minister will confirm the resulting frustration; '95% of government business just keeps on going as a matter of routine, and the Cabinet occasionally shakes up the remaining 5%,' one new, but already disillusioned, Tory Minister told me. Or, as one ex-Minister put it, 'When you become a Minister, you have got to decide what you want to push through. You usually can only push one thing through. So I decided to concentrate on afforestation.'

Often Ministers feel themselves the victims of the system, manipulated by civil servants. For example, the story is told of how Richard Crossman, when he was Minister of Housing, found himself at a Cabinet Committee with a civil service brief making a plea that the supervision of sport should come under his department. Half-way through the meeting he decided that this was nonsense, and that sport should come under Education. The other Ministers agreed. But a few days later Crossman looked at the minutes of the meeting and found that the recorded decision was to give sport to Housing. The civil servants explained to him that a committee of officials had decided that sport should go to Housing, and had not realized that the Minister seriously proposed departing from his brief.

'Civil servants,' according to another ex-Minister, 'give you advice about everything – about whom to talk to, about what toothpaste to use. They try to keep you busy; they will press you to go to the lavatory-brush manufacturers' dinner. And if you are very busy, and if you don't feel very strongly about the issue, you take their advice.' But if some politicians tend to be paranoic about civil servants, civil servants also see themselves as victims of the same system. Giving evidence to the Fulton Committee, one of the few occasions when civil servants were able to speak their minds in public, W. S. Ryrie, an Assistant Secretary at the Treasury, summed up the situation with some acerbity:

'We see our political masters overburdened with detailed work on day-to-day issues, and unable to give proper attention to the basic and long-term issues of policy which should be their main concern. At the same time we feel frustrated. Government departments grow larger and responsibility tends to get pushed up. Officers at the level of Assistant Secretary and Principal feel they have much less responsibility than their predecessors 20 or 30 years ago, and they are right. They are advisers and drafters, yes, and that requires intelligence and conscientiousness. Very few have much sense of responsibility for decisions. The whole ethos of the Civil Service discourages the taking of responsibility. All the pressures are in the direction of referring upwards if in any doubt; anyone who errs on the side of taking too much responsibility will soon discover that everything can be of political interest and need to go to the top. Hardly ever is a civil servant reproved for putting too much up, for not taking enough responsibility.'

Sir George Dunnett, a former senior civil servant, put the same point differently: 'In industry the test is results. . . . In the Service, on the other hand, a man is not so easily judged by the results, but is judged more by style or method; and in so far as he is judged by results the sort of comment made is "So-and-so is a very good negotiator".' These are not just the views of disgruntled or disillusioned insiders. Summing up the contrast between the Government and industry, a group of management consultants reported to the Fulton Committee: 'It is noticeable, compared with big companies, that the long-term planning role of top management is given far less emphasis than dealing with day-to-day matters, many of them relatively trivial. In big firms, the evaluation of different courses based on research is a major concern of top management. In the Civil Service, top management is largely preoccupied with reacting to such immediate pressures as Ministers' cases, Parliamentary debates and questions, reports of Parliamentary committees and deputations.' And what goes for the top civil servants applies even more strongly to Ministers themselves.

What does all this add up to? It is tempting to conclude that government, precisely because it is a political process, is bound to be inefficient by its very nature: that an efficiency drive, such as that launched by the present administration, will soon be bogged down in the sands of political expediency and day-to-day bargaining. But this is excessively pessimistic, just as the view that there is nothing wrong with government that a bit of management expertise cannot cure is wildly over-optimistic. In practice, there are two possible ways of improving efficiency, both of them more complex than appears at first sight, but which need not be ruled out on that account. The first is to try to build in a long-term planning mechanism to check the present bias of government towards dealing with today's problems, and letting the future take care of itself. The second is to try to de-politicize areas of government activity and so ease the pressure on decision-makers, on the principle that the quality of decisions goes in an inverse ratio to their quantity. (It is a fair assumption that the more budgets a Chancellor produces a year, the more he is floundering).

Governments tend to suffer from what could be called the 'Ely syndrome': this is the tendency to rush into policy changes as the result of some sudden crisis or scandal. Thus the recent revelation that patients had been maltreated at Ely Hospital led the Secretary of State for Social Security and Health to issue a circular to all Regional Hospital Boards asking them to reallocate their resources in order to provide more money for the care of the mentally subnormal: a perfectly reasonable decision in itself, but one which made nonsense of the idea of planning the allocation of health resources in a comprehensive, long-term way.

But how can resources be allocated rationally? Here one comes to the mystic initials: PPB – Planning, Programming, Budgeting. Imported from the United States, where Robert MacNamara pioneered the use of this management tool in government, first tried out in the Defence Department in this country, this has now become the new Treasury orthodoxy. PPB, also called output budgeting, is in effect a system for analysing public expenditure and policy in order to achieve a more rational allocation of resources. It involves, according to the Treasury (1) Defining objectives; (2) Analysing existing expenditure to obtain a picture of how resources are being used to achieve these objectives; (3) Obtaining information to check the effectiveness of existing programmes against their objectives; (4) Setting out alternative ways of achieving the same objectives; (5) Planning present policies in the light of future needs; (6) Regularly reviewing plans and programmes in the light of new situations, evaluations and analyses.

As a technique of management this is revolutionary only in the context of the traditions of government. But it does, hopefully, try to remedy two basic weaknesses of governmental management. The first is that the present machinery of control – in Parliament and in Whitehall – is geared to checking whether money is being spent on the purposes to which it was allocated, not to questioning whether those purposes make sense. The Gladstonian emphasis on saving candle-ends lingers on; the question of why the Government should (metaphorically) still be using candles generally remains unasked. The second weakness is that government activities tend to be self-sustaining. If a workshop producing gas mantles finds that it can no longer sell its product, the chances are that it will be closed down. But once a government department has launched out on a project, there is no market which tests whether its product is actually required or not.

Output budgeting is, in effect, an attempt to find some substitute for the market as a test of the rationality of government policies. For example, the conventional way of presenting the Home Office estimates is to show the money spent on the police, on prisons, on the probation service, and so on. The output budgeting technique is to ask how much is spent on particular objectives: e.g., crime prevention. The next step is then to analyse which form of expenditure achieves the best results. In this example, it could turn out that the cheapest form of crime prevention is not spending more on the police or on prisons, but employing more probation officers.

Again, the National Health Service has since its launching been run on the principle that you cannot have too much of a good thing: in other words, that the service will improve as the number of doctors and nurses increases, and with them the number of operations performed and cases dealt with. But this is to confuse the technology of the NHS with its objectives. If the aim of the NHS is defined as maintaining people in good health, then it could turn out on analysis that any money invested would show a higher return if it were devoted to persuading people to eat and smoke less – rather than being spent on doctors and nurses to deal with coronaries and cancer.

Unfortunately, output budgeting is no magic formula for taking politics out of government decisions. As an accounting system it is an extremely helpful tool of management: for instance, a PPB exercise in one police force showed that the cost of its police dogs was £37,900 a year – as against the £1,600 which appeared in the conventional accounts (which included only the costs of feeding and housing the dogs, but excluded the costs of training, handling and transporting the animals). But no PPB system can eliminate the need for judgment in defining the objectives of any programme.

The objective of a shoe factory is to produce shoes at an optimum cost in order to maximize profits (and if that objective cannot be achieved, the management is likely to investigate the possibilities of using its resources in another way – to manufacture slippers, say). But what is the objective of a school? How is its performance in achieving this objective to be measured? If the objective is to produce educated children, what is the criterion of education? Is it the ability to pass examinations, or to be happy human beings?

It is not surprising, therefore, that a recent feasibility study on output budgeting for the Department of Education and Science, drawn up by a Civil Service team, concluded that 'the objectives of education have, of course, always been a subject for debate. They are inextricably bound up with the objectives of society as a whole: and it will be recognized that our society has no clear consensus of opinion on its own objectives or, therefore, on the objectives of education.' In other words, a full-blown PPB exercise is impossible for education, since its aims are the subject of political controversy, and consequently it is impossible to define objectives and monitor performance.

This may be too defeatist a conclusion. In a more limited way, output budgeting may have a useful role in taking some of the guesswork out of management, even in education. For instance, it should be possible to compare the returns of spending any extra resources on nursery education as against devoting them to raising the school leaving age, just as it is possible to compare the likely returns of improving the quality of the product as against spending more on advertising.

Output budgeting is likely to be useful mainly to the extent that its limitations are recognized. Otherwise the inevitable disillusion springing from excessive expectations will kill it in this country, as happened in the US. Daniel Moynihan, the American sociologist who has commuted between academic life and Washington, has written its American epitaph: 'PPB hasn't worked; it's dead – it just isn't there. I left Washington in 1965 full of enthusiasm about it, and when I came back in 1969 it had disappeared. Partly because the people and the concepts it took to run it just didn't exist, partly because the output part of the function just couldn't be defined, much less traced.' With this warning in mind, it is therefore important to be clear about what to expect from PPB. Output budgeting can help to define problems more clearly and can act as the grit in the oyster for producing policy alternatives. But to take some of the muddle out of the decision-making process is a very different matter from taking the politics out of the decisions themselves.

Even though it is not possible to take politics out of the management of government, is it possible to take large areas of activity out of government altogether? This, in effect, is the second leg of the present Government's strategy. 'This Administration believes that government has been attempting to do too much', was the theme of Mr Heath's White Paper on the Re-organization of Central Government; less government means more efficient government. But less government can, of course, mean many different though not incompatible things. It can mean selling off marginal subsidiaries, like state pubs, or closing unprofitable ones, like the agricultural advice services. It can mean a change of managerial style in the way government is conducted. Or it can mean a Government decision to run its business as a holding company by hiving off some of its subsidiaries.

One of the main characteristics of government at present, as already noted, is its nanny-like obsession with details. In its evidence to the Fulton Committee, for instance, the Manchester Regional Hospital Board complained that 'the Board recently had to obtain Ministry approval to pay fees amounting to 45s each for 13 officers of the Board wishing to attend a course of 10 lectures after working hours, designed specifically to illustrate the use of computers in the hospital service. It is not merely difficult but impossible to appreciate the need for Ministry control over a matter of such small moment. . . .' Indeed it is, but this kind of niggling control is exercised not only over hospital boards but local authorities as well, and Manchester's example could be capped a hundred times over.

One solution is to introduce, as proposed by the Fulton Committee, the principle of accountable units of management; that is, administrative units – whether they are hospital boards or civil service units – which can be set financial targets, and judged by their success in reaching them, rather than being subjected to detailed day-to-day scrutiny. It is a solution which Sir William Armstrong and his Civil Service Department are now busy examining, but which again comes up against the rock of Ministerial accountability to MPs.

There are a number of Government enterprises which, in theory at least, could easily function as accountable units of management. Obvious examples are the naval dockyards and the Stationery Office. Units like these are performing functions which can be judged by the normal business criteria of efficiency. And to the extent that they are given non-commercial jobs to do – like printing White Papers, Bills or *Hansards* – it is possible to make allowance for the extra costs and to adjust financial targets accordingly.

But how can the present practice of Ministerial accountability be squared with such an approach? What happens if an MP inquires about the price of Christmas cards produced by the Stationery Office? If accountable management is to make any kind of sense, the Minister should be able to say that it is none of his business to answer questions like this. But who, in that case, is responsible? A company is in the end answerable to the shareholders who provide its capital. Is the Stationery Office not going to be responsible to the shareholders who provide its capital – Parliament? One way out might be for the civil servant responsible for running the Stationery Office to be directly answerable to MPs: for how can one have accountable management without accountable managers? But this would mean abandoning the myth of Ministerial omniscience and omnicompetence.

One way of resolving the conflict between managerial efficiency and political responsibility is the Morrisonian Public Corporation formula: the formula which has given birth to the nationalized industries and, most recently, the hived-off Post Office. Under this Ministers are – in theory at least – responsible and answerable only for setting strategic targets, while individual boards are responsible and answerable for achieving these targets. So why not use this Labour recipe for increasing the power of the State to further the Conservative aim of lessening the role of government – for example, by hiving off the Health Service?

The trouble about the Public Corporation formula is that, while deceptively neat and simple in theory, it has proved extremely difficult to apply in practice. For the nationalized industries do not exist in a non-political stratosphere. If they increase prices, it is a political issue. If they increase wages, it is a political issue. If they wish to close down plant or to expand on a new site, it is a political issue. In effect, therefore, the nationalized corporations are not only a constitutional hybrid, but also an economic hybrid, with severe political constraints on management.

For example, the then Ministry of Power told the 1968 Select Committee on Nationalized Industries that '. . . the Magnox nuclear programme was undertaken, not because it was economic for the Board, but because the

Government of the day favoured it as a means of furthering technical advance. Coal-fired stations continue to be built because it is the Government's policy to protect coal in certain respects, even when the Board's calculations show that coal-fired stations will not be as economic as other types of generating plant. . . . In short, the Board's generating programme is a compromise between what would be most economic for them and what is likely to be acceptable in the light of government policy.' The aircraft procurement policies of the nationalized airlines have been similarly affected by political considerations.

Nor has nationalization insulated the industries concerned from detailed surveillance of their affairs. Ministerial authorization has to be sought for individual projects – often of a relatively minor kind, like the installation of new £600,000 escalators at Waterloo Station – and detailed Ministerial inquiries frequently follow. For example, in 1966 a British Railways Board proposal to purchase 250 new passenger coaches over a 10-year period produced a 19-point questionnaire from the Ministry of Transport. Formal surveillance is reinforced by informal pressure or 'arm twisting', as Lord Robens described it in giving evidence to the Select Committee. Asked why the chairmen of nationalized industries do not resist such pressure, Sir Stanley Raymond, the soon-to-be-dropped head of British Railways, said quite simply: 'My banker is the Minister of Transport'. In short, while the nationalized industries are dependent on the Government for finance, they are not likely to be independent in their policies.

Many attempts have been made to square this circle. The 1968 Select Committee itself propounded the doctrine that Ministerial supervision should be limited to setting financial targets and checking the accountancy methods used. If in addition the Government wishes these industries to do anything for political or social reasons, the Committee recommended that it should say so clearly – and subsidize the specific activity (acquiring a commerically uneconomic aircraft or power station) accordingly.

Like PPB, this formula skates over some of the real difficulties. How is efficiency to be measured in the nationalized industries? By return on capital, comes back the answer. But how is return on capital decided in the case of the nationalized industries? By the prices charged – and so the argument comes full circle, since it is the Government which largely determines what are the prices charged. If the nationalized industries had won complete freedom to fix their prices over the past 25 years, they could now be the most 'efficient' businesses in the country – if efficiency is to be determined by return on capital. But how, given their near-monopoly position, could they be allowed such freedom?

Again, it may be argued that the nationalized industries should have to raise money for investment on the market, instead of having privileged access to the Treasury. This, too, could make them more independent of government, more 'businesslike' in their approach. But this comes up against the same snag: after all, ICI and Unilever would not be particularly exciting investment prospects if their prices were subject to government control. Thus, market criteria for efficiency in the nationalized industries will not work, with the possible exception of a concern like BOAC which operates in an area where prices are fixed by international agreement, not government decree. If efficiency is to be measured, new indices will have to be invented: output per man (though that begs the question of capital investment), the performance of certain functions (though that raises the difficult problem of whether quantity is more important than quality), and so on.

So it is not surprising that despite the Select Committee report, and despite a growing mountain of academic treatises, the dilemma of the relationship between the Government and the nationalized industries remains unsolved. When I asked Nicholas Ridley, a member of the 1968 Select Committee, who has since been translated to the new-style Department of Trade and Industry, whether he had found any changes on taking office from the situation described in the report, he said 'not one iota'. Indeed the recent episode of Lord Hall's dismissal from the Post Office has only underlined the difficulties which a Conservative Administration faces in trying to sterilize the nationalized industries politically. Clearly if there is to be efficient management, there must be freedom to appoint and sack managers. But this assumes both that Ministers know whom to appoint and the existence of generally acceptable criteria of efficiency.

Both assumptions are questionable. Appearing before the Select Committee, a succession of Ministers publicly lamented their ignorance of suitable candidates. Equally, given the absence of agreed criteria (would Lord Hall have been a more successful head of the Post Office if he had been allowed to increase postage charges by 2d and so produced higher profit figures?), changes are likely to be attacked as politically motivated. The Post Office controversy also points up an ironical shift in attitudes. The Labour Party, which launched the whole concept of nationalization precisely because it saw State ownership as the antithesis of commercially-motivated management, is now the champion of commerical freedom in its advocacy of diversification. The Conservatives, who have traditionally opposed nationalization because of its non-commercial character, now argue against State industries acting as business animals and diversifying into any branch of business where they see a profit to be made. 'The Coal Board at the present rate will end up producing everything except coal', one Conservative Minister bitterly told me. The State-owned mines in capitalist Holland have done precisely this.

The Conservative suspicion of diversification is perfectly logical if it is assumed that nationalized industries, because of their peculiar nature, can never be wholly commerical profit-maximizing animals. But if that assumption is correct, then clearly there are going to be severe limits to the process of hiving-off. Such a process may be desirable from the point of view of improving administrative efficiency, because it helps to free Ministers and civil servants to spend more time on making strategic decisions – assisted perhaps by Lord Rothschild and his brains trust. It is not, however, going to produce 'efficient' government in the normal business sense. There will still have to be a clear distinction between the essentially and inescapably political function of setting objectives and the managerial role of monitoring the way in which those objectives are being achieved.

In one respect, however, Mr Heath and his Administration should perhaps lean more on business techniques than they have done so far. As industry has discovered, it is no use improving the production process if your marketing is inadequate. Policies, like goods, have to be sold. If they are wrongly designed for the market, if they are inadequately pre-sented or if excessive claims are made for them, then customers are going to reject them – however efficient the production line. So although there is undoubtedly scope for greater business efficiency in government, it will need considerable political efficiency if Mr Heath's managerial revolu-tion is not to go the way of Mr Wilson's technological revolution – promising too much and delivering too little.

37

Growth and Its Enemies

COMMENTARY
June 1972

One of the characteristics of the human race, a look at current bookstore displays would suggest, is that it is the only species of animal which worries obsessively about its own future. What religious prophecy was to the past, social prophecy has become to the present: predicting the future of man in this life as distinct from the next – a sort of communal fortune-telling. Any roll call of contemporary exponents of the art would include Herman Kahn, Herbert Marcuse, John Kenneth Galbraith, Marshall McLuhan, among others. Mostly, there is a thin dividing line between prediction and prescription, prophecy and propaganda; between those who purport to be neutrally observing events and those committed to preaching what ought to be happening.

Although prediction appears to be a growth share on the cultural stock exchange, interest in the future is obviously not a new phenomenon. Leaving religious prophecy aside, even the secular variety can be traced back for some centuries. What appears to be new is the intellectual industrialization of social prophecy which, like some other forms of research, is rapidly entering the mass-production stage. On the one hand, there are the academics in search of as yet unclaimed territories to stake out. On the other, there are the mass media, hungry for new ideas to transmit before they are worn out by overexposure. So futurology becomes a new academic discipline, with its own institutions, and its own products displayed in the windows of the press and television.

It is as the latest model off this assembly line that *The Limits to Growth·ꞏ A Report for the Club of Rome's Project on the Predicament of Mankind**

---

*Donnella H. Meadows, Dennis L. Meadows, Jorgen Randers, William W. Behrens III, Universe Books, 205 pp., $6.50 clothbound ($2.75 paper).

is of some significance. By now its recommendations are familiar. To avoid a "global crisis" within the next hundred years or so, both the world population and the world economy must be stabilized within the next few decades. If control by eventual catastrophe is to be avoided, a "global equilibrium" must be achieved, with the world population fixed at roughly its present size and the average income per head at about $1,800 a year – half the present U.S. income and roughly equal to the current European income. Otherwise an overpopulated world, corrupting its environment and exhausting its resources, faces an inevitable cataclysm.

Dramatic though these recommendations are, paradoxically they are the least interesting aspect of this study. It is as a variation peculiar to our own times and culture on what is a long tradition of social prophecy that *The Limits to Growth* deserves looking at: less for what it tells us about the future than for what it shows us about the present.

To start with, *The Limits to Growth* is itself an example of the intellectual industrialization of social prophecy. Commissioned by the Club of Rome – an international consortium of intellectuals concerned to "foster understanding of the varied but independent components . . . that make up the global system" – the study was financed by the Volkswagen Foundation and carried out by an MIT team under the direction of Dr. Dennis L. Meadows. It involved systems analysis – that is constructing a highly simplified model of the "real" world and expressing in a series of mathematical equations the relationship among the factors selected. The study also, inevitably, used a computer. So the book is the product of a process which shares many of the characteristics of the industrial system: in particular, the specialization of labour and the use of mechanical tools.

So much for what is new about the technology of this particular study. But it ought to be seen also in the context of the Western prophetic tradition – with which it has more in common than its manner of production might suggest. This tradition has two main themes which comes together in a somewhat unexpected way in *The Limits to Growth*. There is the theme of apocalyptic catastrophe: the threat of doom to come. And there is the theme of millennial hope: the promise of eventual human perfectibility.

The theme of apocalyptic catastrophe runs through the history of Western Europe in the Middle Ages and beyond. There were regular prophecies of approaching devastation by wind and storm, drought and famine, pestilence and earthquake; often, indeed, a precise date was given for the impending catastrophe and when the Antichrist, the Red Dragon with Seven Heads and Ten Horns, or the Tyrant of the Last Days would appear. Equally regularly sects and movements would arise of the select who knew both how to avoid the doom and how to achieve the millennium: the 13th-century Pastoureaux who impartially killed Jews and clergy, the 14th-century flagellants, and over several centuries, various varieties of the Free Spirits. The doctrine of this last sect, a sort of mystical anarchism, has some curiously modern overtones: "When a man has truly reached the great and high knowledge, he is no longer bound to observe any law or any command, for he has become one with God. . . . He shall take from all creatures as much as nature desires and craves and shall have no scruples of conscience about it, for all created things are his property." The property included women: one of the signs of being a member of the elect was the ability to indulge in promiscuity without qualms of conscience.

The historian of this dark, prophetic tradition, Norman Cohn, in *The Pursuit of the Millennium*, also described the social conditions which bred the various movements. It was not the often starving but secure peasants who provided the raw material for the prophetic movements. It was the townspeople of the prosperous belts of Western Europe where, even in the Middle Ages, some of the features usually associated with modern industrial society were found: great inequalities of wealth, unemployment, and insecurity.

The other tradition of prophecy is more recent, the product of the last three or four centuries of scientific and economic development. It is basically optimistic, relying for its appeal not on fear but on hope. Man's history is a progression from ignorance to knowledge, from being the victim of his environment to being its master. Clearly this tradition casts the intellectual or scientist in a central role – since it is his knowledge which gives mankind its tools and his skills which allow it to steer an untroubled course into the already mapped waters of the future.

It is in this optimistic intellectual climate that futurology has flourished. It is difficult to draw a clear distinction between utopianism (an ideal future world) and futurology (a probable future world). Given sufficient optimism – and there was an abundance of it in the 18th and 19th centuries – the ideal easily shades off into the probable. Thus in 1770 Sébastien Mercier, in his *L'an 2440*, anticipated many 20th-century works of futurology by predicting a world in which man would only work for a few hours a day, and (more acutely) in which the study of classical languages would disappear and that of history be neglected, since it records "the disgrace of humanity, every page being crowded with crimes and follies." But although there was great faith in civic and intellectual progress, the emphasis on material progress – economic growth – was not to come before the second half of the 19th century; only then did the possibility of rubbing the magic lamp of technology to produce unlimited prosperity become one of the main props of social prophecy. This theme survived even the world Depression of the 20's and 30's. In

1930 John Maynard Keynes, in his essay, "Economic Possibilities for our Grandchildren," celebrated the approaching solution of the "economic problem" and announced the impending arrival of the problems of technological unemployment and leisure.

To look at the prophetic tradition historically is to realize that futurology may be revealing chiefly of the social and cultural assumptions of its authors: that one of the best guides to the preoccupations of any generation or any society may be its fears and hopes about the future. Indeed, just to glance at some recent products is to realize how quickly intellectual fashions now oscillate: man's future (if one is to believe the professional social prophets) is changing almost on a year-to-year basis. Dennis Gabor, in his unassuming but shrewd *Inventing the Future*, published in 1963, concentrated largely on following the trail laid by Keynes. He explored some of the social implications of technology and automation. In 1967 Herman Kahn and Anthony J. Wiener in their *The Year 2000* – modestly subtitled a "Framework for Speculation on the Next Thirty-Three Years" – dealt with politico-social developments but also put much emphasis on the nuclear balance and its consequences for the world military situation. Both books discussed population increases. Neither book as much as mentioned, let alone discussed, pollution, and only Gabor referred to the drain on the world's natural resources of raw materials, and that very briefly.

Now, five years later, it appears that the world's long-term future has suddenly changed. We no longer live under the shadow of nuclear war. We no longer live under the threat of enforced idleness brought about by automation. We are no longer faced by the danger of domination by an all-knowing because all-computerized bureaucracy or by a military-industrial power elite (to quote some other prophetic visions of the recent past). Instead we are told that we are living in the shadow of an overpopulated, overexploited, overproducing, and overconsuming world. Tell me who your futurologist is, one is tempted to conclude, and I will tell you what your future is.

Is this too facile or cynical a view? Futurology is, after all, one of the social sciences now. It is practiced by reputable academics. It uses all the paraphernalia of science, mathematical models, and computers. This is neither the nightmare world of the medieval prophets of doom nor the inspired guesswork of dilettante essayists. To try to dismiss *The Limits to Growth* as an example of cultural fashion may therefore be a sign of an unwillingness to face up to the "predicament of mankind" (to quote the portentous title of the Club of Rome's project), evidence of moral cowardice hiding behind a parade of historical knowledge.

Hence the importance of looking at the methods used in *The Limits to Growth*. For what makes it distinctive, after all, is its claim to have found some sort of scientific basis for its social prophecies. If its recommendations had been put forward by an old gentleman with a white beard parading up and down Times Square carrying tablets of stone, no one would have paid any attention. It is because this study typifies what is very much the approach of the 70's – and is by no means the worst example of methods being applied wholesale to predict the future of industries, cities, and the world – that it is worth analyzing in detail the way in which it reaches its conclusions.

This emphasis on the *how* of futurology may seem like unnecessary pedantry. However, it is no more pedantic than asking how Roman soothsayers arrived at their prophecies. To discover that they consulted the entrails of a slaughtered ox is to put the value of their prophecies into perspective. The fact that modern social scientists tend to consult the entrails of computers hardly changes the principle of the situation. This is all the more so since the attraction of *The Limits to Growth*, the reason it has provoked so much discussion, lies in its claim to be able to put figures to its prophecies – much as in the Middle Ages prophecy tried to reinforce its credibility by naming a specific year for the coming of the Antichrist, or the end of the world. It is this which largely distinguishes it from most previous exercises of the same kind.

For although recent exercises in prediction have tended, like Kahn's and Gabor's, to prophesy rather different futures, all the specific themes of *The Limits to Growth* have predecessors. The emphasis on the need to prevent population growth goes back at least to Malthus, in 1803. The emphasis on the dangers of unlimited economic growth was contemporaneous with the first signs that mankind could even contemplate emancipation from subsistence living: "He who has enough to satisfy his wants," wrote a medieval scholar of the 14th century, "and nevertheless ceaselessly labors to acquire riches . . . all such are incited by damnable avarice, sensuality, or pride." More recently, this theme has been taken up by Galbraith and E. J. Mishan, among others. Finally, warnings about the threat to the world's resources also have a long ancestry. Interest in ecology is not an invention of the 70's: in 1949, Fairfield Osborn wrote his *Our Plundered Planet*, calling for a "complete revolution in man's point of view toward the earth's resources and toward the methods he employs in drawing upon them," as well as prophesying disaster if the exploitation of nature continued unchecked. So, all in all, no sort of originality can be claimed for any of the predictions in *The Limits to Growth*, but only for its manner of making them.

How, in fact, are these predictions made? The MIT team which produced the study devised a "world model . . . to investigate five major trends of global concern – accelerating industrialization, rapid population growth, widespread malnutrition, depletion of nonrenewable resources, and a deteriorating environment." The model, they concede modestly, is "like every other model, imperfect, oversimplified, and unfinished." However, less modestly, they announce it to be "the only formal model in existence that is truly global in scope" and "that has a time horizon longer than thirty years."

But no model is better than the assumptions on which it is based. The actual physiology of any model – the mathematical equations expressing the relationships among the different factors being analyzed which are then fed into a computer – is a matter for experts to discuss. But its flesh-and-bone structure – the facts and theories on which these relationships are based – is comprehensible by the layman. Basically the whole exercise revolves around looking at past trends and projecting them into the future, on the assumption that these trends and the interaction among them will remain unchanged. Thus, if it is found that a particular factor has been growing exponentially or geometrically, i.e., doubling itself every few years or decades, it is assumed that this will continue. Population is a case in point: it is currently doubling itself every 33 years, with the result that the present world population of 3.6 billion is expected to be 7 billion by the year 2000.

Trends, however, are not immutable. Anyone trying to carry out the same sort of exercise in population predicting in 1940, on the basis of the trend of the previous decade, would have come a cropper. Extrapolating that trend would have produced a world population of 4.4 billion by the end of the century. The same is true of the other factors in *The Limits to Growth* model. Again, predictions about the point in time at which the world's resources of either food or raw materials will be exhausted, assume constant trends on both the demand and the supply side, a very bold assumption indeed. Anyone writing in the late 19th century, it has been pointed out, might well have argued that the production of fodder for transport animals put a limit to the growth of the United States economy. Similarly, extrapolating existing trends is an entertaining parlor game which (if one chooses one's base year carefully) can be designed to produce almost any wished-for result. It would not be too difficult to show that at the present rate of growth, by the year 2000 every new graduate student will be either an ecologist or a futurologist. It is perfectly legitimate, of course, to use the technique of extrapolating as a demonstration of what might happen, without any pretense of predicting what will happen – simply as an illustration of the kind of changes that are likely to be required to prevent present-day trends from causing possibly undesirable or disastrous consequences. And if *The Limits to Growth* were presented simply as an exercise of this kind, and no more, it would be difficult to quarrel with it.

But if it had been presented in this tentative way, it would not have gained the attention and publicity it has already attracted. As it is, the text veers disconcertingly between warning the reader against taking it too literally and then ignoring its own cautions. Thus at one point we read of "the inexorable progress of exponential growth." It is almost as though exponential growth has suddenly become the Red Dragon ravaging the earth in some apocalyptic vision. Later on, we learn that the growth curve of resource consumption "is driven by both the positive feedback loops of population growth and of capital growth." This time feedback loops appear to have taken on a life of their own like the Tyrant of the Last Days. As in Marx and other social prophets, history itself is on the march.

More seriously, *The Limits to Growth* deals in aggregates: that is, global statistics about population, production, and so on. But global statistics can be actively misleading. For instance, the brute statistics of the Gross National Product (GNP) can conceal as much as they reveal. These statistics tell us the income-per-head of population. But they tell us very little else. They do not tell us how that income is distributed. They can be actively misleading about comparative standards of living. For example, a country where children under five are looked after in nursery schools would appear to have a higher standard of living than a country where they are looked after at home, since teachers' salaries are recorded in the GNP statistics but the efforts of mothers are not. Also, global GNP figures mask what may turn out to be crucial trends for the future. Thus, unless the GNP figures are broken down, it is quite possible to miss the trend in advanced industrial countries away from manufacturing and toward service industries, a development which is surely crucial for future prospects. Again, *The Limits to Growth* ignores the growth in the proportion of the GNP spent on health and education in the North American and Western European countries: trends which (if one were to use the same technique as *The Limits to Growth* does) would lead to the conclusion that soon after the year 2000 the entire population of these countries would be either in the hospital or in school.

In fact, it is tempting to go much further still in drawing up an alternative exponential vision. In place of an apocalyptic view of a globe ravaged by famine and environmental decay, it would not be too difficult to sketch out a vision of a world where the main problem was to persuade people to work in factories – where the revolt against materialism had gone so far as to produce a pot-smoking population too dozy to engage in either procreation or production. Looking at the phenomenal increase in conviction rates for pot-smoking in recent years, any schoolchild – let alone a computer – could produce the appropriate statistics to support the alternative vision. It would, of course, be an utterly absurd one. But why assume that it is any more absurd than the one sketched in *The Limits to Growth*? Arguably, it is less so. For the MIT team viewed as historic and immutable some trends which may already be changing: indeed, the whole exercise is itself part of this reaction – one of many symptoms of the current interest in ecology, the environment, and so on. If anything, then, it would be more reasonable to look at the beginnings of what might be the trends of the future than at what could conceivably be the exhausted trends of the past. (This is exactly what Kahn and Wiener did in their futurological exercise. Taking their cue from Keynes, they speculated about the possible evolution of a society where the "puritan ethic" has become "superfluous for the functioning of the economy" and as a result "the conscience-dominated character type associated with it would also tend to disappear. Parents would no longer be strongly motivated to inculcate traits such as diligence, punctuality, willingness to postpone or forgo satisfaction. . . .")

There is another oddity about *The Limits to Growth*: typically, it conveys a medieval sense of doom about the environmental plagues that are foreordained to descend on mankind unless we quickly repent and repudiate the false god of economic growth; there is no truck with technological toys like nuclear fusion or solar energy which might rescue mankind from this cruel choice; for once technology is now the wild card in the pack of cosmological poker.

Yet in sharp contrast to all this, the unspoken assumptions built into *The Limits to Growth* reflect a quite astonishing optimism: a belief in the perfectibility of man which belongs to the heyday of 18th-century optimistic rationalism. Thus its projections assume that there will be no major world war – to kill off some of the surplus millions – in the next 130 years: in short, the book's calculations are based on the belief that, for the first time in centuries, the world will live in peace. More fundamental still, while rejecting scientific technology as the savior-to-be, the study characteristically shows an infinite and pathetic faith in mankind's social technology. It assumes that, once its warning is heeded, mankind will be able to carry out the social revolution demanded to implement its recommendations.

Is there any reason, though, for taking these recommendations any more seriously than the methods used to support them? If futurology appears to be closely related to astrology or medieval prophecy, why bother to discuss its conclusions at all? The answer is that to ignore the future implications of present-day trends is as irrational as to assume that these trends will continue unchanged. To dismiss the need for some sort of futurology – even if we repudiate the name and the excesses of some of its popularizers – is to assume that there is some cosmic self-steering mechanism which will see us right in the end.

Many personal decisions and nearly all public-policy decisions are an attempt to shape the future, using some sort of crystal ball: whether it is investing in savings for a comfortable old age (implicit in which is a prediction that state pensions will be inadequate) or investing in highways (implicit in which is a prediction that the automobile is here to stay). The trouble with this sort of instinctive futurology or prediction by hunch is that, inevitably, it does not make its assumptions explicit. And because the assumptions are not clearly spelled out, they are usually not discussed but taken for granted, although they may turn out to be unrealistic or unrealizable hopes. This sort of approach can easily slip into the Panglossian view that everything will eventually turn out for the best in the best of all possible worlds. The kind of social prophecy epitomized by *The Limits to Growth* is a reaction to this approach. It reacts by swinging in the opposite direction, and by assuming that mankind has the knowledge, will, and ability to engage in social engineering on a global scale. In doing so, it oversimplifies as much as those who reject the need for any sort of attempt to look at future options.

In fact, futurological studies are of value, provided that they are seen as sketches of one (among many) possible options. Kahn and Wiener adopted this approach in their book, where they presented a number of speculative, alternative futures. This method allows us to examine the implications of alternative policies and avoids the trap of confusing what *might* conceivably happen with predictions about what *will* happen. It also permits us to acknowledge the complexity of social engineering – to take into account that policy decisions often produce unexpected side-results – instead of forcing everything into the mold of prophetic oversimplification. In contrast, *The Limits of Growth* assumes that while the side-effects of technological change can be assumed to be harmful (in terms, for example, of increasing pollution or depleting resources of raw materials) the side-effects of social change can be assumed to be neutral or beneficial.

Take the case of population policy, where *The Limits to Growth* does little more than express the consensus of most Western opinion. In practice, the case for limiting population – for adopting zero population growth as the object of policy – rests much more on value judgments about what makes for a tolerable life-style than on pseudo-scientific predictions. Hence, the real difficulties faced by governments in underdeveloped countries which wish to bring the birth rate down: these difficulties reflect not so much technical problems about diffusing birth-control methods as the existence of social values which put more emphasis on large families than on rising living standards.

It is not necessarily impossible to change social values: for example, in the grossly overcrowded island of Mauritius, there has been a 40 per cent fall in fertility in the last five years. However, the unfortunate paradox – from the point of view of the "global equilibrium" thesis – is that it may well be possible to limit population growth in the underdeveloped countries of the world only by inculcating precisely those values which the developed countries are being adjured to abandon; that is, by offering the prospect of ever-growing material prosperity and by preaching the importance of rising living standards and showing that birth control is the means to achieve them. Arguably, the best weapons in the battle against overpopulation are precisely those products of Western civilization – television sets, washing machines, and cars – which are often seen by the prophets (none of whom has as yet, though, abandoned detergents in favour of beating his washing with flat stones in the local stream) as undesirable luxuries, foisted upon an innocent public through the machinations of Madison Avenue advertising agents.

But introducing new ideas about the possibility of rising standards of living is rather like introducing rabbits into a new continent. Ideas also breed, and once established may prove difficult to eradicate. Why should we assume that it is possible to carry out two major social revolutions in the space of a few decades, first to establish a culture of material progress and then to replace it with one of non-growth? Yet this is the astonishingly naive assumption buried in the equilibrium model. A successful population-control policy could conceivably have other undesirable side-effects as well. In practice it means exploiting the revolution of rising expectations. But there can be absolutely no assurance that a population policy can by itself satisfy the expectations aroused. Prosperity achieved usually tends to fall short of prosperity hoped for. If so, it may well be that the cultural changes required in a successful population policy will also increase political instability in developing countries. Standards of living will rise as birth rates fall, but will they rise fast enough to satisfy the new-found appetite for economic growth? And if not, will the often rather fragile political structures be able to deal with the resulting discontents? Once politicians there begin to auction off promises of faster economic growth – on the Western model – will there not be increased friction, resulting perhaps in revolutions and periodic *coups d'état?* This already seems the pattern in many developing countries. It could well become accentuated.

To make this point is not to indulge in a prediction that it is bound to happen. It is simply to suggest that it could happen. Again, to say that population equilibrium could result in political and social disequilibrium is not to argue against adopting population-control policies. It is to indicate that there may be a price to pay. For there is little point in constructing a global model which ignores the possibility (it is no more) that achieving an ecological balance may cause a social imbalance. This is to leave out of account the complexity of the real world and, by doing so, to lose what is surely the real point of futurology: not to predict the future but to encourage thought and thus prepare people for the many possible and plausible eventualities.

If there is a fairly widespread consensus about the desirability of limiting the world's population – despite the lack of knowledge about all the potential consequences – there is no such agreement about the proposal for seeking to stabilize economic growth within the next two decades. Here *The Limits to Growth* crystallizes what is very much a mood of the 70's and has clothed in statistical language the emotional vocabulary of the revolt against the cult of economic growth.

This revolt was entirely predictable. The circumstances which provided the soil of the cult – the years of Depression and mass unemployment – are now part of historical folklore. For anyone under forty they are no longer part of felt experience. More important still, perhaps, it has become apparent that economic growth is no cure-all. It does not in itself guarantee an end to poverty. It does not cure racial stress and conflict. What is more, it has unpleasant side-effects: congested streets, blighted city centers, polluted lakes and rivers.

Accepting all this, it is possible to draw two quite different conclusions. The first is that the emphasis on economic growth was exaggerated, that too much was hoped for from it, and that, however desirable, its benefits must be seen alongside its debits in a complex socioeconomic balance sheet. The other is that economic growth is positively undesirable, that the damage it inflicts quite clearly outweighs the possible advantages.

The sort of ecological doomsday approach typified by *The Limits to Growth* tends to support the second view. Just as growth was once seen as the magic formula, so now non-growth replaces it: one oversimplification takes over from another in a depressing dialectic of slogans. The emphasis on repudiating worldly goods is, of course, drawing on a very deep well of Western tradition – and the final irony is perhaps that what is basically a religious impulse now feels obliged to reinforce itself with "scientific" predictions from a computer, the 20th-century version of the apocalyptic vision. But in the past the choice was seen as a personal one. It was the individual who chose to join a mendicant order of friars or give a part of his income to the poor. Now, however, the choice is presented as a communal one. It is society as a whole which is expected to take a pledge of voluntary poverty (or, more accurately, to abstain from enriching itself still further). And the sanction is not the traditional one of retribution in the next life but ecological catastrophe in this one: present affluence and future squalor, the contemporary version of visiting the sins of the fathers on the sons.

All this may seem exaggerated. The proposed "stable state" average income per head of population – $1,800 a year – is well on the comfort side of poverty. But unfortunately the habit of the social prophets of talking in global terms conceals, as usual, some of the very real problems involved. As *The Limits to Growth* coyly puts it: "A draw-back of this approach is of course that – given the heterogeneity of world society, national political structure, and levels of development – the conclusions of the study, although valid for our planet as a whole, do not apply in detail to any particular country or region." Yet if they cannot be applied to "any particular country or region," it is difficult to see their usefulness, particularly in the case of something as specific as the average income of the world's inhabitants. For how is the "average" to be arrived at? Extrapolating existing trends, the world average income would indeed be about $1,800 by the year 2000 or shortly before then: however, this would range from well over $6,000 per head in North America to less than one-tenth of that figure in Africa and Asia (which will contain two-thirds of the total population).

In short, to talk of aiming at an economic equilibrium without discussing its political and social implications, is to indulge in meaningless rhetoric. Such an equilibrium could be achieved with only two alternative sets of assumptions. The first is that, broadly speaking, the global distribution of income will remain in the future much what it is now. The other is that there will be a massive redistribution of income from the rich nations to the poor nations. It is difficult to know which is the more unrealistic.

Leaving all moral arguments aside, it is not conceivable that the developing countries would be prepared to bring their growth rate to a halt while enormous disparities remained between their standards of living and those of the advanced Western nations. So the latter would either have to tolerate continuing growth in other countries or repress it in much the same way as traditional colonial powers dealt with native rebellions. Alternatively, the Western nations would deliberately have to cut back on their own standard of living in order to lessen the gap. Just to state these implications is to suggest that the advocates of the stable state are engaging in the luxury of mental self-flagellation, publicly confessing their own sins in the sure knowledge that they will not be asked to travel along the road of repentance themselves (the religious phraseology comes naturally in discussing what is essentially a neo-religious phenomenon).

Of course it may be unfair to push the arguments of the stable-state advocates to their extremes. However, even assuming charitably that they do not really mean all that they say, assuming also that they are simply using their slogans to dramatize the case for less emphasis on economic growth rather than for total abstention, assuming finally that they realize that most of their arguments will sound like a blasphemy to two-thirds of the world's population, it is worth looking at some counter-speculations. For after all, there may be some disbenefits to non-growth, just as there are some disbenefits to growth.

Here, writing from Britain has its advantages. For Britain is not only a country which is currently enjoying the "stable state" standard of living – that is, an average income-per-head not too far away from $1,800 a year. Equally it is an example of a society which, quite involuntarily, has for the past few years had a non-growth economy (only now is the economy picking itself up from the floor where it has been for so long). What is more, it is a society which has a strong political system, a homogeneous social culture, and despite the presence of colored immigrants, no racial conflicts on the United States scale. Here, if anywhere, there should be the model of the global-equilibrium society.

But if Britain is indeed to be taken as a model, then the prospect is gloomy. The experience of Britain would suggest that a non-growth society can produce as many and as unpleasant stresses on the social and political economy as industrial growth can impose on the ecological and natural resources of the globe. The stable-state advocates argue that growth does not guarantee greater social equality or justice. But the experience of Britain shows that stagnation (even under a Labour government ideologically sympathetic to equality) is no more helpful. Resentment of continuing inequalities is compounded by resentment of unemployment and of the failure of living standards to rise. For poverty is not just relative. Rising standards can and do mean better food, better housing, and better clothes for people. And at the current British standard of living – the "standard" for the future, let it be remembered – these sorts of improvements still matter very much. Although Britain probably has better housing conditions than most Western European countries, 13 per cent of households still lack private bathrooms and 12 per cent still live in houses or flats officially classified as unfit for human habitation. More than a third of households have no refrigerator or cooling machine, 55 per cent have no car, 65 per cent have no telephone, and 70 per cent have no central heating.

By the standards of Africa and Asia these are not symptoms of deprivation. But neither are they symptoms of an over-gadgeted, over-cosseted society. More important, the experience of the 1964–70 Labour government suggests that if the aims of policy are to be to increase equality and to spend more on social services like health and education, then it is only politically possible to achieve them at a time of economic growth (which is not to suggest that economic growth in itself guarantees more radical social policies; it may be a necessary, but is certainly not a sufficient, condition). The Labour government did not manage to achieve growth, failed to secure its other aims, and was defeated at the polls. What is more, there was a noticeable crisis of confidence in the political system as such and some signs of rising social tension, as shown in the increased number of strikes.

It is, of course, possible to argue that such social stresses reflect the pains of growth and not of stagnation. This is the position of E. J. Mishan, for example, who maintains that the British people were happier and more contented in 1951 while still in the postwar era of rationing and austerity. This, as he himself recognizes, is an unresolvable argument since no one is in a position to measure happiness and contentment. However, there are some points which need stressing. The first is that it is clearly nonsense to present the argument as though it were a straight choice between growth and non-growth. Growth in Britain, as everywhere else, has had many unpleasant effects: the destruction of old buildings and communities, pollution by noise and fume, and, possibly, the introduction of a more hectic and therefore less satisfying life-style for some people. But it is perfectly logical to concede all this to Mishan and yet to repudiate his conclusion, since equally clearly growth has brought many advantages to a great many people in Britain. The real question is whether the penalties of growth outweigh the advantages. Here it is worth stressing that the majority of the British people have repudiated the anti-growth verdict: over the past 20 years at successive general elections they have consistently voted for the party which, in their view, would deliver the fastest growth rate. It may be that the British voters are misguided about what makes them happy and contented; equally, though, it may be that they are better placed to know than Mr. Mishan. The other point that needs stressing is that the balance sheet of advantages and penalties of growth may well work out differently for different sections of a community. Thus growth tends to threaten traditional middle-class values: it is felt to be disruptive and unpleasant precisely because it turns minority privileges into majority ones – because it means crowded roads, crowded beaches, and so on.

To share these traditional values – and to fear their erosion – should not necessarily mean accepting the anti-growth argument, though. Arguably, only when the majority of a population have achieved middle-class standards of values – and be prepared to give priority to, say, anti-pollution measures over consumer durables. In the mean-time, lamenting the consequences of the popularization of prosperity begs precisely the same questions on a domestic scale as it does on the international scale. Do the anti-growth advocates assume that the existing social and economic structure of society will somehow be frozen – and that the present inequalities (which in Britain, as elsewhere, are considerable) will become happily accepted? Or do they assume a political system which insures that non-growth does not become a synonym for perpetuating existing inequalities – that economic stagnation can be reconciled with social change?

It is at this point in the argument that the advocates of global equilibrium throw up their hands in horror at the assumption that such minor political problems as the distribution of income among countries or within individual societies cannot be overcome under the threat of catastrophe. Suddenly it appears that although the technologists and scientists cannot solve the problems of increasing food yields, recycling raw materials, or stopping pollution, politicians can square the circle of reconciling everyone to the social and economic consequences of global equilibrium.

This, of course, is a nonsense assumption. If anything it would, on past experience, be much more plausible to make the opposite assumption: that the social consequences of trying to achieve a global equilibrium would lead to conflict, the collapse of existing political systems, and, most likely, war between societies competing for their rations of fixed resources. Even conceding that eventually it might be possible to enforce an equilibrium, the costs of doing so might well be heavier than the (in any case problematic and uncertain) costs of refusing to be panicked into taking the ecological doomsday slogans at face value.

No one can be certain that these slogans are wrong, any more than their proponents can be certain that they are right. Indeed it is probably worth taking out a collective insurance policy on their turning out to be at least partially right: by taxing polluters, by spending more on environmental preservation, and so on (all policies, it must be stressed, which are urgently desirable in themselves and worth pursuing in order to make life more pleasant here and now even if there were no threat of ultimate catastrophe). What is really wrong – alarmingly wrong – is the fact that they are slogans, and no more. Just as the 50's and 60's spawned the slogans reflecting the fear of a nuclear holocaust, so now the 70's have produced the slogans born of the fears of an ecological cataclysm, and no doubt the 80's will make their own, distinctive contribution.

It is not ignoble to be afraid of being blown up by an H-bomb, any more than it is ignoble to fear the degeneration of the physical world in which our children will live. Indeed it is right to be angry and aroused. But it is desperately important that complex problems should not be reduced to the simple symmetry required of systems analysis. This is, if anything, the final surrender to technology – to adjust our own vision of our problems to the technical necessities of feeding them into a computer. For the inevitable result is to produce an equally simple answer, whose very simplicity makes it unfit as a guide to action. To the extent that the complex interaction of economic, ecological, social, and political factors makes prediction hazardous, the best prophets are those who allow for uncertainty: who do not sell the future like a patent medicine but persuade mankind to make continual running adjustments to what, after all, is a continually changing future.

38

The Stalemate Society

COMMENTARY
November 1973

At the beginning of this century, most people living in America worked with their hands, either in factories or on the land. By the middle of the century barely half did so. By 1980, little more than a third will do so if present trends continue. During the same period, the proportion of white-collar workers rose from one in six of the total manpower force to one in three in 1950. By the end of this decade, the figure is expected to be one in two. From being an industrial society, America has become a service society. From being a society in which the ability to read and write was the main qualification required of new entrants into the labour force, the country seems to be moving to the point where anyone who hasn't been to college will be barely employable in any except the most menial tasks. (Indeed, using the methodology of extrapolation from recent trends, so popular among the prophets of ecological doom, one should be able to demonstrate that soon after the year 2000 a Ph.D. will have become essential to anyone looking for work.) What is more, all economically developed nations appear to be moving in the same direction – with the United States, as the richest and most developed country, simply moving ahead of the rest of the pack. The imperatives of modern technology seem to be creating a new sort of society, transforming social structure as much as physical environment.

Neither the recognition of these trends nor debate over their possible implications is a recent phenomenon. A vast speculative literature has collected on the fly-paper of this particular subject, which offers lush opportunities for do-it-yourself sermonizing. Thus, there are those who foresee a world dominated by "knowledge-capitalism" (Ivan Illich's phrase) or by the technostructure (John Kenneth Galbraith's). Others, more hopefully, see a forced convergence of capitalist and communist societies, with technology making a monkey of ideology and politics. Indeed the rapidity with which such ideas are diffused – often in a very simplified form – is in itself a tribute to the powers of the technology of communication; sometimes it seems as though ideas were now manufactured on much the same principle as consumer durables – that is, with a view to appealing to the largest possible market and having the shortest possible life before being thrown away to be replaced by a new model.

In all this, however, there is a danger that ideas may become accepted as part of the conventional wisdom long before they have been fully argued out or developed. Thus, it is only ten years since Daniel Bell, one of the most eminent of the social analysts who have devoted themselves to these issues, first began to explore the emergence of what he called the "post-industrial society." Now that he has put together in book form* his various writing on the theme, he runs the risk of paying the usual penalty of the pioneer. So many others have dipped their buckets into this particular intellectual well that the shock of novelty has, to a large extent, worn off. Familiarity with simplified, secondhand versions of Bell's ideas may tempt some to believe they have already read the sophisticated complexities of the original. This would be a pity. For in a sense the importance of Bell's work lies less in his conclusions – which are interesting precisely because they stimulate disagreement – than in his way of working toward them.

The occupational disease of those who, like Bell, write about the future is prophecy. On the whole, Bell himself is immune to the bacillus – an immunity that springs from his recognition of the complexity of social forces and the consequent danger of deducing what will happen or what might happen from what has happened, assuming (a very big and very frequent assumption) that no new, entirely unforeseen factor will come into play. Similarly, he is aware that there are many ways of slicing the analytic cake. Looking at the impact of technology on the social structure is only one of these; it is equally important to examine the impact of changing attitudes on the political structure and on the culture. And what actually happens will depend – as Bell stresses – on the social chemistry of the reaction among all three elements, the political, the social, and the cultural. It is possible to speculate intelligently about the outcome of this reaction; indeed, it is highly desirable to do so in order to equip ourselves intellectually to meet the unexpected. But speculation about the possible must not be confused with prediction.

---

*The Coming of Post-Industrial Society: A Venture in Social Forecasting, Basic Books, 528 pp., $12.50.

Bell is cautious, then, in forecasting what *will* happen, but he is emphatic in his diagnosis of what *has* happened: the basic change, as he sees it, in the structure of American society that will determine future options. Knowledge has replaced property, in his view, as the primary source of power. The scarce commodity in post-industrial societies is not capital or goods but expertise.

> In the post-industrial society, the chief problem is the organization of science, and the primary institution the university or the research institute where such work is carried out. In the 19th and early 20th centuries the strength of nations was their industrial capacity, the chief index of which was steel production. . . . After the Second World War, the scientific capacity of a country has become a determinant of its potential and power, and research-and-development has replaced steel as a comparative measure of the strength of the powers.

At the same time, there have been a number of other crucial developments, according to Bell. Chief among these is a shift in emphasis from profit-maximization to welfare-maximization. Abundance has produced precisely those problems (pollution, traffic jams) and wants (health care, education) which call for a collective approach. Hence the phenomenon, common to all highly developed economies, irrespective of the prevailing ideology, of an expansion in state activity, whether measured by the proportion of the Gross National Product spent by government or by the amount of direct intervention and regulation. Hence, also, the gradual transformation of the business corporation, in which not only is control being divorced increasingly from the ownership of capital but the interests of both the community at large and of those actually working for the corporation may well come to prevail over the interests of the stockholders. More and more, Bell argues, corporations are becoming like universities, in the sense of being primarily responsible to their own members and to the wider community: self-preservation and self-perpetuation, as distinct from profit-making, become the main driving forces.

In this process, the role of the new scientific, professional, and technical "estates" is crucial. Power is passing to them, and not only because of their rapidly growing numbers (by 1975, they will account for nearly a fifth of the total work force in the United States). The growth in their numbers simply reflects, after all, the growth of certain types of activity. It is because society is increasingly coming to depend on (or value) these activities – research, development, health care, education, social work – that the knowledge "estates" are gaining in power. Equally important, these "estates" tend to straddle the traditional demarcation lines between public and private power (between government and business). There is not only the fact, noted by Galbraith, that the same sorts of people, with the same sorts of values, work in both spheres: a scientist moves from a government laboratory to a private firm's laboratory, and vice versa. But, in addition, the nature of technological activity, in particular its cost, means that both laboratories are in any case likely to be financed by the taxpayer.

In short, as one analyzes the emergent social structure, one sees that the traditional ways of dissection are becoming rather meaningless; the distribution of scientific, professional, and technical manpower has become an increasingly helpful way of explaining both the articulation of society's skeleton and the flow of its blood. And the new social anatomy, moreover, begins to look remarkably like a kind of feudalism,* with power in the hands of the "estates" controlling the key institutions: universities, corporations, research institutes.

II

There are a number of real difficulties in trying to present Bell's argument concerning the change in the distribution of power in post-industrial society. One is that Bell assumes the change, rather than demonstrating it; another is that he fails to define what he means by power. Thus, the fact that society increasingly depends on the "estates" does not necessarily prove that the "estates" are gaining power. It might similarly be argued that, given the complexity of our cities, we are becoming increasingly dependent on street cleaners, sewage workers, and rubbish movers: a reasonable enough proposition, but one from which it does not follow that these workers are gaining in power (except perhaps in the power to demand and get higher wages). There are many dimensions of power, and the ability to gain higher rewards is only one. There is the power to regulate one's own life or work; the power to control other people's lives or work; the power to influence policy decisions at various levels of national or local government. The list is not meant to be exhaustive, only to show that it is quite conceivable that the "estates" may lose out on some aspects of power while gaining on others; scientists, for example, may forfeit autonomy and control over their own activities by becoming government employees, while at the same time obtaining access to, and influence over, governmental decision-making.

It is necessary, moreover, to distinguish among the different "estates." On the whole, in his discussion of the changing balance of power in post-industrial societies, Bell tends to lump together scientists, professionals, and technicians. He analyzes the scientific community at some length

---

*The term is Theodore J. Lowi's, used in his onslaught on pluralism, *The End of Liberalism.*

since he believes (in a rare lapse into jargon) that "the scientific estate – its ethos and its organization – is the monad that contains within itself the imago of the future society." The implication is that what holds for science also holds for professionals and for technicians like engineers. But does it? If science is indeed a special kind of social arrangement designed to achieve, by a process of free inquiry and peer judgment, "a consensus of rational opinion," is the same true to anything like the same extent of medicine, of teaching, of social work? Michael Oakeshott's distinction between two sorts of knowledge seems particularly relevant here:

> The first sort of knowledge I . . . call technical knowledge or knowledge of technique. . . . The technique (or part of it) of driving a motor car on English roads is to be found in the Highway Code, the technique of discovery in natural science or in history is in their rules of research, of observation and verification. The second sort of knowledge I . . . call practical, because it exists only in use, is not reflective, and (unlike technique) cannot be formulated into rules (*Rationalism in Politics*, 1962).

All Bell's "estates" use both sorts of knowledge, but in different measure. Their organization, their ethos, and their methods of work will vary according to the precise nature of the mix. Thus, the professions tend to place more emphasis on the second kind of knowledge, while technicians tend to stress the first. Even within the same profession, there will be variations: in medicine, for example, the surgeon may see himself as a technician using scientific methods based on "a consensus of rational opinion," while the psychiatrist may depend heavily on charismatic authority. Indeed there would seem to be a significant distinction to be made, as far as society is concerned, between those "estates" which (like scientists) seek to explore natural phenomena and those which (like social workers, teachers, and doctors in varying degrees) are engaged in a form of social control over people.

Similarly, in any discussion of scientific method and "the consensus of rational opinion" it is important to distinguish between rationality of means and rationality of ends. Consider in illustration the recently published report of the British government's inquiry into the reasons Rolls-Royce went bankrupt after it undertook to supply aircraft engines for Lockheed.* Here was a company that might be taken as a prototype of the corporation in the post-industrial society: dominated by engineers, subsidized by government money, engaged in pushing forward the fron-

---

*R. A. MacCrindle and P. Godfrey, *Rolls-Royce Limited: An Investigation under Section 165 (a)(1) of the Companies Act 1948.* HMSO (London), 1973.

tiers of the technically feasible. It went bankrupt because the development of technology became an end in itself and because, as a consequence, an *irrational* commitment was undertaken:

> The board, as it appears to us, treated this essentially as a matter upon which it should be guided by the assessment of those experienced aero-engineers from among its members who were most closely concerned with the project. . . . Their standing in Rolls-Royce was such that they could and did influence the decisions of their colleagues in this matter. Their knowledge and experience should have enabled them to recognize the awesome dangers of the venture. But they shared an abiding conviction that without an involvement in this sector of the aero-engine market the future of Rolls-Royce would be but a shadow of its past. . . . To conclude a contract with a U.S. manufacturer had become for them not merely a consummation devoutly to be wished, but a task in which failure would be unthinkable. This is not an attitude of mind best calculated to produce the most objective analysis of the risks involved. Nor did it. The terms ultimately negotiated meant a commitment for Rolls-Royce which placed at hazard its continued existence.

The quotation illustrates a number of points. It provides evidence for the Bell thesis of the power of the "estates": a power which in this case (as in many others) seems to have rested on the incapacity or unwillingness of laymen to challenge technical expertise – a sort of deference to the authority of the new technological priesthood. It indicates also, however, that this particular power can all too easily be abused when technical development becomes an end in itself: it suggests the need for some form of control. And this is where politics comes in.

III

In effect, as I have noted, Bell's analysis of the changes that have taken place in the organization and distribution of power in society assumes a new sort of feudalism, with the "estates" controlling the key institutions of the university, the corporations, and so forth. Inevitably the question arises as to what the relationship will be between the "estates" and the political structure of society – to what extent their power will be independent of that structure and to what extent subordinated to it. Yet to this question Bell gives no clear answer. By controlling the techniques of governmental management, including especially the intellectual machinery of decision-making – itself transformed by the development of systems analysis and the computer simulation of problem situations – it would seem that the "estates" will simply be the ultimate holders of power in society. As Bell concludes at one point, "It is clear that in the

society of the future, however one defines it, the scientist, the professional, the technician and the technocrat will play a predominant role in
the political life of the society." Elsewhere and repeatedly, however, he
recoils from the full implications of this statement. The reasons for Bell's
hesitancy on this crucial point are themselves worth examining for the
light they shed on the relation between the "estates" and politics.

Bell rightly points out that science and politics have different styles:
"In science, 'truth' is achieved through controversy and criticism, in which
a single answer has to be forthcoming. In the polity, a consensus is
achieved through bargaining and trade-offs, and the answers are a compromise." To this extent, then, improving the technology of decision-
making leaves open the question of *who* makes the final decision, and
for what reasons. Greater knowledge can improve decision-making in
the sense of creating new perceptions about the nature of problems and
the available options for solving them; this, however, does not remove
politics – construed as judgments about what is right or possible – from
the process. (It does not, for example, tell us what a desirable distribution
of income is.) So Bell concludes, rightly in my view, but inconsistently
with some of his other statements, "In the end, the technocratic mind-
view necessarily falls before politics; the hopes of rationality – or, of a
particular kind of rationality – necessarily fade. . . . Politics, in the sense
that we understand it, is always prior to the rational, and often the
upsetting of the rational." This is a long way from the assumption that
the emergence of a knowledge society in itself determines the power
structure, rather than being one of the elements within it, creating new
tensions, new coalitions, and new outcomes in the determination of
priorities and policies.

The real difficulty in trying to speculate intelligently about the future
is knowing how large a role will be played by the various elements in the
social equation. Will the scientists and professionals play a "predominant"
role, as Bell suggests? Or will they simply play a large role, alongside
other social groupings, as he also implies? Are they a new class, or are
they merely a new, if powerful, pressure group?

It would clearly be absurd to be dogmatic on this point. But there is
much evidence – some of it provided by Bell himself – to suggest that
it might be a mistake to regard the emergence of the "estates" in the
same terms as the emergence, say, of the entrepreneurial middle class
in the late 18th century – to assume that the former will put their imprint
on post-industrial society in the same way the latter put their impression
on industrial society. To begin with, there must be some question, as I
have already noted, about equating the growth in numbers of scientists
and technicians with that of teachers and doctors, many of whom may
well be anti-technological in their ethos and attitudes. Nor does it follow,

as Bell recognizes, that the "estates" will necessarily be internally coherent: their members may be torn in their loyalties between their own
reference group and the demands of their organizations (but this in itself
is to concede that the organizations, whether profit-making or not, may
have different aims from those of the supposedly dominating professions).

More interesting still, to compound perplexity about the future, change
is not one-directional. That is, the explosion in the numbers of the
"estates" affects them as well as society. Thus, the old entrepreneurial
values – whose obituaries have filled so many books and articles – seem
to be creeping back, and finding new life, in precisely those institutions
that are supposed to be transforming society in the reverse direction.
The academy, where a large part of the average faculty member's time
is spent preparing applications for grants, is perhaps the most striking
case in point. To an extent Bell recognizes this trend when he points
out that the new "estates" are increasingly becoming client groups, ham-
mering on the doors of government for more funds. But he fails to give
sufficient weight to this development or explore its implications fully.
For the relationship between client and donor – whether the client be a
university or a corporation seeking development funds – is a subtle and
complex one. Governments come to be dependent on pressure groups for
information and, provided the constituency is big enough, are reluctant to
cut off their funds. But to a considerable degree the client is even more
dependent in the relation, not only because he needs government money
to continue his work, but because the terms on which the money is given
(or withheld) have a decisive influence on the kind of work he will
do. The relationship, in other words, tends to become one of mutual
readjustment, and need not necessarily result in the imposition of one
set of values on another.

Then there is the matter of participation in the political process. Bell
argues that as professionalism becomes a criterion of position it clashes
with the populism which is generated by the claims for more rights and
greater participation in the society. "If the struggle between capitalist
and worker, in the locus of the factory, was the hallmark of industrial
society, the clash between the professional and the populace, in the
organization and in the community, is the hallmark of conflict in the
post-industrial society." And elsewhere he asserts: "To a considerable
extent, the participation revolution is one of the forms of reaction against
the 'professionalization' of society and the emergent technocratic decision-making of a post-industrial society". But it seems to me that the
phenomenon of professionalization and that of participation in the political process are cause-and-effect in a rather different sense from that
implied by Bell. The important contrast may be not between professionals

and the general population, but between professionals *qua* professionals and professionals *qua* citizens. In other words, the most committed participant may be the professional *after* he steps out of his working role and into his role as citizen, where he finds himself cast as a passive consumer of decisions made for him by others. Real participation is a high-cost activity in terms of the information required and the time spent, and it would be surprising to find that this too, though certainly not exclusively, were to become a professional activity; indeed, a recent study* suggests that protest itself is becoming highly professionalized.

To make this point is, if anything, to reinforce Bell's conclusion that the main problem for the future in the political sphere is going to be the "relation between the desire for popular participation and bureaucracy." But it is also to stress that the coming clash should be seen not merely as a popular reaction to the professionalization of society – though that is certainly one element – but as a product of professionalism itself. Indeed, it is surprising in this connection that Bell does not appear to attach very much importance to the possibility that a frustrated intellectual proletariat, excluded from participation in decision-making and condemned to routine work, may develop *within* the "estates": that these, far from being cohesive and homogeneous groups, may become microcosms of conflict within the society as everyone seeks to "participate." Could it be that professionalization creates new expectations in this direction, just as prosperity creates new expectations about standards of living?

IV

In any case, it may be that at present there is too much emphasis on participation and too little on accountability. (The two are, of course, linked.) This is another question to which Bell has no clear answer: to what extent and by what means will the "estates" be controlled or held accountable? Already a great many decisions – and there will be a great many more, if indeed the intellectual sophistication of the process grows – are extremely difficult for the layman (for example, the consumer of a professional service like medicine) to grasp or "participate in" in any meaningful sense. This is particularly true of those areas where science has, in Bell's terms, a charismatic aspect. But it is also true of a great many routine cost-benefit exercises in which the recommended outcome may depend on which factors are included and how they are weighted

---

*John D. McCarthy and Mayer N. Zald, *The Trend of Social Movements in America: Professionalization and Resource Mobilization*, General Learning Press, 1973.

in the analysis: how, for instance, leisure time is valued, what importance is attached to amenity factors like noise and privacy, and so on. It is difficult to see anything except sham participation in circumstances like these unless and until some form of accountability is developed; until, in short, it becomes possible to scrutinize the way the expertise of the "estates" is being applied. In the last resort, it seems to me, participation depends on evolving forms of counter-expertise in the service of the "populace," to use Bell's word.

The problem of accountability also arises in the case of the new centers of power as delineated by Bell: the corporation, the university, and the research institute. If profit ceases to be the yardstick of corporation performance, what should replace it? As universities become quasi-entrepreneurial institutions, seeking to maximize not knowledge but their own activities, who will decide what resources should be allocated to them and how they should be used? A case could be made here for much stronger political institutions, capable of carrying out forms of control which have yet to be devised, let alone executed. To introduce this consideration is to recognize a paradox underlined by the experience of those European countries where government already plays an even larger role than it does in America. This is that state control – for example, in industries like steel, coal, and the railways in Britain – cannot be equated in any sense with participatory or popular control. The larger the area of intervention by government, the greater the role of the administrative technocracy. The pressure to delegate power to the bureaucracy, and, if need be, to create new, semi-autonomous, quasi-governmental institutions, has the effect of actually reducing the power exercised by elected governors or representatives. The more we seek to control technology, the greater becomes the temptation to extend the power of the "estates" in the process.

Bell does not provide a shopping-list of solutions for problems like these (or, one might add, to others of the many issues he raises and deals with here: the development of a new culture, no longer supportive of the work ethos, increasingly at odds with the social structure; or the tension between the demands of technology for a meritocracy and the populist demand for equality of results as distinct from equality of opportunity and esteem – a theme he handles with particular brilliance). His book, with its remarkable richness of scholarship, is designed to stretch the reader's intellectual imagination, not to supply a set of ready-made recipes for action. Yet, in a way, it conveys a more urgent message for precisely this reason. Perhaps the main conclusion to be drawn from the work is not that America and other post-industrial societies must prepare to meet certain specific crises, but that they must develop a more generalized political and institutional capacity to meet difficulties and cope with issues which cannot even be specified at this particular moment in time. The post-industrial society, as Bell emphasizes again and again, creates the opportunity and the need for more conscious social policies in the largest sense. But it may also, one pessimistically concludes from reading his book, make it more difficult to implement those policies.

For there seems to be a real possibility that the post-industrial society will also turn out to be a stalemate society. If, indeed, we are moving toward a new feudalism – in which power is becoming concentrated in self-regulating corporations and academic institutions – then it is the capacity for collective action which may suffer. And if we are indeed entering an era in which the main emphasis is on political participation – which, by definition, means the ability to stop things from getting done – then it may become more, not less, difficult to move beyond the lowest common denominator of political action. Technology may give society some of the tools required to shape its own future; it may also create a social situation in which it will become impossible to use those tools effectively.

39

The Politics of Public Expenditure: American Theory and British Practice

BRITISH JOURNAL OF POLITICAL SCIENCE
1976

Public expenditure is quite the most visible and quantifiable measure of government activity. It is therefore surprising that in Britain, as distinct from the United States, this area has been massively neglected by political scientists.[1] This neglect is all the odder since public expenditure in Britain – comprehensively and conventionally defined to include all spending by central and local government, as well as capital investment by public corporations[2] – has been increasing rapidly both in absolute terms and as a proportion of the national income: between the early 1960s and the middle 'seventies, it rose from just under two-fifths to almost three-fifths

---

[1] The only major study of public expenditure in Britain is by two economists: Alan T. Peacock and Jack Wiseman, *The Growth of Public Expenditure in the United Kingdom* (London: Oxford University Press, 1961). More recently the Centre for Studies in Social Policy has published analyses of the Public Expenditure White Papers whose focus of interest has, however, been on the content of spending decisions rather than on the factors shaping them: Rudolf Klein *et al.*, *Social Policy and Public Expenditure, 1974*, and Rudolf Klein, ed., *Inflation and Priorities, 1975* (London: Centre for Studies in Social Policy, 1974 and 1975 respectively).

[2] For the Treasury definition of public expenditure, see *Public Expenditure White Papers: Handbook on Methodology* (London: HMSO, 1972).

of the Gross National Product. So, in effect, the scope of political decision-making about the distribution of national resources has grown considerably, reflecting the changing balance between the political market and the economic market. The dynamics of this process are highly relevant for an understanding of the British political system.

What follows is in the nature of a preliminary exploration, designed to map out the territory, to identify the problems of analysis and to produce some tentative, interim conclusions about the factors that appear to affect the size and pattern of public expenditure in Britain – conclusions which, however, are in the nature of hypotheses requiring further, more rigorous testing. For this paper is in no sense a statistical analysis. The method used is rather different. The first part of the paper reviews selectively some of the main explanatory modes developed primarily in the American literature on public expenditure, with only tangential references to the British experience; the second concentrates on a more detailed and specific analysis of British public expenditure in the light of this ground-clearing discussion.

To simplify the task of presentation, the various explanatory modes are set out in three groups in a descending order of generality. In the first group are those that try to explain trends in public expenditure by changes in the societal system. In the second are those that concentrate on the political system. In the third are those that look predominantly at the governmental system. As the area of inquiry narrows, so the focus of attention shifts. The first mode of explanation puts the emphasis on the structual determinants, economic and demographic, of public expenditure. The second stresses factors specific to the political system, like party competition and the role of ideology. The third concentrates on the organizational setting within which public expenditure decisions are made.

In reviewing these different modes of explanation, it seems more interesting to define which particular aspects of public expenditure are illuminated by them than to attempt to arrange them in some hierarchical order. The appeal of public expenditure as a subject of inquiry is that it sums up a mass of very different decisions and developments – with very different implications for the political and social order – in a common unit of currency. The corresponding danger, however, is that the appearance of homogeneity will be mistaken for the reality. The starting assumption of this paper is, therefore, that a variety of analytic tools is required when it comes to trying to explain something as complex as changes and movements in public expenditure, where a seductively quantitative face conceals some tough, unyielding questions about what the figures signify.

I. The Modes of Explanation

(a) The Societal System Approach

Looking at the societal system and at the structural determinants of public expenditure must logically be the first step in an analysis of public expenditure. If in fact changes in public expenditure reflect environmental changes in society at large, then it is redundant to seek an explanation in political or organizational demands or processes. To discuss the political factors affecting public expenditure decisions may be to fall into the trap of discussing the illusions of policy-makers who believe in their own freedom of action when in reality they are being driven by forces outside their control. Or, to take a weaker version of this approach, the discretion of the policy-makers may be limited to their ability to adjust to such forces – in which case the problem of studying trends in public expenditure becomes one of identifying the areas of discretion and defining the differential scope for adjustment. On either assumption, it would be misleading to concentrate exclusively on what the men in the life-boat are doing, without taking into account the sea current or the direction of the wind.

The evidence that it is socio-economic rather than political factors that influence movements in public expenditure is strong. This indeed is one of the main themes to emerge from the American literature on variations in state spending.[3] There is, of course, a problem about generalizing from such studies: they may be more significant as a statement about the limited range of political variations within the United States than as a finding about the behaviour of public expenditure. However, the importance of societal factors is also confirmed by a series of comparative studies of international expenditure trends. For example, one of the most recent of these concludes that social security spending as a proportion of GNP is correlated most strongly with population structure, with the

[3]This literature is both vast and far from unanimous in its conclusions. But for a general review, see John H. Fenton and Donald W. Chamberlayne, 'The Literature Dealing with the Relationship between Political Processes, Socio-economic Conditions and Public Policies in the American States', *Polity*, I (1968–69), 388–404. For a more recent statement of his views by one of the main protagonists in the debate, see Thomas R. Dye, *Understanding Public Policy* (Englewood Cliffs, N.J.: Prentice-Hall, 1972). A 'significant direct relationship between inter-party competition and welfare expenditures' has been claimed by Gary L. Tompkins, 'A Causal Model of State Welfare Expenditures', *Journal of Politics*, II (1975), p. 392–416.

age of the social security system itself and with *per capita* GNP but that elite ideology has no effect.[4]

This point can be further illustrated by looking at the experience of the twenty-three member states of the Organization for Economic Co-operation and Development.[5] This again indicates that the rising trend in public expenditure (both in total and as a proportion of GNP) is not a peculiarly British phenomenon, to be explained in terms of the British political system alone. Taking all the OECD countries, government expenditure rose from 27 per cent to 32.5 per cent of GNP between 1955 and 1969. Comparing the six major countries – the United States, Canada, Japan, France, Germany, Italy and Britain – there are slight differences but the trend is unaffected; for example, the figures for Britain are 27.9 per cent and 33.0 per cent respectively, while those for Germany are 28.9 per cent and 32.7 per cent.

Within this overall expansion, there were similarities in the way in which the components of public expenditure moved. On the one side of the balance sheet, defence expenditure as a proportion of GNP fell in the OECD countries taken as a group: from 7.1 per cent in 1955/7 to 6.2 per cent in 1967/9. On the other side, expenditure on transfer payments (pensions and other cash benefits) rose from 6.0 to 8.5 per cent. So the British figures – of a fall from 7.3 to 5.4 per cent for defence expenditure and a rise from 5.3 to 8.4 per cent for transfer payments – must be seen as part of this wider trend. Such international trends do not of course, explain what is happening in a particular country. They can only suggest that the explanation lies in factors, like economic development and demographic change, shared by various nations. The fact that there is an overall correlation does not mean that any one country at any specific point in time may not be above or below the point that would be predicted on the basis of such factors, and it is precisely these divergences which may be politically relevant.

A further variant on the structural-determinist mode of explanation differs in both its initial assumptions and final conclusions from the studies so far mentioned. This is the Marxist analysis of public expenditure. Here

---

[4]Harold L. Wilensky, *The Welfare State and Equality: Structural and Ideological Roots of Public Expenditure* (Berkeley: University of California Press, 1975). This usefully complements, and also reviews, the previous literature on the subject, notably Frederic L. Pryor, *Public Expenditures in Communist and Capitalist Nations* (London: Allen and Unwin, 1968).

[5]Organization for Economic Co-operation and Development, *Expenditure Trends in OECD Countries, 1960–1980* (Paris: OECD, 1972). The figures drawn from this report are used illustratively only: the OECD definition of government expenditure is different from the British Public Expenditure White Paper definition.

the central assumption is that expenditure is rising because of the specific characteristics of capitalist society. The main contention is that the 'growth of the state sector is indispensable to the expansion of private industry, particularly monopoly industries' and that welfare expenditure should be seen as an investment in social control made necessary by the disruptive impact of capitalism.[6]

Up to a point, it is impossible to disagree with this sort of approach. It could well be subsumed under an Easton-style of analysis,[7] which treats public expenditure as systems-maintenance. The problem is that, while there is little difficulty – as the evidence already cited shows – in demonstrating that systems-maintenance becomes more expensive as the society and economy become more complex, it is quite another matter to demonstrate that this is true only of capitalist societies. Nor is there any evidence that the mix of expenditures in capitalist societies will necessarily be different because it reflects their repressive character and their need for social control.[8] But the Marxist approach is a useful reminder that the analysis of public expenditure can also be an analysis of conflict. To the extent that the political system is under pressure from demands that it cannot meet in full, so it can react either by trying to reduce overall expectations or by satisfying some at the expense of others.[9]

(b) The Political System Approach

So far the emphasis has been on the pressures on the political system. Inevitably, given the perspective of the structural determinist approach, the role of party competition, ideology and other political factors is seen as, at best, secondary and reactive – responding to demands rather than generating them. Theories of public expenditure which treat the political system as an autonomous actor unsurprisingly provide a different mode of explanation. The emphasis then shifts to pressures generated by the political system.

---

[6]Perhaps the best known Marxist analysis is J. O'Connor, *The Fiscal Crisis of the State* (New York: St Martin's Press, 1973). For a sympathetic British critique, see Ian Gough, 'State Expenditure in Advanced Capitalism', *New Left Review*, 92 (1975), 53–92.

[7]David Easton, *A Systems Analysis of Political Life* (New York: Wiley, 1965).

[8]For example, Gough, in 'State Expenditure in Advanced Capitalism', cites the growth of expenditure on police and prisons in Britain as an example of a repressive response to the 'growing class and other antagonisms'. In fact, taking the period 1953–73, expenditure on the law, order and protective services went up by 106.3 per cent as against 265.6 per cent for education, 138.7 per cent for the National Health Service and 527.3 per cent for the personal social services.

[9]Anthony King, 'Overload: Problems of Governing in the 1970s', *Political Studies*, XXIII (1975), 284–96.

This point can perhaps best be illustrated by examining the model devised by Anthony Downs to explain public expenditure as a function of party competition.[10] In the Downs model, each party pursues whatever policies it believes will gain the support required to defeat its opponents and 'Since expenditures and taxes are two of the principal policies of government, they are set so as to maximize political support.' This means maximizing the visible benefits from expenditure and minimizing the visible costs of taxation. Since Downs assumes that voters are more ignorant about the benefits than about the costs of public expenditure, he concludes that the size of government budgets in a democracy will be less than optimal – in the sense of being smaller than it would be if all citizens had perfect information.

This may appear a somewhat perverse theory to consider in the context of a discussion of rising public expenditure; but in fact the Downs model is helpful – provided that its empirical assumption about the relative visibility of costs and benefits is reversed. As he himself points out: 'insofar as taxation can be concealed from the electorate, the government budget will tend to be larger than the "correct" one. Voters will underestimate the costs they are paying for special benefits received, and parties will build this bias into their budget.'

In fact, what little evidence there is about information levels in Britain suggests that voters are at least as ignorant about tax costs as about public expenditure benefits.[11] So although the fact of rising public expenditure

---

[10]Anthony Downs, 'Why the Government Budget Is Too Small in a Democracy', *World Politics*, XII (1960), 541–63, p. 542. See also the same author's *An Economic Theory of Democracy* (New York: Harper and Row, 1957). For a contrasting analysis of the effects of party competition, see Samuel Brittan, 'The Economic Contradictions of Democracy', *British Journal of Political Science*, v (1975), 129–59, where the argument is that this competition will produce a budget that is too big because of 'the lack of a budget constraint among voters'. Here the empirical assumption is the reverse of that made by Downs: i.e. that voters will be more aware of the benefits (real or imagined) of government activity than of the costs.

[11]For a review of the evidence about the widespread ignorance about the impact even of direct taxation on personal incomes (let alone indirect taxation), see C. V. Brown and D. A. Dawson, *Personal Taxation, Incentives and Tax Reform* (London: Political and Economic Planning, 1969). This might appear to support, in the British context, the Brittan as against the Downs view. However, the available, if rather thin, evidence suggests that the ignorance is symmetrical: i.e. that people are as ill-informed about the benefits they receive as they are about the taxes they pay. See Ralph Harris and Arthur Seldon, *Choice in Welfare* (London: Institute of Economic Affairs, 1965). The survey described in this study showed that 'few people have an accurate impression of the value of the social benefits they receive', and that over half underestimated the benefits they got (since there are severe problems about apportioning these benefits to particular

is consistent with the view that the parties compete in terms of increasing spending – on the assumption that the benefits are more visible than the taxes – it would be rash to assume that this proves the point: this would be to ignore the evidence, rehearsed in the previous section, of environmental pressures. Perhaps the interest of the Downs model lies more in its implications for the way in which governments will raise and spend their money than in its assumptions about the size of the budget. For example, his model might suggest (although he himself does not draw this particular conclusion) that the 'purer' the public good, in the economist's sense of the term, the less attractive it will be for governments to spend money on it since it is very difficult for a voter to assign a particular benefit to himself from expenditure on, say, defence or the police.[12] In contrast, it will be much more attractive for governments to spend money on those services where there is a clearly visible benefit – in particular, measureable cash payments – to defined groups.

In addition, the Downs model suggests that these groups should be politically purchasable at a reasonable price. In other words, one would not expect a Labour Government to try to buy the votes of property speculators or a Tory Government to attempt to buy the votes of Rhondda miners. Instead, one would expect governments to plan public expenditure rather like an investment portfolio and concentrate marginal extra spending in those areas where it brings the highest marginal political support. This would mean concentrating benefits on those groups – ex-party supporters, floating voters, waverers and potential defectors – that need least persuading rather than trying to buy over committed opponents.

This last point raises a larger question about the Downs model. Like most models which treat voters as though they were consumers shopping

households, it is difficult to give precise figures: however, a figure of 54 per cent would seem to be a fairly conservative interpretation of the results). For a theoretical discussion of the problem of lack of information, in the context of public expenditure, see Gordon Tullock, *Private Wants, Public Means* (New York: Basic Books, 1970), p. 117–21.

[12]This is to ignore the effect on behaviour of both altruism and the need for symbolic reassurance. Thus the former might explain why societies spend money looking after the mentally handicapped, and the latter might account for expenditure on such services as mountain rescue teams. Most of us are unlikely to benefit from either type of provision but we might feel happier as a result of living in what is visibly a 'caring' society. Empirical evidence on this point is sadly lacking; but in the only analysis I have been able to find of voting behaviour bearing directly on this question – Mickey Levy, 'Voting on California's Tax and Expenditure Limitation Initiative,' *National Tax Journal*, IV (1975), 427–35 – the finding is that 'the electorate behaves largely in accordance with narrow self-interest'.

around for the best buy in the market place, it ignores the role of party 'ideology'. (The word is used here non-technically, to describe policy predilections and general attitudes about social priorities – whether or not these are organized into a coherent ideological system.) Instead it is designed to explain why parties will behave in the same way, regardless of ideology. But in the case of public expenditure it can be argued that parties ought to behave ideologically in their own self-interest. To the extent that their predilections and priorities reflect a link with or bias towards certain group interests – whether the trade unions or small shopkeepers – it may be rational for them to concentrate benefits on these interests. For instance, it may be cheaper for parties to invest in reinforcing 'loyalty' or preventing 'exit' than to devote resources to advertising campaigns or special policy offers designed to attract new customers.[13] Thus, while party competition might help to explain a general trend towards rising public expenditure, there might well be different, ideologically-based priorities within such an increasing total depending on the politics of the specific government in office.

The other difficulty about the Downs model lies in the assumptions it makes (or rather the lack of them) about the information available to parties and governments as distinct from voters. Implicit in its whole approach is the assumption of knowledge by the parties about voter preferences as regards benefits – and, more problematic still, about the intensity of public wants. Thus I may well want the government to provide free seats at Covent Garden, and if I were asked in a public opinion poll whether I favoured spending government money in this way I would emphatically reply 'yes'. But I would not necessarily be prepared to translate this sort of day-dream want into a political demand – that is, I would not make the necessary investment of time and interest to try to enter the political market – unless, perhaps, I could minimize my costs by subscribing to some on-going campaign. In short, a demand is a want which I feel sufficiently strongly to invest some effort and perhaps even money in trying to exert pressure on the government.

This suggests that the competition-push model of public expenditure developed by Downs ought to be complemented, though not replaced, by a more traditional demand-pull model. This approach looks at the organization of the political market,[14] in which various interest groups

---

[13]The terms, though not the gloss on them, are of course from Albert O. Hirschman, *Exit Voice, and Loyalty* (Cambridge, Mass.: Harvard University Press, 1970).

[14]This concept, building on the work of Downs, has been developed by Albert Breton in his 'A Theory of the Demand for Public Goods', *Canadian Journal of Economic and Political Science*, XXXII (1966), 455–67.

collect, order and articulate voter preferences – and in which, allowing for the imperfections of this market in terms of the differential ability of various groups to organize themselves and to gain access, their activities provide information about the intensity of public wants. Using this model one might try to explore, for example, whether the changing pattern of expenditure on farming subsidies reflects changes in the power of the farming lobby: whether, furthermore, such a lobby has greater access and buying power in the political market (as measured by public expenditure benefits) under a Conservative than under a Labour Government. This is a reminder, again, that there is not only competition between political parties but also between different groups of the population for scarce resources. However, limiting the usefulness of this approach is the implicit assumption that all demands are generated within the political system. It tends to concentrate on the horse (the pressure groups) while ignoring the driver (the governmental system), so it is to the latter that the next section addresses itself.

(c) The Governmental System Approach

Both of the modes of explanation considered so far tend to deny, if only implicitly, an independent role to the governmental system: by this I mean, in the British context, the administrative network embracing ministers, civil servants and those responsible for running and delivering public services like education and health care – some 7,000,000 people in all, of whom just over one-tenth are civil servants directly employed by central government. Thus one of the weaknesses of the party-competition model of public expenditure is the assumption that the only role of governments is to win the next election; this is to overlook the fact that the prior concern of any government must be to retain sufficient control over the means of governing to function effectively as an autonomous decision-maker. Similarly, to talk about demands for public expenditure as though these were extraneous to the governmental system is to ignore the possibility that they may be generated within it.

The governmental systems approach corrects this bias. In particular, it brings the bureaucratic actors out to the centre of the stage. Thus, it has been argued by Downs and other American authors that bureaucracies will measure their success by their own expansion and that, consequently, public expenditure will go up because of the internal pressure to increase the scale of public activity.[15] This is consistent with such

---

[15]Anthony Downs, *Insider Bureaucracy* (Boston: Little, Brown, 1969) and William A. Niskanen, *Bureaucracy and Representative Government* (New York: Aldine-Atherton, 1971).

findings as Pryor's that 'the primary determinant of the ratios of public consumption expenditures for welfare to the GNP at a single point in time is the length of time that the social insurance system for old age pensions has been in operation'.[16] This is what might be expected, assuming that any administrative agency seeks to attract extra resources and is thus likely to extract more funds as time goes on.

There is another reason for expecting demands for higher expenditure to be generated by the public services themselves. The introduction of a particular service or benefit both marks the acceptance of responsibility by society in a new area and provides an opportunity to contrast the aims of policy (expandably vague) and the means provided (inevitably limited). Since many expenditure policies tend to be ill-defined, with no precise indication of the output to be achieved or the impact to be made,[17] it can be taken as almost axiomatic that the expenditure will appear to be inadequate on one interpretation or other of what the objectives are supposed to be. Those responsible for running the service can argue that they can only improve quality and effectiveness by increasing resources: that better education means more teachers, that a better health service means more doctors. Altruistic advocacy on behalf of the service being administered – and the clients being served – can push expenditure in the same direction as bureaucratic self-interest.

Apart from pressing for an expansion of the scale of governmental activity, those running the public services may press for better pay and conditions for themselves. Public expenditure will then go up because each unit of 'output' becomes relatively more expensive. This point will be developed more fully in the context of the British experience, but it is worth stressing at this point in the argument because it draws attention to the differential bargaining power of various groups within the governmental system. It suggests also that some forms of expenditure can be seen as compensation payments to particular, strategic groups within the

---

[16]Pryor, *Public Expenditures in Communist and Capitalist Nations*, p. 147.

[17]A characteristically vague and all-embracing statement of policy aims can be taken from Treasury, *Public Expenditure to 1978–79* (London: HMSO, Cmnd. 5879, 1975). Defining the objectives of the expenditure on health and personal social services, this states: 'The aim of the programme is to provide, within the resources available, health and personal social services for the whole population, with particular emphasis on helping people who have special needs, such as the elderly, the mentally ill and handicapped and the young.' This, clearly, can mean both everything and nothing and makes no specific commitment as to what services will be available, at what level and to whom, while yet raising expectations all round. Nor does it suggest any indicators which would show progress towards the achievement of the policy aims – unsurprisingly since such vague aims do not lend themselves to any sort of monitoring.

system. For example, defence would seem to be an exception to the observation that services tend to generate pressure for their own expansion. But while governments may cut defence expenditure, they tend not to cut the number of civil servants, generals and admirals proportionately. This is precisely what would be expected if expenditure is used to bribe elite groups within the governmental system.

The importance of organizational factors is even more central to another governmental system approach to the problem of explaining public expenditure increases. This is the theory of budgetary incrementalism. The father of this theory was the Italian public finance economist Maffeo Pantaleoni, writing at the beginning of this century.[18] More recently it has been developed and amplified by Wildavsky, who sums up its main theme as follows: 'Budgets are almost never actively reviewed as a whole in the sense of considering at once the value of all existing programs as compared to all possible alternatives. Instead, this year's budget is based on last year's budget, with special attention given to a narrow range of increase or decrease'.[19] From the incrementalist perspective, it is the interaction between organizational routine and the inherited pattern of public expenditure that is the key – and the residual problem is to identify the economic, social and political factors which help to influence the gradual modification of the historical legacy.[20]

The value of this approach is that it underlines the constraints within which public expenditure decisions are made and the limits on the options for change. But it also presents some problems. The first is to give some operational definition to the term 'incremental'. When does a

---

[18]Maffeo Pantaleoni, 'Contribution to the Theory of the Distribution of Public Expenditure' in Richard A. Musgrave and Alan T. Peacock, eds., *Classics in the Theory of Public Finance* (London: Macmillan, 1964), pp. 16–28.

[19]The quotation comes from Otto A. Davis, M. A. H. Dempster and Aaron Wildavsky, 'A Theory of the Budgetary Process', *American Political Science Review*, LX (1966), 529-42. The theory of incrementalism is most fully developed in Aaron Wildavsky, *The Politics of the Budgetary Process* (Boston, Mass.: Little, Brown, 1964).

[20]For the most sophisticated attempt to do so, see Otto A. Davis, M. A. H. Dempster and Aaron Wildavsky, 'Towards a Predictive Theory of Government Expenditure: US Domestic Appropriations', *British Journal of Political Science*, IV (1974), 419–52. It would be misleading to try to apply its findings to Britain if only because Congress plays a very different, and more active, role in the process than Parliament. However, it is worth noting its conclusion that 'an examination of exogenous variables shows that, when they do exert an influence, it is over the most vulnerable agencies ... For the most part, however, our agencies live in worlds of their own, worlds which are fully comprehensible to them but not yet to us.' For the extent to which this conclusion may reflect the method of analysis, see below.

public expenditure change stop being incremental – if there is a decrease/ increase of more than 10 or 20 or 30 per cent in a year? To bracket increases of, say, 2.5 and 25 per cent under the same 'incremental' heading is to risk depriving the whole mode of analysis of explanatory power, since the same process appears to be producing such different results.[21]

The second problem is to be sure that incrementalism is not just a function of the size of the unit of expenditure chosen for analysis. On *a priori* grounds, it would seem reasonable to assume that change will become more pronouncedly incremental – in the sense of representing only a marginal adjustment of inherited commitments – as the size of the unit of expenditure increases. Thus, given that even a 10 per cent increase at constant prices in British public expenditure implies shifting 5 per cent of the GNP from the private to the public sector, it is clear that the sheer scale of national budgets now imposes severe inhibitions on the rate of change feasible in any one year. So there may well be economic and political constraints on movements in total public spending which have little or nothing to do with the organizational processes within the governmental system – and it is these constraints, rather than the nature of the processes, that produce an incremental result. Conversely, disaggregating expenditure data ought to show a more volatile behaviour. This indeed is the finding of an American study of the US Atomic Energy Commission's budget.[22] While changes in the Commission's overall expenditure conformed to the incrementalist thesis, there were violent changes within the total – with some programmes adding greatly to their budget while others were being cancelled.

---

[21]For a critique of the Davis, Dempster and Wildavsky approach along these lines, see John J. Bailey and Robert J. O'Connor, 'Operationalising Incrementalism: Measuring the Muddles', *Public Administration Review*, XXXV (1975), 60–6. Reviewing the literature, these authors conclude that 'it appears that incrementalism has expanded to the point where it is an open-ended concept, explaining everything with little rigor.'

[22]Peter B. Natchez and Irvin C. Bupp, 'Policy and Priority in the Budgetary Process', *American Political Science Review*, LXVII (1973), 951–63. Note their conclusion: 'Priority setting in the federal bureaucracy resembles nineteenth century capitalism: priorities are established by aggressive entrepreneurs at the operating levels of government.' See also, John Wanat, 'Bases of Budgetary Incrementalism', *American Political Science Review*, LXVIII (1974), 1221–8. This criticizes the statistical foundations of the conclusion reached in 1966 by Davis, Dempster and Wildavsky in 'A Theory of the Budgetary Process' on the grounds that:

the correlations are of the same magnitude as those generated by random data under budgetary constraints. This is not to say that the Davis, Dempster and Wildavsky characterization of budgetary decision rules is inaccurate. It may very well be that those decision models are true representations of budgetary decision phenomena, but such a judgment cannot be made solely on the basis of high correlation coefficients.

To put the emphasis on organizational processes – that is, on the way in which decisions are taken – may also risk neglecting another aspect of public expenditure policies: the administrative characteristics of the programmes themselves. The raw material coming into the policy machine is not homogeneous, in the sense that different types of expenditure commitments vary in their malleability, vulnerability and responsiveness to change. The importance of taking the characteristics of individual programmes into account will be illustrated in the next section, which looks in more detail at the pattern of recent public spending in Britain and which examines trends and changes in terms of the utility or otherwise of the various modes of explanation discussed so far.

II. The British Experience

(a) Main Trends in Expenditure

In trying to explain why Britain is devoting more than half of its national income to public expenditure, there is a danger of trying to explain too much. In the case of overall public expenditure, the most powerful determinant of the present is the past – as was noted above – and it is only too easy to be trapped into an ever-receding inquiry into history. It seems more useful therefore to test the various modes of explanation discussed so far first by identifying discontinuities in historical trends and then by applying the various approaches to the task of trying to account for these changes. In other words, the focus of this analysis – which concentrates first on the total of public expenditure before turning subsequently to its composition – is on the dynamics of spending: the process of change rather than the stage reached at any one point in time.

Concern about rising public expenditure, whether in total or as a proportion of national income, is not a new phenomenon. In his budget speech of 1860, Gladstone pointed out that between 1853 and 1859 the national wealth had grown by only $16^{1}/_2$ per cent while public expenditure had increased by 58 per cent.[23] 'I may at once venture to state frankly that I am not satisfied with the state of public expenditure and the rapid rate of its growth. I trust, therefore, that we mean in a great degree to retrace our steps,' he concluded. In fact, public expenditure was 11 per cent of GNP at the time, and decline as a proportion (while rising in

[23]Quoted in Lord Bridges, *The Treasury*, 2nd edn. (London: Allen and Unwin, 1966).

total) for the rest of the nineteeth century.[24] It was not until the outbreak of the Boer War that there was another leap forward (just as the rise in expenditure, lamented by Gladstone, has been caused by the Crimean War). Moving into the twentieth century, the major changes in public expenditure trends have again been associated with times of war. In 1910 public expenditure was 12.8 per cent of GNP – not so very far off the figure in Gladstone's day – but by 1920 it had risen to 26.1 per cent. Therefore it fell marginally, only to increase slightly in the late 1930s, when rearmament got under way. In 1938, the figure was 20.1 per cent; by 1950 it was 39.5 per cent.

Looking at these trends over a century, Peacock and Wiseman concluded that the 'displacement effect' of war and the changes in social policies associated with war have been the main factors which explain the rising proportion of national income devoted to public expenditure.[25] Their analysis tended to reject Wagner's Law – an early form of the structural-determinist approach – which asserted that public expenditure would inevitably rise at a faster rate than output because government activity was bound to increase in line with the growing economic, administrative and social complexity of modern industrial states.[26] Writing in 1961 and basing themselves on the trends of the 1950s, Peacock and Wiseman argued that – looking twenty years ahead – it would be sensible to expect the total of public expenditure to go on growing but not to increase substantially as a proportion of national income. This conclusion, they stressed, was in no sense a prediction since it was contingent on a number of assumptions such as the absence of major social disturbances. Other studies of public expenditure published either before or after Peacock and Wiseman tended to confirm their conclusions.[27]

---

[24]Peacock and Wiseman, *Growth of Public Expenditure*. This book most valuably provides constant-price series of public expenditure figures from 1792 to 1955. However, these are not always strictly comparable with those quoted elsewhere in this paper since they use a different price base (1900 prices) and also use a price index calculated separately for the various programme ingredients of the total – something that it has not been possible to do for the tables based on the National Income and Expenditure Blue Book, desirable though this would be.

[25]Peacock and Wiseman, *Growth of Public Expenditure*, p. xxiv. The displacement effect, the authors argue, has two aspects. On the one hand, 'large-scale social disturbances, such as major wars' make new, and higher, levels of taxation acceptable. On the other hand, they direct attention to new social problems and make new forms of social action acceptable to governments and public.

[26]Adolph Wagner, *Finanzwissenschaft* (Leipzig, 1890). Quoted in Peacock and Wiseman, *Growth of Public Expenditure*, pp. 17–20.

[27]For example, B. Abel-Smith and R. M. Titmuss, *The Cost of the National Health Service* (Cambridge: Cambridge University Press, 1956) seriously under-

In practice, as Table 1 shows, the 1960s and 'seventies have turned out to be different from the 'fifties. Instead of falling as a proportion of national income, as in the 'fifties, public expenditure has increased. In terms of the overall increase, this is as much a 'displacement effect' as the increase in the two war periods, 1914–18 and 1939–45. This would seem to suggest that something was happening in the recent period that could not have been predicted simply by extrapolating from the past and that there was indeed some form of social, political or economic discontinuity.

Given that the upward trend in British public expenditure in the 1960s appears to have been part of a general movement in advanced industrial

TABLE 1   Public Expenditure as a Percentage of Gross National Product at Factor Cost*

	%		%
1952	41.8	1964	43.0
1953	40.8	1965	44.7
1954	38.0	1966	45.7
1955	37.0	1967	49.6
1956	36.8	1968	50.6
1957	36.0	1969	49.6
1958	36.5	1970	49.9
1959	36.9	1971	49.4
1960	37.3	1972	49.6
1961	38.3	1973	50.0
1962	39.6	1974	56.2
1963	42.8		

*This has been used to make this table comparable with the data in Peacock and Wiseman, *Growth of Public Expenditure.*
Source: Central Statistical Office, *National Income and Expenditure, 1964–1974* (London: HMSO, 1975) and previous editions as required (known as the Blue Books).

estimated the growth of spending on health, on the basis of using demographic data (though also warning that this might be an inadequate basis for forecasting). Similarly, W. Beckerman and Associates, *The British Economy in 1975* (Cambridge: Cambridge University Press, 1965) under-estimated the rate of growth in public expenditure, though it rightly anticipated an acceleration. Thus it assumed (p. 283) that public expenditure would rise to about 42 per cent of the national income in 1975. Partly this reflects, of course, an over-estimate of the growth in the national income as much as an underestimate of public spending growth rates.

societies, as was noted earlier, it is natural to start by seeking the reasons for this displacement in structural-determinist factors common to them all. But attempting to do so immediately draws attention to the problems involved in trying to apply this mode of analysis. What were the drastic socio-economic changes which produced the public expenditure growth? In the absence of a model specifying causal relationships, it is impossible to know; but certainly there is not reason to think that the 1960s differed from the 'fifties in terms of demographic or technological change on the same scale as the two decades differed in terms of expenditure change. Certainly in the case of Britain, projections of public expenditure based on demographic factors invariably under-estimated future spending.[28]

The Marxist version of this approach again raises as many difficulties as it solves. On the one hand, the 1960s in Britain did see the beginnings of a crisis of low profitability in private industry,[29] and therefore to some extent at least it is possible to view rising public expenditure as a response to this (although alternatively it can be seen as a cause). On the other hand, the 1960s were a period of low, if rising, unemployment and, by recent standards, mild inflation. Moreover, although the Marxist approach seems more convincing when it comes to trying to explain the acceleration of public expenditure after 1973 as a crisis of capitalism, this in turn only raises the question of why such dissimilar decades as the 'sixties and 'seventies (in terms of the economic and social situation) should seemingly have produced the same outcome.[30] Once again, the Marxist mode of explanation proves too much in general and too little in particular.

Much the same problem is encountered in trying to apply the party-competition model – reversing the Downsian assumptions about information and assuming that the parties will compete in terms of increasing

---

[28]One of the earliest post-war examples of this kind of calculation can be found in F. W. Paish and A. T. Peacock, 'Economics of Dependence (1952–82)', *Economica*, XXI (1954), 279–99.

[29]For a general review of trends in profitability, see M. Panic and R. E. Close, 'Profitability of British Manufacturing Industry', *Lloyds Bank Review*, 109 (1973), 17–31. This argues that while there was indeed a decline in profitability in the 1960s – which was widely perceived as a crisis – this was part of a secular trend, not confined to Britain.

[30]The analysis of this paper stops at 1973, for two reasons. First, the end of 1973 conveniently marks the end also of the Heath Conservative Government – which lingered on into the beginning of 1974 but cannot be held responsible for most of the expenditure decisions in that year. Second, the effects of the oil crisis – and the consequent world-wide inflation and recession – seem to me to mark the beginning of a new and still developing era for public expenditure policies everywhere, requiring separate analysis.

expenditure. This explanation is certainly consistent with the general upward trend; but it provides no basis for predicting or explaining the sort of discontinuity in this trend that was found in the 1960s. There seems to be a case, therefore, for seeking an explanation in the specific political circumstances of Britain and, in particular, for asking whether the weakness of the party-competition model lies in its neglect of party ideology. The acceleration of the 'sixties might well reflect the fact that a Labour Government was in power for the second half of the decade, while the Conservatives were in office for virtually the whole of the 1950s; and traditionally Labour is the party of public spending, while the Conservatives are the party of retrenchment and tax-cutting.[31]

At first sight, a comparison of the public expenditure record of the 1951–64 Conservative Governments with that of the 1964–70 Labour Government seems to confirm the importance of party. Immediately after the Conservatives took office in 1951 public expenditure rose sharply, as a result mainly of increases in defence spending planned by the outgoing Labour Government. In order to avoid distortion by this once-and-for-all effect, the average annual increase in public expenditure has therefore been calculated for the years 1953–64.[32] During this period of Conservative Government, the rate was 2.75 per cent at constant 1970 prices. During the period of the 1964–70 Labour Government, however, it was 4.18 per cent. But the neat symmetry of this contrast is spoiled when the record of the 1970–74 Conservative Government is included in the comparison. During this period the average annual rate of increase was 5.02 per cent.[33]

---

[31]For the party rhetoric, see F. W. S. Craig, *British General Election Manifestos 1900–1974* (London: Macmillan, 1975). The pattern shows some sign of convergence. For example, in the 1966 manifestos the Tories warned that 'no programme worthy of this country can be cheap' while Labour promised 'urgent measures to stop the waste of taxpayer's money'. But in the 1970 election the Tories again put the emphasis on controlling government spending.

[32]The decision risks, of course, another sort of distortion: it masks the ability of the Conservatives to increase civil expenditure in the post-Korean years when defence spending was declining and it was therefore possible to keep the total almost static. However, when the average annual rate of increase is re-calculated with 1951 as the base year, the main conclusions drawn in the text are not affected. Between 1951 and 1964 the rate was 3.34 per cent (as against 2.75 per cent for 1953–64), and between 1951 and 1957 it was 2.37 per cent (as against 0.26 per cent for 1953–57). Even the latter, quite considerable, difference leaves the pre- and post-Macmillan contrast intact, although less glaring. Choosing 1953 has the additional advantage of making it easier to construct time-series for individual programmes.

[33]In interpreting these figures, care must be taken not to over-emphasize the importance of small differences – which might well reflect classification and book-keeping changes. Thus the 1964–70 Labour Government changed investment

The picture becomes even more complex when the records of the 1953–64 Conservative Government and of the 1964–70 Labour Administration are analysed in more detail. As far as the first post-war Conservative Government was concerned, the main landmark in the management of public expenditure was the resignation of Peter Thorneycroft as Chancellor of the Exchequer in 1958.[34] Thorneycroft was a monetarist, who believed in the strict control of public expenditure; in effect, he was prepared to accept rising unemployment rather than rising prices. The Prime Minister, Harold Macmillan, did not share his view.[35] Rather than accept the expenditure cuts demanded by Thorneycroft, he was prepared to let the Chancellor and his whole team of Treasury ministers depart. It therefore seems sensible to compare the pre- and post-Macmillan years of Conservative Government. And at once a startling difference emerges. Between 1953 and 1957, the average annual rate of increase was only 0.26 per cent. Between 1957 and 1964, it was 4.18 per cent – virtually the same figure as for the Wilson Government that succeeded Macmillan's. However, the record of the Wilson Government can again usefully be looked at as falling into two distinct periods: pre- and post- the 1967 devaluation, which marked the defeat of the Government's initial economic strategy. Between 1964 and 1967, the average annual rate of increase was 6.66 per cent. Between 1967 and 1970, it was only 1.78 per cent.

These figures suggest two conclusions. The first is that there is indeed a slight political or ideological effect: this is suggested by the record of the Wilson Government in its first three years. The second, however, is that this effect tends to be swamped by the responses of governments to economic circumstances. If there is convergence, it is because all governments – irrespective of party and ideology – use public expenditure as a tool of economic management.

But this conclusion, in turn, needs qualifying for it contains two separate assumptions. The first is that the political parties are agreed about the

---

allowances to industry (which, being a tax concession, do not appear in the public expenditure statistics) into investment grants (which, being cash payments, do appear in these statistics). The succeeding Conservative Administration reversed this decision.

[34]As my main sources for the post-war history of economic management, I have used Andrew Shonfield, *British Economic Policy since the War* (Harmondsworth, Middx.: Penguin, 1958) and J. C. R. Dow, *The Management of the British Economy 1945–60* (Cambridge: Cambridge University Press, 1965) for the 'fifties and, for the 'sixties, Samuel Brittan, *Steering the Economy*) London: Macmillan, 1969).

[35]For Macmillan's own account of this episode, see Harold Macmillan, *Riding the Storm* (London: Macmillan, 1971), pp. 363–73; also, Donald Winch, *Economics and Policy* (London: Collins/Fontana, 1972), pp. 301–2.

aims of policy: in this case, that they share roughly the same view about the trade-off between maintaining full employment, on the one hand, and preventing balance of payments or inflationary crises, on the other hand. The second is that they are also agreed about the means of working towards these aims: in this case, that they are prepared to use public expenditure as an economic regulator by increasing spending at times of recession and cutting it at times of inflationary or balance-of-payments crises. For example, the changes from the pre- to the post-1957 Conservative strategy revolved as much around an argument about the techniques of economic management – the rejection of Thorneycroft's monetarist approach – as around the aims of policy. In respect of the latter, there may well have been a change in emphasis, in that Macmillan was particularly sensitive to rising unemployment figures, but there was certainly no change in direction. So the convergence of the two parties depends on agreement not only about policy aims but also about the techniques of economic management – about what is technically possible.

This is why, although it is easy enough to demonstrate the impact of economic circumstances on changes in the level of public expenditure, the relationship is not always easy to analyse: the intervening variable is the changing perception of how to cope, technically, with a specific economic situation. The complexity of the relationship between political ideology, economic circumstances and the perception of the technical means for dealing with a specific situation is, however, emphasized even more by the second example: the expenditure policies of the 1970–74 Conservative Government. On coming to office, the Heath Government announced plans for drastic cuts in spending, in line with what might be called the ideological model.[36] But with rising unemployment, the direction of change went into reverse, and the rate of increase accelerated. This, in turn, would seem to be in line with the consensus model of agreement about the aim of policy. But, crucially, this change reflected in turn new assumptions about the techniques for dealing with what was also a new economic phenomenon: a combination of rising unemployment and a worsening balance-of-payments position, with inflation also on the increase. The Government's decision was to allow the exchange rate to take the strain rather than to contain public expenditure. In other words, both the Labour Government in 1967–70 and the Conservative Government in 1971–73 behaved in ways that would seem to run counter to their political bias, because the former took an orthodox view of what

---

[36]Treasury, *New Policies for Public Spending* (London: HMSO, Cmnd. 4515, 1970).

was possible or desirable in the way of economic management, while the latter took a radical view.[37]

In trying to explain the rising percentage of the national income absorbed by public expenditure, our discussion has concentrated so far on analysing the spending records of successive governments. But this is only one factor in determining the relationship between the national income and public expenditure. The other, obviously, is the rate of growth in the national income itself. The Governments of Macmillan, Wilson and Heath did not say to themselves that they would increase the percentage of national income devoted to public expenditure; rather, they assumed that they could square the circle and maintain public expenditure as a steady proportion of national income by paying for rising spending out of economic growth. This was the theme of the first Public Expenditure White Paper to be published by the Conservatives in 1963 and continued to be the theme of its successors.[38] The 1975 White Paper was the first to concede that private consumption might have to be sacrificed to public consumption.[39] If the question is why public expenditure has grown as a percentage of national income, as distinct from its growth in absolute terms, then the answer appears to be comparatively simple: because successive governments got their sums wrong and assumed that the underlying growth potential of the economy (as calculated by their Treasury advisers) could actually be achieved. This is to underline the danger of analysing public expenditure trends as though they are invariably the product of intended effects: they may also be the product of miscalculations.

But this only prompts a further question: why did governments not act to correct their errors by cutting the planned expansion rate of public expenditure to take account of the failure to reach the hoped-for economic growth target? This failure is all the more remarkable in that the period of optimism about the possibility of paying for rising public expenditure out of economic growth coincided with the strengthening of

[37]The most notorious example in British politics of the importance of economic theory determining public expenditure decisions is, of course, to be found in the history of the 1929–31 Labour Government. In effect, this fell because the Chancellor of the Exchequer (and the Treasury) rejected Keynesian economics and decided to take the conventional view that cutting spending was the right response to recession. See Robert Skidelsky, *Politicians and the Slump* (Harmondsworth, Middx.: Penguin, 1970).

[38]Treasury, *Public Expenditure in 1963–64 and 1967–68* (London: HMSO, Cmnd. 2235, 1963).

[39]Treasury, *Public Expenditure to 1978–79*.

the machinery of control over public expenditure;[40] the two developments were closely related, in that they both reflected the general enthusiasm about economic planning evident from the beginning of the 1960s onwards. When the assumptions about economic growth turned out to be wrong, the institutional machinery for adjusting public expenditure plans was thus already available and tested: the PESC system first introduced in 1961. Yet, paradoxically, the development of this machinery coincided with a rising imbalance between economic growth and public expenditure growth and a major shift in the balance between the private and public sectors – a trend which was certainly not consciously intended and which the PESC system was designed to control, if not to prevent. Why did this happen?

One reason may lie in a perverse side-effect of the PESC system of control, unintended and unforeseen by its main authors. By projecting expenditure plans for each programme on a five-year basis, the annual Public Expenditure White Papers give public visibility to the relative position of each department by providing a league table of relative priorities – i.e. the average annual percentage increase. This may well be a misleading measure of priorities;[41] but both within Whitehall and outside there is pressure on civil servants and ministers to demonstrate their effectiveness in terms of getting at least the average share of increases for their department and, better still, an above-average increase.[42] This is not to imply that there was no competition between ministers and civil servants before the introduction of the PESC system. But the system has formalized the institutional framework for competition between ministers

---

[40]Sir Samuel Goldman, *The Developing System of Public Expenditure Management and Control* (London: HMSO, 1973).

[41]Expenditure Committee, Session 1970–71, Third Report, *Command Papers on Public Expenditure* (London: HMSO, HC 545, 1971). Note the reply to Q. 263 of J. J. B. Hunt of the Treasury: 'The percentage increase or decrease is clearly very interesting but it is not necessarily a measure of priority. If, for example, you take an entirely new programme, this will show a very big percentage increase. Also comparing some programmes you may have a relatively level figure, whereas within the programme there has been both a real increase and a real decrease.'

[42]See the Treasury official quoted in Hugh Heclo and Aaron Wildavsky, *The Private Government of Public Money* (London: Macmillan, 1974), p 239: 'PESC has simply enforced an earlier tendency for each dog to get its share. Thus, each permanent secretary can test his virility for next year by seeing whether he got the required x plus percentage like everyone else.' In what follows, I have also drawn on conversations with ex-civil servants and Treasury ministers who would not, however, thank me if I expressed my gratitude for their help by quoting them.

while giving the spending ministers a shared interest in persuading the Chancellor of the Exchequer to increase the total so as to avoid having to cut each other's throats.[43]

The introduction of the PESC system, and the annual publication of the Expenditure White Paper, may also have had another perverse consequence. The forward look in public expenditure is, essentially, a planning exercise; the system was designed by civil servants who, as was shown in the Plowden Report, were concerned to achieve stability – a framework within which they could get on with the business of planning the development of government services without too much interference from the politicians.[44] But, being a planning exercise, the forward look is chiefly concerned with resource allocation. This is why its detailed projections are published – a technical point of some political significance – in volume terms which measure 'the scale of provision of a particular service'.[45] But in fact the costs of providing a particular level of service may rise even while the level of service remains unchanged. This is because of the so-called 'relative price effect', which measures the extent to which the costs of public services are rising relative to costs in the rest of the economy. In fact, over the past twenty years public services have tended to get more expensive for any given level of services provided, largely because, while productivity gains offset to some extent the rising price of labour in the private sector, economists conventionally do not allow for such compensatory gains in the public sector. Spending has grown as much

---

[43]For an example of a Cabinet conflict over expenditure being resolved by increasing the previously agreed total, see Richard Crossman, *The Diaries of a Cabinet Minister*, Vol. I (London: Hamish Hamilton and Jonathan Cape, 1975), pp. 555–6. Crossman wanted an extra £31 million for his department, housing, but the consequent Cabinet resistance was overcome by a decision not to take his sum away from any other ministry but to add it to the previously settled PESC total.

[44]Treasury, *Control of Public Expenditure* (London: HMSO, Cmnd, 1432, 1961). Although chaired by Lord Plowden, the recommendations of this committee largely reflected the views of a Treasury official, Sir Richard 'Otto' Clarke. Note the emphasis in para. 18: 'There is no doubt from the evidence that we have received that chopping and changing in Government expenditure policy is frustrating to efficiency and economy in the running of the public services . . . The experience of recent years, both in the Treasury and in the Departments, and in the wide circles of local government and nationalised industries outside them, is that short-term "economy campaigns" and "stop-and-go" are damaging to the real effectiveness of control of public expenditure.' For a review of recent examples of 'chopping and changing', uninhibited by the PESC machinery, see: Expenditure Committee, Session 1972–73, Fifth Report, *The White Paper Public Expenditure to 1976–77* (London: HMSO, HC 149, 1973), para. 13.

[45]*Public Expenditure White Papers: Handbook on Methodology*. See paras. 65–71 for a definition of 'volume terms' and also the 'relative price effect'.

because the costs of providing public services have risen as because of conscious decisions to expand the scale of those services. This indeed is one of the reasons why public expenditure has risen not only in Britain but in other advanced industrial countries as well; the relative price effect is international.

There is, in a sense, nothing 'inevitable' about such increasing costs: government could decide to keep public sector wages and salaries below those in the private sector – even if this meant manpower shortages in the public sector. For short periods, at various times, this has happened; some of the short-term fluctuations in the cost of individual programmes can in fact be attributed to changes in relative labour costs rather than to policy decisions about the level of service. But most governments seem to have decided that the political costs of trying to keep down the economic cost of public services are too great. They may well have been encouraged in this decision by the failure of the planning figures used for most public-expenditure projections to take full account of the likely rise in prices.

(b) Benefits and Costs

The discussion so far has looked at the party-competition model in terms of its ability to explain the underlying upward trend in public expenditure and, in particular, the acceleration that took place in the 1960s and early 1970s. In this respect, it appears to lack explanatory power – at least in a direct sense. Other modes of explanation – especially those which take the organizational processes of the governmental system into account – appear to be more powerful. Furthermore, the British evidence suggests that the competition between the parties is in terms of their rival claims to effectiveness in managing the economy as a whole, not in terms of increasing the benefits of public expenditure.[46]

But the interest of the Downs approach does not end here. Unlike many modes of explanation, it is specific enough to allow testing against data. One of its crucial assumptions, it will be remembered, is about the relative visibility of benefits and costs. It suggests that public expenditure will go up only if the benefits are more visible than the costs, i.e. taxes. Has this in fact been happening? There is obviously a problem about giving a precise definition to the 'visibility' of public spending. However, there would probably be little argument that the most visible items of public expenditure are straight social security cash payments to individuals. Have these in fact grown as a proportion of all public expenditure?

---

[46]David Butler and Donald Stokes, *Political Change in Britain*, 2nd edn. (London: Macmillan, 1974).

Indeed they have, from 13.3 per cent of the total in 1953 to 17.2 per cent in 1973 (see Table 2). In contrast, defence spending, which offers no visible benefits to any one person, declined from 24.5 per cent of the total to 10.6 per cent over the same period. Complicating the picture somewhat, and illustrating the difficulties of this kind of exercise, is the fact that the growth rate of social security payments has been slower than that of some other government programmes: an increase of 157.8 per cent in constant price terms over the same twenty-year period as against 265.6 per cent for education and 259.1 per cent for subsidies and other forms of expenditure on industry, nationalized and private. Clearly, all of these services also provide some form of benefit, but it would seem that the concept of visibility is either less important than was assumed initially or needs refining – a point that will be explored further in the more detailed analysis below of the comparative performance of individual programmes.

On the other side of the balance sheet, the picture is equally complex. It might be assumed that the most visible form of paying for public benefits – which would thus be avoided by governments – is direct taxation.[47] As public expenditure rises so the proportion raised by direct taxation (including national insurance contributions) might be expected to fall. In fact, the trends are confused. In 1900 central government raised £42 million by way of taxes on income and capital as against £74 million by way of taxes on expenditure; the former accounted for just over one-third of the total raised in revenue. The 'displacement effect' of war also had its effect on the pattern of taxation; by 1920 roughly twice as much was being raised by direct than by indirect taxation. Between 1920 and 1939 indirect taxation rose as a proportion of the total, but by 1945 the two-to-one relationship was again evident. After 1945 however, the trend was once more towards increasing the proportion of total revenue raised by indirect taxation, until by 1970 for every £5 raised by direct taxation £3 was raised by indirect taxation.[48] Thus far the post-1945 trends are in

---

[47]'The best taxes are such as are levied upon consumption, especially those of luxury; because such taxes are least felt by the people. They seem, in some measure, voluntary; since a man may chuse how far he will use the commodity which is taxed: they are paid gradually and insensibly: they naturally produce sobriety and frugality, if judiciously imposed: and being confounded with the natural price of the commodity, they are scarcely perceived by the consumers.' David Hume, 'Of Taxes', *Essays, Literary, Moral and Political* (London: Routledge, 1894), Essay XXX, pp. 203–7.

[48]For the period before 1964, the figures come from the London and Cambridge Economic Service, *The British Economy: Key Statistics 1900–1966* (London: The Times, n.d.). For subsequent years, the source (as for all public expenditure

the predicted direction; but after 1970 they go into reverse. By 1973 almost twice as much was being raised by direct as by indirect taxation. It thus seems impossible to come to any clear-cut conclusion about the trend in the type of costs imposed on the public to pay for rising public expenditure – at any rate on the basis of the sort of rough-and-ready analysis attempted here.

In any case, two cautions are indicated. First, the equation of direct taxation with visibility may be over-simple. Not only is there widespread ignorance about marginal tax rates.[49] More important, the phenomenon of fiscal drag – the fact that with inflation and the delay in adjusting tax allowances to take account of the fall in their real value people's rate of taxation tends to increase without their realizing it – may give a degree of invisibility to income tax. Second, and following on from this point, the degree of invisibility obviously rises with the rate of inflation – so it is perhaps not surprising that the proportion of revenue raised by direct taxation rose in the 'seventies with increasing speed while indirect taxes became unpopular with governments because they raised the cost of living.[50]

The problem of analysis is further compounded because the politics of revenue raising are affected by considerations that have nothing to do with the visibility or otherwise of various taxes. They also involve a judgement about the distribution of the burden. It may well be that a highly visible tax is also judged to be a highly acceptable tax because it will fall on a minority of taxpayers to the advantage (real or apparent) of the majority of consumers of public services and benefits. In the case of taxes on capital, it may be precisely their visibility – rather than their revenue raising capacity – which appeals to governments of the left. Additionally, direct taxes on income tend to be progressive while taxes on expenditure tend to be regressive, so it is possible that governments

---

figures for calendar as distinct from financial years) is Central Statistical Office, *National Income and Expenditure 1964–1974* (London: HMSO, 1975). The Blue Book groups rates under the heading of taxes on expenditure. From the point of view of political visibility it seems wrong, however, to include rates among indirect taxes so I have excluded them from the calculations made. If they were included among the direct taxes (as they should be, I believe, for the purposes of this analysis), the broad trends revealed would not be changed. I have, however, included national insurance contribution under direct taxation.

[49] See fn. 11, above.

[50] Peacock and Wiseman, *Growth of Public Expenditure*, for instance, discuss the possibility that inflation might create the sort of social disturbance that is reflected in the 'displacement effect' but find none attributable to this source in the period covered by their analysis.

TABLE 2   Public Expenditure, 1953–1973, at 1970 Constant Prices*

Programmes	Expenditure in £ million (and as % of total)		Total % increase	Average annual percentage rate of increase:					Range of annual change (% rise or fall)	
	1953	1973	1953–1973	1953–64	1953–57	1957–64	1964–70	1970–73	Max.	Min.
Military defence	3,112(24.5)	2,675(10.6)	–14.0	–1.37	–4.33	0.33	–1.27	2.75	6.1	–11.1
External relations	165(1.3)	504(2.0)	205.5	7.10	6.09	7.69	–0.79	14.70	53.2	–22.1
Roads, transport and communications	564(4.4)	1,947(7.7)	245.2	7.40	9.98	5.99	5.78	3.87	31.6	–7.7
Industry and trade incl. employment services	631(5.0)	2,266(8.9)	259.1	6.49	9.46	4.86	8.48	3.27	38.6	–11.4
Research	42(0.3)	212(0.8)	404.8	14.39	21.32	10.58	3.94	–2.94	27.0	–5.8
Agriculture, forestry, fishing and foods	602(4.7)	391(1.5)	–35.0	–2.62	–2.10	–2.96	–1.84	–0.73	44.4	–33.5
Housing	1,078(8.5)	1,771(7.0)	64.3	0.10	–8.34	5.28	2.57	11.69	43.9	–14.2
Environmental services	428(3.4)	1,327(5.2)	210.0	4.91	0.52	7.50	5.83	9.17	14.1	–2.0
Libraries, museums and arts	27(0.2)	137(0.5)	407.4	8.01	7.46	8.32	7.26	12.58	18.1	1.5
Law, order and protective services	381(3.0)	786(3.1)	106.3	1.44	–11.28	9.52	5.99	7.55	29.6	–21.6
Education	877(6.9)	3,206(12.7)	265.6	7.26	7.61	7.08	5.65	6.68	11.3	1.9
N.H.S.	987(7.8)	2,356(9.3)	138.7	3.99	2.93	4.57	4.91	5.30	7.8	–0.8
Personal social services	66(0.5)	414(1.6)	527.3	5.83	3.59	7.12	14.41	14.48	31.8	1.0
School meals, milk and welfare foods	148(1.2)	159(0.6)	7.4	0.30	–1.73	1.48	2.16	–2.94	10.9	–13.8

TABLE 2   Public Expenditure, 1953–1973, at 1970 Constant Prices*

Programmes	Expenditure in £ million (and as % of total)		Total % increase	Average annual percentage rate of increase:					Range of annual change (% rise or fall)	
	1953	1973	1953–1973	1953–64	1953–57	1957–64	1964–70	1970–73	Max.	Min.
Social security benefits	1,691(13.3)	4,359(17.2)	157.8	4.75	1.67	6.53	5.70	3.58	15.9	–1.3
Other public services	390(3.1)	506(2.0)	29.7	–2.16	–3.37	–1.49	6.95	3.39	27.7	–19.8
Debt interest	1,521(12.0)	2,322(9.2)	52.7	1.62	0.26	2.40	2.82	2.67	12.0	–5.3
Total	12,708(100.0)	25,338(100.0)	99.4	2.75	0.26	4.18	4.19	5.02	11.1	–2.6

*Source: National Income and Expenditure Blue Books. The constant price series has been calculated using the GDP deflator.

may consider that the disadvantages of visibility in the former case are outweighed by their perceived fairness.[51]

Given the inconclusiveness of the evidence about the balance of visibility between the benefits and costs, it remains something of a puzzle why the British parties do not compete by cutting taxes rather than by increasing expenditure[52] – the assumption of the original Downs model. To try to meet this point, it may be useful to return to the concept of organizational pressure: to the role of the governmental system in its widest sense, including service-providers as well as service-administrators. If it is accepted that the governmental system is a factor in determining the level of public expenditure, then the reluctance of successive ministries to cut spending becomes much more comprehensible. Such cuts, to the extent that they are a reduction in the level of services provided, as distinct from cash payments or subsidies, pose a direct threat to jobs in the public sector. It is therefore not surprising that teachers, doctors and others employed in public services have traditionally taken the lead in protesting against reductions even in the planned rate of growth in public expenditure – though, significantly, they have usually done so in a way calculated to enlarge the arena of controversy from the governmental system to the political system as a whole by invoking the interests of their clients (a reminder that, while it is analytically useful to distinguish between these two systems, in practice much of the power of governmental interest groups may derive from and depend upon their ability to mobilize support from other interests). Thus organizational pressure may help to explain why the movement in public expenditure tends to be in one direction only.[53]

The public demand model may also be of some assistance in this connection. The desire for lower taxes, while no doubt widespread, is

---

[51]Royal Commission on the Distribution of Income and Wealth, *Report No. 1* (London: HMSO, Cmnd. 6171, 1975).

[52]This is not to say that governments never cut taxes: the Conservatives did so after coming into office in 1970. But cutting taxes is not seen as an alternative to increasing expenditure: the two have gone together, with the resulting deficit being met by government borrowing – which rose sharply, as a proportion of total public expenditure, in the 1970s.

[53]In support of this contention, it is possible to invoke the views of Lord Diamond who was Chief Secretary to the Treasury in the Labour Cabinet of 1964 to 1970 and as such the minister most directly concerned with the control of public expenditure:

'It is very difficult indeed to halt an old-established programme; the forces making for its continuation seem to grow stronger with every year that passes. Programmes which, if they did not exist, would not secure ministerial approval will nevertheless be able to secure ministerial approval to their continuation, and departments tend to fight hard to maintain that continuity for reasons other also in the nature of a want (see above): that is, a vague aspiration, a generalized hope. But the organizational machinery for translating it into a political demand does not exist: even those groups that call for cuts in public expenditure with one voice tend with another to ask for specific forms of subsidies or help; industry is a case in point. There is no organized group dedicated to the single aim of cutting taxes; the opposition to high taxes is diffuse.[54] In contrast, there are any number of pressure groups – from the aircraft industry lobby to the National Farmers' Union – that exist to translate wants for more spending into concentrated political demands.[55] This would suggest that there is a basic asymmetry in the universe of politically articulated demands in favour of higher public expenditure. What is more, while taxpayers cannot – emigration apart – exit from the political system, as distinct from individual parties, some organized groups in society can effectively do so: that is, they can withhold their co-operation from the government. The fact that governments in complex modern societies increasingly depend on the co-operation of organized groups – for information, for participation in economic planning, for support in the operation of incomes policies, and so on – has by now become somewhat of a cliché in political analysis. But the implications of accepting this view for public expenditure have been less discussed: they are, surely, that governments may have to spend more in order to buy co-operation from certain strategic groups (although obviously the price of co-operation may be laws passed or repealed, as much as subsidies paid or services expanded).

The first half of this proposition – that government expenditure rises as governments have to buy more support – would seem to be consistent with the British experience. The turning point in the post-war history of public expenditure came, as we saw, in 1957, which also marked the adoption of markedly more interventionist policies by the Conservative Government of Harold Macmillan. Since then the emphasis on economic

---

than the intrinsic merits of the programme.' Lord Diamond, *Public Expenditure in Practice* (London: Allen and Unwin, 1975), p. 92.

[54]'Although everybody grumbles all the time about the burden of taxation – and a lively democracy requires a harmless safety valve like this for letting off steam – it is usually the case that bitter complaints about particular tax proposals are fairly short-lived. They represent the kind of pressures that governments have learnt to face' (Diamond, *Public Expenditure in Practice*, p. 27).

[55]The concentration may, of course, be geographical as well as interest-centered. Thus one of the most powerful arguments for securing funds for a particular industry may be that it is heavily concentrated in one particular place, where unemployment would have both political visibility and impact. This may help to explain, for example, government financial support (irrespective of political party) for Concorde, Rolls-Royce and the car industry.

planning – on involving trade-unions and industry – in the process of decision-making has been accompanied by rising public expenditure. Logically there need be no connection between increasing state regulatory activity (e.g. incomes policy) and increasing government expenditure. But politically, as was suggested, there may well be a link: governments may be compelled to spend more in order to secure the co-operation of the groups involved in the regulatory or planning process. As the system changes, so the price of maintaining it rises.

In any case, there is a danger, apparent in the discussion so far, of analysing public expenditure as if all decisions were taken in terms of the total and as though the significance of changes in public policy could be assessed exclusively in terms of the final out-turn. This is a necessary simplifying assumption when discussing broad trends, but it may nevertheless be misleading. Political factors may be of significance in influencing changes in the detailed composition of public expenditure as well as in its total, and it is with this issue that the last section of this paper deals.

(c) The Composition of Public Expenditure

One of the problems in trying to analyse the political factors affecting changes in the composition of public expenditure is that all spending is expressed in terms of pounds. Just because the budgets of two programmes can be measured in terms of the same currency, it does not follow that the two programmes are strictly comparable. They vary in their economic significance, in their administrative flexibility, in the degree of commitment they represent, and in the scope for change they offer. The first stage in any analysis must therefore be to try to differentiate between programmes in these respects.

Public expenditure policies, as has already been noted, are closely linked to the management of the economy. Their impact on the economy is therefore likely to influence the decisions taken, and to the extent that different programmes have different kinds of impact so these decisions are likely to vary. The most basic distinction is that between programmes that pre-empt resources and those that transfer them: between those, like health and education, that employ people or buy goods and those, like social security, that merely shuffle money from the taxpayer to the beneficiary. To quote the Treasury:

> A major consideration in planning public expenditure is the extent to which spending by the public sector involves claims on the supply of resources ... Different kinds of expenditure may have dissimilar implications in this respect. Thus when public expenditure puts a direct demand on resources, as it does for example when a department buys good or employs people,

the expenditure is a fairly good measure of the resources used. But when the government helps to finance personal consumption, by transferring money, the amount of money transferred may be a poor guide to the resulting demand on resources. One reason for this is that the government automatically recoups some of its expenditure in taxation, either by direct taxes, as, for example, income tax on family allowances, or by indirect taxes on expenditure. . . .[56]

So one public expenditure pound is not necessarily the same as another public expenditure pound.

Equally, different public expenditure options have different degrees of administrative feasibility and different time-horizons.[57] For example, programmes that simply involve transferring money can be implemented more quickly than programmes that involve hiring people or putting up buildings. Again, capital spending plans can be changed more easily than on-going services: cancelling a contract is easier than laying off employees. Hence the frequency with which successive governments have changed the capital investment programme.[58] This last point links administrative feasibility with political expediency; it is less invidious for ministers to export unemployment into the private building industry, where their responsibility will be less visible, than directly to dismiss public employees.

Different programmes can also be distinguished by the extent to which they commit governments to spend more in response to circumstances outside their control. For example, paying old-age pensions is a very precise commitment, while providing a health service is not. In the former case, expenditure is bound to go up if the number of people over the retirement age increases: in the latter case, demographic change may increase the strain on the service – in the sense, for example, that the

---

[56]Expenditure Committee, Session 1971–72, Seventh Report, *Public Expenditure and Economic Management* (London: HMSO, HC 450, 1972). See *Memorandum* by the Treasury 'Public Expenditure and Demand on Real Resources'.

[57]Select Committee on Procedure, Session 1968–69, First Report (London: HMSO, HC 410, 1969). See *Memorandum* by the Treasury 'The Planning and Control of Public Expenditure', and subsequent questioning of Sir William Armstrong and other Treasury officials.

[58]For a critique of this emphasis on capital cuts, see Expenditure Committee, Session 1974–75, Ninth Report, *The Public Expenditure Implications of the April, 1975, Budget* (London: HMSO, HC 474, 1975). Note the reply of a Treasury official to Q. 49, where he was asked why successive governments preferred to make the public sector more labour intensive in relation to the available capital investment, while the private sector was moving in the opposite direction: 'It may be that when faced with the practical problems of cutting expenditure, governments take into account similar factors.'

demand for health care rises with age – but need not necessarily affect its scale. However, commitment ought not to be interpreted in a crudely deterministic way: an undertaking to pay old-age pensions is not a pledge to pay it at a particular level. Thus, while changes in the structure of society do have implications for services specific to particular groups of the population like the elderly, they do not explain the decision to increase the real value of benefits like pensions in line with rising standards of living. In other words, changes in the societal system may produce the policy cues but they do not necessarily explain the policy reactions. To do this, it may be necessary to look at the role of the political system.

When the focus of analysis was total public expenditure, the evidence suggested that the similarities in the behaviour of the political parties were more important than their ideological differences – in line with the predictions of the party-competition model. But it does not follow that the same would be true of their priorities within the total: their policy reactions to particular cues might well be shaped by their values and by their links with particular interest groups. However, the growth rates for individual programmes in Table 2 once again indicate that there is no simple or direct relationship. The average annual rise in spending on social security was 1.67 per cent between 1953 and 1957 (the pre-Macmillan Conservative Government), 6.53 per cent between 1957 and 1964 (the Macmillan era), 5.7 per cent between 1964 and 1970 (the Labour Government) and 3.58 per cent between 1970 and 1973 (the Heath Conservative Administration). Thus the rate of increase was higher under Labour than in two out of three periods of Conservative Government. The same is true of expenditure on the National Health Service. But in the case of education the rate of increase was slightly lower under Labour than under all three Conservative Governments while in the case of housing, where spending tends to move erratically, two out of the three Conservative Administrations produced a much higher growth rate than the Labour Government.

It would be difficult to draw a confident conclusion from these trends, except tentatively that the 1953–57 Conservative Government does seem to have had a different approach to social spending – education excepted – than any of its successors of either party. It exploited the scope for manoeuvre created by declining spending on defence to hold back total public expenditure instead of using the funds so freed to accelerate the expansion of social programmes.

All this is not to claim that political or ideological considerations are irrelevant when it comes to determining public expenditure priorities. It is rather to suggest that these may well be masked either by programme characteristics or by economic circumstances and often by both; for example, the apparent priority given to housing by the Heath Administration largely reflects the upward leap in spending in 1973 as a result of the inflationary pressures to which this programme is exceptionally sensitive.[59] In particular, the evidence presented underlines the need for a more fine-mesh approach to the analysis of public expenditure patterns. For, clearly, the ability of ministers to influence expenditure patterns is in an inverse relationship to the size of the programme in question: their apparent lack of influence may be largely a reflection of the fact that the time-series of expenditure are published by programmes rather than being broken down into their components.[60] So there is an obvious danger that any conclusions reached will simply be an artefact of inadequate statistics over-confidently used. A new policy commitment may grow much faster than the programme of which it is part, without greatly affecting the overall rate of increase.[61]

Historically, too, it is possible to illustrate the inverse relationship between the size of the expenditure unit chosen for analysis and the role of political ideology. Take, for instance, a programme that is both financially modest and politically sensitive: subsidies for school meals and welfare food. Two out of the three Conservative periods of government actually showed cuts – an average annual fall of 1.73 per cent between 1953 and 1957 and of 2.94 per cent between 1970 to 1973 – and the third, 1957 to 1964, showed only a modest average annual rise, of 1.48 per cent. As against this, expenditure went up by 2.16 per cent a year during the Labour Government of 1964–70. On the whole, despite the

---

[59]For a discussion of housing and inflation, see Edward Craven, 'Housing' in Klein, ed., *Inflation and Priorities, 1975.*

[60]Only broad programme categories, as shown in Table 2, are available from the Blue Books for the entire post-war period: the more detailed information provided by the Expenditure White Papers only starts in 1968–69. Work urgently requires doing to put the information available in the Blue Book, the Supply Estimates the local authority return on a basis which would allow detailed expenditure comparisons for the entire post-war period. In the absence of such work, it may prove impossible to advance to a more sophisticated analysis of public expenditure patterns over time.

[61]For example, attendance allowances first feature in the social security programme of the 1970 White Paper: Treasury, *Public Expenditure 1969–70 to 1974–75* (London: HMSO, Cmnd. 4578, 1975). This provided for spending £3,000,000 in 1971/2 to rise to £10 million by 1974–75 (both at 1970 71 outturn prices). In fact, the commitment having been once made – and the government having been seen to assume a new sort of responsibility – pressure to increase the scale and the scope of the policy grew rapidly and successfully. The 1975 White Paper, Treasury, *Public Expenditure to 1978–79,* shows that – at 1974 Survey prices – expenditure rose from £9,000,000 in 1971–72 to £61 million in 1974–75. Even so, it represented only 1 per cent of the total social security expenditure.

aberration of the Macmillan premiership, this pattern is what might have been expected from the ideological predilections of the two parties.

Changes over time in individual programmes also allow some of the other explanatory modes, discussed in the first part of the paper, to be tested. To begin with, as the final two columns of Table 2 show, the incremental approach has only limited explanatory power. Even leaving aside the problem of giving precise definition to what is meant by incremental rate of change, it is quite clear that even the most generous interpretation of this term would not explain what happened in some of the major programmes. Thus, agriculture (which includes food subsidies as well as farm support payments) shows variations from −33.5 per cent to +44.4 per cent; in housing the range is from −14.2 per cent to +43.9 per cent; and in industry and trade the swing is from −11.4 per cent to +38.6 per cent.

These fluctuations suggest that the incremental approach has only a limited usefulness in explaining budgetary, organizational and political processes – in Britain at any rate. But the figures do tell us something about programme characteristics. All the three programmes chosen to demonstrate non-incremental fluctuations have certain characteristics in common. First, they have a large cash content: that is, they represent decisions about channelling money, not about providing services. They are therefore exceptionally flexible. Second, they represent commitments which – to varying degrees – are outside the control of governments; for example, fluctuations in farm support payments to a large extent reflect (particularly in the period before Britain's entry into the Common Market) variations in world food prices. This is less true of housing and industry, but even here the cost of government commitments is to a large extent shaped by such factors as the take-up of grants by local authorities or individual firms and movements in interest rates. Third, in the case of housing and industry though not of agriculture, these programmes tend to have a large investment content and therefore to be vulnerable to the tendency of governments to use capital expenditure as an economic regulator.

In contrast, the programmes that do show an incremental pattern of change have characteristics that tend to be the mirror-image of the programmes discussed so far. For example, the range of change for education is from +1.9 per cent to +11.3 per cent and that for the National Health Service is from −0.8 per cent to +7.8 per cent. Both these are manpower-intensive services, where something like three-fifths of the total-budget is represented by labour costs. They are also extremely large consumers of funds, so that very considerable sums would be required to make marginal adjustments in any one year. It is therefore not surprising that changes tend to conform to the incrementalist prediction: arguably, the policy changes would be even less than implied by the figures in the table if allowance were made for the distorting effects in any one year either of large wage and salary settlements or of pay freezes.

The direction, as well as the rate, of change seems to be of some significance. The manpower-intensive services tend to move in one direction only: upwards. The main exceptions – defence and law and order – are interesting in that they are examples of 'pure' public goods; the fall in spending on the former and the relatively volatile performance of the latter would seem therefore to confirm the Downsian theory that spending will be a function of visible benefits. Generally, however, the pattern is consistent. Education has never had its spending reduced; National Health Service expenditure has fallen in only one year, and then marginally. This would seem to confirm the importance of the organizational factor. There would appear to be a built-in resistance from within the services to any threat of losing any achieved gains. The tendency is to defend the existing budget, to hoard the resources already allocated to the service, even when the demands that originally generated the expenditure diminish. The point can be illustrated from the experience of the education service. In the 1960s expenditure on education rose largely because the number of young people in the relevant age cohort increased. In the 1970s, however, a fall in the birth rate has brought about a decline in the pressure of demand, mainly at the primary-school stage. There could therefore have been a matching reduction in expenditure. In fact, the opportunity was used not to cut expenditure but to expand the programme: i.e., to ensure that the existing resources would be used by inventing new demands on them – notably by launching the nursery school programme.[62] Politically, too, it is of course attractive to be able to offer a new service without seemingly imposing extra costs: the political benefits are visible while the opportunity costs are not.

So far our emphasis had been on looking at change on a government-by-government basis. But this may be to miss underlying trends, and the analysis therefore concludes by examining changes over the whole 1953–74 period. The most immediate conclusion to be drawn from looking at the figures in column 3 of Table 2 is that rate of growth varies inversely with size of programme. The three services that show the biggest increase – research (404.8 per cent), libraries, museums and the arts (407.4 per cent) and the personal social services (527.3 per cent) – all had budgets of less than £100 million in 1953. But, though unsurprising,

---

[62]For the relevant statement of government policy, see Department of Education and Science, *Education: a Framework for Expansion* (London: HMSO, Cmnd. 5174, 1972). For an interpretation of this in public expenditure terms, see Jack Barnes, 'Schools' in Rudolf Klein, ed., *Inflation and Priorities, 1975.*

this finding is not unimportant: it once again emphasizes that the picture of slow change would be greatly modified if it were possible to disaggregate the data.

But even among the major programmes – and even excluding defence and law and order as special cases – significant differences emerge over the twenty-one year period. There is, for example, a conspicuous difference between the experience of health and education. The former recorded an increase of 138.7 per cent, while the latter showed a rise of 265.6 per cent – and, while in 1953 the former's budget was bigger than the latter's, by 1973 the position had been reversed. A comparison between these two services may therefore be helpful in generating some possible explanations about the factors likely to influence the expenditure patterns of different services.

In trying to account for their different rates of expansion, the obvious starting point is the societal system. If the contrasting performance of the two services reflects contrasting structural factors, then it would be redundant to seek other explanations. The increasing expenditure on education, it may be argued, was determined partly by the growth in the number of children within the school age – the population of under-15s rose from 11.4 million in the census year 1951 to 13.4 million in 1971 – and partly by the requirements of a technologically more complex society. But while this helps to account for the rise in spending on education in Britain – as in other countries – at best it only partly solves our problem. It does not explain the dramatically lower figures for health. For in the case of health, too, it is possible to invoke structural factors: the number of the elderly, the most heavy users of the service, increased from 6.9 million in 1951 to 9.1 million in 1971. Equally, it could be argued that the growing complexity of society may, on the one hand, create extra stresses while, on the other, requiring a healthy as well as an educated labour force. As before, the conclusion appears to be that, while structural factors may explain many of the pressures for higher public expenditure, they do not account for the way in which those pressures are accommodated by the political and governmental systems.

One obvious difference is that health is the responsibility of central government while education (with the exception of the university sector) is the responsibility of local authorities. The difference in the expenditure patterns might therefore reflect either that central government finds it more difficult to control the expenditure of a multiplicity of local authorities than it does its own or that this multiplicity in itself creates pressures for extra spending.[63] Certainly international comparisons suggest that

---

[63]R. Joseph Monsen and Anthony Downs, 'Public Goods and Private States', *The Public Interest*, XXIII (1971), 64–76.

nations with a relatively large central government role in education spend less of their national wealth on this programme than those where sub-national units or local governments have predominant financial responsibility.[64] But the British experience is ambiguous. To take the case of two other local authority services, the experience of personal social services would appear to reinforce the hypothesis that decentralization means higher spending, while that of the law, order and protective services (which show a smaller increase over the period than health) would seem to point in the opposite direction – although this may, of course, be because of its other characteristics, already discussed.

What evidence there is suggests that the differences in the growth records of education and health cannot be explained by differences in the system of administration as distinct from differences in the political environment or programme characteristics. If the crucial factor were the problem of control – i.e. the fact that the Treasury can exercise tighter financial discipline over a centralized service than over a decentralized one – then it would be reasonable to expect larger divergences between targets for expenditure and actual out-turns for local government services. But this does not appear to be the case. Expenditure White Paper projections for expenditure on education are almost as 'accurate' as those for health.[65] So it would appear that, if the diffusion of financial control has any influence over expenditure, then in the case of education at least it is because of political rather than administrative factors. The role of the local authorities is significant to the extent that they succeed in creating a constituency of pressure groups, organizing and articulating demands for higher spending.

Looking at the institutions that translate wants into demands and then demands into political pressures seems in any case to be more helpful than trying to apply the crude public demands model. Public opinion may not be irrelevant over issues of detail: i.e. about the form taken by public expenditure benefits. For example, the level of family allowances seems to have been traditionally depressed by the awareness of politicians that they are far less popular than, say, pensions. But there is no evidence that, to take the examples of education and health, public opinion has been consistently in favour of expanding the former rather than the latter. Indeed both sectors appear to have little salience in people's minds and

---

[64]David R. Cameron and Richard I. Hofferbert, 'The Impact of Federalism on Education Finance: A Comparative Analysis', *European Journal of Political Research*, II (1974), 225–58.

[65]Quentin Outram, *The Significance of Public Expenditure Plans* (London: Centre for Studies in Social Policy, 1975).

the general impression is of a high degree of satisfaction with existing levels of service rather than of pressure to improve on them.[66]

Yet again the missing links between structural factors, political variables and expenditure patterns can perhaps most usefully be sought in the characteristics of the programmes themselves. In the first place, there is a crucial difference in the administrative visibility of the demand for education as compared with the demand for health. In the case of education, there is fairly widespread agreement about the currency of demand – children – and the means for meeting it – teachers. Deciding on how to react to rising demand is then a relatively simple task, revolving on the desirable ratio between pupils and teachers (the sum gets a bit more complicated in the case of higher education, but the nature of the exercise does not change). In the case of health, there is no agreement either about how to measure demand or about formulae for meeting it. There is a widespread consensus that more old people means greater burdens on the health service, but no way of translating that consensus into the specific number of doctors, nurses or beds required. In the case of education, therefore, any apparent drop in standards is clearly visible: the number of pupils per teacher rises. In the case of health, the absence of any target makes it impossible to monitor success or failure.[67]

But the whole concept of political visibility – so crucial when one tries to apply the political competition model – requires further analysis. In particular, it may be useful to try to imagine the various programmes of public expenditure arranged along two axes: the first indicating the programme's degree of 'generality', the other indicating its degree of 'certainty'. The first axis measures the beneficiaries of the service: is it the population at large or a specific group? The second axis measures the certainty or otherwise of anyone's receiving the benefits: are they automatic or are they contingent on something happening and, if the latter, what are the odds on that contingency in fact happening?

The idea is illustrated in the figure. Thus the health service rates high on generality but rather lower on certainty (benefits being contingent on illness). In contrast, education presents the reverse situation since it offers certain benefits to a specific, if large, group of the population (benefits flowing automatically from the fact of birth). But educational expenditure is, of course, a very heterogeneous category and a distinction ought to

---

[66]For a general review of this area, see Rudolf Klein, 'The Case for Elitism: Public Opinion and Public Policy', *The Political Quarterly*, XLV (1974), 406–17.

[67]The tenuous relationship between expenditure decisions and indicators of need or performance is best illustrated by the evidence of the Department of Health and Social Security in Expenditure Committee, Session 1971–72, Eighth Report, *Relationship of Expenditure to Needs* (London: HMSO, HC 515, 1972).

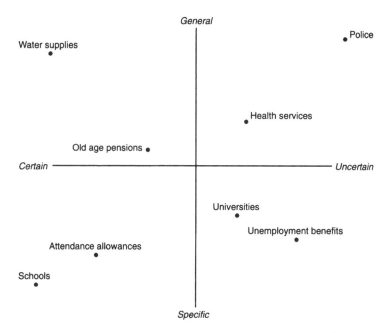

FIGURE I

be drawn between spending on schooling and on universities: in the former case, the benefits are certain because the law compels every child below a specified age to attend school, while in the latter case there is much less certainty as to who will benefit. Again, different sorts of social security payments vary in terms of both certainty and generality. Old-age pensions are both general and reasonably certain (in the sense that everyone over retirement age will get them, but not everyone will necessarily live to reach that age). Unemployment benefits, on the other hand, are both extremely uncertain – since it is difficult to predict who will fall into this category – and very specific. It would therefore be reasonable to assume that expenditure policies will be different for these two types of social security benefits, and this is indeed what has happened in Britain where the *per capita* level of old age pensions has risen faster than that of unemployment benefits.[68] Lastly, the law and order services – which, as already noted, have had a conspicuously low rate of expansion – are different from the others so far discussed in that they are even less certain in presenting the assurance of benefits to come than health, while also

---

[68]Rudolf Klein, Martin Buxton and Quentin Outram, *Constraints and Choices* (London: Centre for Studies in Social Policy, 1976).

being even more general. Indeed the political definition of a pure public good might be that it offers totally uncertain benefits to the entire population, the benefits being entirely contingent on events that the expenditure is designed to prevent from happening in the first place (in the case of the police and the military).

The suggestion that expenditure will be highest on those services that offer certain benefits to specific groups is certainly in line with what might be predicted from the political competition model, since this is based on the assumption that public benefits can be offered to particular sections of the population – so allowing a political choice as to where the investment will pay off. Thus it could be argued that the beneficiaries of education are a politically more attractive target group than the beneficiaries of health treatment; parents belong to the politically active generations while the most intensive users of health services are the elderly who tend to be politically passive.

The concepts of visibility, certainty and generality – and the trade-offs between them – are also useful in explaining the form, as well as the level, of expenditure on different programmes. For, by giving a high degree of visibility to expenditure on a clearly defined and concentrated group of the population, governments may be able to spend less to achieve a given political impact than if they chose a more diffuse, less easily identifiable form of spending. Aid to industry provides an example: concentrating funds on a particular region or on a particular industry may be both cheaper and politically attractive than general subsidies. Some forms of expenditure may thus have a demonstration effect – symbolizing the determination of government to help a particular section of the population – that cannot be measured by the size of the financial commitment. Once again the conclusion must be that, just as one public expenditure pound cannot be equated with another public expenditure pound in terms of their economic impact, so they are likely to vary, too, in their political impact.

Some Speculative Conclusions

Public expenditure is the outcome of many decisions. It reflects decisions about the desirable total of expenditure, taken in the light of changing economic circumstances. It is shaped by decisions about how that expenditure should be distributed among competing groups, whether geographically concentrated or aggregated in organized interests. In turn, these decisions are taken under pressure from a variety of sources. Some of these pressures reflect changes in society. Others reflect the influence of political parties, service-clients or service-providers. Different decisions may therefore be taken for different reasons, with a variety of commitments and constraints inhibiting the freedom of manoeuvre in each particular case.

It is therefore not surprising that this discussion of the British experience has found no one mode of explanation capable of accounting for the pattern of public expenditure. But what our analysis does suggest is that the limitations of each mode of explanation largely reflect the fact that each is anchored in a particular definition of the relevant universe, when it is the interaction between the societal, political and governmental systems taken together that largely determines the outcome. Furthermore, the explanatory power of the various approaches is likely to vary, depending on whether the focus of analysis is on total public expenditure, on individual programmes or on still smaller categories. The problem then is not to decide which is the single most useful mode of explanation but how the various approaches should be fitted together. The British experience also suggests that the public expenditure should be seen not just as a measure of governmental activity but, in part, as the outcome of such activity: that regulatory activities by the State, like economic planning and incomes policy, may have political consequences that in turn generate spending.

To advance beyond these very general conclusions would require two developments. On the side of theory, it is clear that most of the modes of explanation need to be made more specific in terms of making explicit their assumptions about the relationship between causes and effects. Thus the structural-determinist approach begs the question of just what social, economic and demographic changes are supposed to affect public expenditure, and how. Similarly, the party competition approach offers no criteria that allow conclusions about when the competition is more or less intense. In neither case is it possible therefore to use these models to explain discontinuities in expenditure trends. On the side of practice, much work clearly requires to be done on public expenditure data, partly to distinguish those increases that are due to relative price movements from those that reflect rises in the volume of resources, and partly to break down the available information to the level of sub-programmes. Finally, linking theory and practice, there is a need to move towards a typology of public expenditure which would distinguish different programmes on a variety of criteria: economic, administrative and political – a theme that has emerged with particular clarity from this analysis of the British record, since it suggests that the policy reaction to a given policy cue may depend as much on the characteristics of particular types of expenditure as on other factors.

40

Universities in the Market Place

NEW UNIVERSITIES QUARTERLY
Summer 1979

One of the advantages of becoming a university professor in mid-career is that of retaining the capacity for being surprised by what life-long academics take for granted. The reflections of an academic innocent that follow, based on my first year's experience of the university world, are therefore an attempt to capitalize on this fast-fading ability to react with a sense of discovery and shock to a new environment.

Since becoming a university professor, I have been struck by the number of different roles I have to play. I teach. I research. I sit on committees. So far no surprises. But in addition, I have to be a commercial traveller and a public relations officer. If I want to develop a research programme, I have to go out and sell the ideas: actually doing research is both fun and easy – the real sweat and tiresome toil lies in raising funds. If I want to attract students, I have to spread the message in the world at large: again, trying to develop interesting courses is stimulating, while the real drudgery lies in trying to make sure that potential students are actually aware of what is on offer. In all this, I am of course in no way exceptional. But the discovery came as something of a cultural shock, since I was brought up as a student in an era, an institution and a discipline where the academic ideal (and to a large extent the reality) was that of the solitary scholar quietly getting on with his work, needing no more than a well-equipped library by way of back-up facilities

This suggests that we need to replace the traditional collegial model of the university teacher as a detached, gentlemanly scholar by one which recognizes his increasing role as an entrepreneur: that we need to develop a political economy model of academia. The university world is becoming increasingly like the competitive, individualistic market economy of early capitalism described by Marx and other nineteenth-century observers. The campus, as Jacques Barzun has observed,[1] has moved into the market; and although his remark was made about American universities, it also applies to the British scene. Individual academics compete with each other for prestige, and the promotion or resources that go with prestige. University departments compete with each other, again for both prestige and resources. The competition goes on both within and between universities. Finally, and perhaps most important, the universities collectively must compete for public funds against a multitude of other claims within the framework of the annual public expenditure allocation exercise. The parallel with the early nineteenth-century market economy of small entrepreneurial firms fiercely competing with each other is not, of course, complete. There is no academic equivalent of bankruptcy; unsuccessful universities are not closed down, though unsuccessful departments may shrink into invisibility. So competition is tempered by the knowledge that even the unfittest will somehow survive.

In stressing the role of the academic as an entrepreneur – in drawing a picture of the university world as the last refuge of genuine competition in an increasingly planned economy – I am, of course, deliberately exaggerating. Many of my colleagues would not recognize the picture I have drawn of them – and would indeed recoil in horror from it. However, my caricature may help to draw attention to future tensions and problems. For the forces which have helped to create the present situation – which are transforming the ivory tower into the competitive firm – are likely to grow in strength.

First of all, British universities taken as a whole are no longer a small collection of elite institutions. They cannot command deference by virtue of scarcity. Moreover, in some important respects, their collective monopoly has been broken. They cannot claim to be unique in terms of either research or teaching (though they may still hope to show that they continue to be unique in their ability to combine the two). Other institutions, e.g. the polytechnics, provide courses which may be very like those in universities. Research goes on in independent institutes and in industry. The days when all the Vice-Chancellors could squeeze into a taxi-cab have gone; nowadays, a fleet of charabancs would be needed to accommodate them all. In all these respects, there has been a transformation over the past 30 or so years: oligopoly has been turned into competitive pluralism – though, as so often, the accepted mythology, so powerful in shaping attitudes, continues to lag behind the reality.

---

[1]Jacques Barzun, *The American University*, 1969.

One reason why recognition of the new reality has been so slow is that until the last few years, the competition has been taking place in an exceptionally benevolent climate. The economy – even the British economy – was expanding. Within an expanding economy, furthermore, the proportion devoted to public expenditure was growing. More money for the universities did not, therefore, necessarily mean less money for other, competing programmes. Within the universities, everybody could expect to get something extra in an expanding market. Moreover, the prevailing conventional wisdom was exceptionally favourable to higher education. For the universities (among other institutions of higher education) were the beneficiaries of economic growth largely because they were seen as the key to still higher growth rates. Even though the Robbins Report carefully avoided basing its arguments for expansion on such narrowly utilitarian grounds, it is clear that investment in higher education was widely seen as part of the process of modernizing Britain.

In turn, all three of the props supporting an expanding higher education programme have been knocked down. First, Britain's economic growth rate has slumped. Second, the Government's policy is to reduce the proportion of the national income devoted to public expenditure. Third, scepticism about the contribution of higher education to economic growth has increased. This is most obviously so in the case of those subjects which, like the Humanities or Social Sciences, appear to have no direct contribution to make to industrial performance. But there is also a growing awareness that even in areas like technology – where research and training would appear to have a directly relevant role – the relationship between investment in the universities and economic growth is a complex one: that a great deal depends on the general economic climate, the social structure and attitudes in industry. In turn this might suggest that those disciplines which deal with the social and economic environment within which science and technology operate may be more relevant and perhaps even directly useful than is usually assumed.

In this new and much chillier climate, the always present undertow of suspicion towards academics has tended to surface. Expansion of the higher education sector has robbed it of its protective mystique; professors are two a penny; academics as a body tend to be regarded increasingly in much the same way as clergymen in an age of agnosticism. Nor do the bad news for the universities end there. Even the birth rate is conspiring against them; as we all know, universities will be fishing from a shrinking pool of eligible young men and women in the 'eighties. And although there are in theory plenty of policy options for taking up any slack – such as increasing the proportion of the relevant age group in higher education or expanding postgraduate education – it cannot be assumed that, given current economic trends and attitudes, these will necessarily be adopted. Further, we cannot even be certain that such policies – if adopted – would work. There are already signs that universities may be losing some of their attraction, at least for those who see a university education in straight cost-benefit terms for themselves. Some American studies have suggested that the return – in the shape of increased life-time income – of a university degree is dwindling.[2] Moreover producing an expanding number of graduates for what may be a contracting or stationery number of public sector jobs could be a formula for manufacturing social frustration and discontent.

In any case, there is an alternative option: to cut back the resources allocated to the higher education sector. And if that were adopted, my comparison with the nineteenth-century world of cut-throat business would be complete; some institutions of higher education might follow the way of teacher training colleges, and we would have the institutional equivalent of bankruptcy. In the United States, perhaps ominously, there is growing interest in the academic study of what is called 'policy termination' – i.e. the study of how, and in what circumstances, it is possible to liquidate existing commitments.

Conceivably this is too pessimistic a picture. Using a different palette, it would be possible to paint a Renoir rather than a Rembrandt canvas; all glowing, optimistic colours. The optimistic picture might take the following form: assume a society which no longer puts such a high value on economic growth, and assume also that such a society (whether of choice or of necessity) puts the emphasis on educating people for leisure and removing them from the labour market in order to reduce the unemployment figures. In such circumstances, it would be possible to imagine yet another golden age of expansion for the universities. From being the instruments of growth, they could become part of a programme of consolation or compensation for non-growth. Creating more places in higher education may, after all, be cheaper than creating jobs – particularly in the case of arts, humanities and social studies, where there is no need for expensive equipment.

Futurology is a dangerous sport, a landscape littered with the broken reputations of those who have embarked on the Cresta run of prediction in the past. It would therefore be rash of me to make a dogmatic choice as between the Rembrandt (or pessimistic) and the Renoir (or optimistic) canvasses. However, the odds seem to be stacked against optimism. Assuming that the dominant social and political problem of the 'eighties will be a continuing high level of unemployment – an assumption which

---

[2]R. Freeman, 'Overinvestment in College Training?' *Journal of Human Resources*, vol. 10, pp. 212–31, 1975.

seems all too plausible – then it seems unlikely that the universities will benefit from such a situation. On the contrary, such a social development may increase the pressures – already evident – for what might be called 'de-professionalization'. In other words, there may be a growing demand to substitute a lot of (fairly) cheap unskilled labour for (relatively) expensive skilled labour; for having fewer doctors, fewer teachers and fewer social workers, and more nurses, more teachers' aides and more child minders. If this new social division of labour were to materialize, there would still be a need to train the extra staff – but very little case for providing them with a university education.

So, overall, it seems sensible to investigate further the metaphor of the university world as a market in which the competition for both students and research funds is likely to become, if anything, more sharp still. First, what strategies are available to the universities to reduce the damaging effects of such competition? Second, what is the currency of the competition; what, in other words, are the criteria used in defining success or failure in this particular, and very peculiar, market?

Starting with the strategies available for reducing the damaging effects of competition, it is worth developing the example of the market economy in the nineteenth century. One strategy might be to open up new markets abroad; to find an academic equivalent of the African continent, where the Victorian explorers opened the way for the Victorian exporters. British academic labour is cheap; the product appears to be attractive. Even if British industry is no longer very successful at exporting goods, we may still therefore be able to import paying students. To an extent, this is happening already: the question is whether it will be able to survive as a viable long-term strategy in the face of increasingly stiff competition from other countries, such as the United States (where universities rival with each other for organizing special courses for Arabs from the oil-rich countries). Perhaps the Government will have to recognize that the universities – like the hotel trade and other service industries – can be an important source of foreign currency earnings, and give them equivalent financial incentives and subsidies.

The other way of reducing the impact of competition is what is known, euphemistically as 'rationalization'. In other words, competition can be reduced by limiting the numbers of units engaged in it. In the case of industry, mergers produce fewer but bigger firms: the small entrepreneur disappears and is replaced by the ICIs and Unilevers of this world. In the case of universities (to pursue the parallel) the equivalent development would be for university departments to be amalgamated, so that particular subjects would increasingly be offered by only a handful of institutions in the country instead of being widely available. Given such a strategy, the University Grants Committee – which at present can only exercise birth-control over new developments – might also acquire powers of euthanasia. Indeed it might emerge in the kind of role played by the various Boards that have been set up to rationalize declining industries like cotton or shipbuilding. Given the expense involved in such exercises, this may not be an altogether attractive prospect for Governments – even leaving side the unpalatable implications for the universities themselves. Even the traumas of competition may be preferable to such forced marriages.

This brings me to my second question: the nature of the competition in the university market. So far I have only referred to the fierce individualism of academics and the competition for prestige and resources. Now let me try to put some flesh on this metaphor, to examine what I have called the 'currency' of competition. Specifically, and rather selectively, I propose to look at three aspects of this competition: (1) the competition between academics as individuals, (2) the competition between academic departments within universities and (3) the competition for students between universities.

The Competition Between Individual Academics

Assuming that the universities are not going to expand, it seems reasonable to predict also that competition among academics will intensify. The point is obvious enough. The 'sixties saw a large increase in the numbers of recruits to the academic profession; the prospect of stagnation in the 'eighties means that promotion prospects are bleak. Admittedly, the incentives to seek promotion may not be so very great in all cases, given shrinking salary differentials. Still, even so it seems likely that competition will intensify, and that the currency of this competition will be research publications. For one of the oddities about the academic profession is the lack of any means for assessing teaching abilities. Of course it is possible to get some idea of a colleague's teaching capacity from students, whether indirectly through written examination work or directly by listening to what they have to say. But, for the most part, both what is taught – and how it is taught – remains something of a mystery; academic autonomy is too often translated to mean the academic's right to teach exactly what he or she wants. Indeed proposals for taking teaching abilities into account, such as those put forward by the Prices and Incomes Board in the 'sixties,[3] tend to be fiercely resisted.

If we cannot easily assess an academic's teaching capacity, it follows that we must inevitably place all the more emphasis on research publica-

---

[3]National Board for Prices and Incomes Report No. 98. *Standing Reference on the pay of University Teachers in Great Britain*, HMSO, 1968.

tions. Reinforcing this trend is another factor. If the Americans have always placed more emphasis on publication, this is not only because their academic system has always been more competitive. It is also because the sheer size of their higher education system makes it that much more difficult to rely on informal networks; the casual telephone conversation between professorial colleagues who trust each other's judgment. Something similar may be happening in this country. As the system has expanded, so it becomes less easy to rely on personal contacts – though British methods of appointment are still far more amateurish, and less stringent, than those used in the United States.

Let me speculate about the possible consequences of these trends. Traditionally, the British academic has placed at least as much emphasis on his teaching responsibilities as on his research. In the mid 'sixties, when Halsey and Trow carried out their survey of academics,[4] only just over a third of those interviewed saw research as their first duty. When the results of the latest survey carried out by Halsey become available, it would not be surprising to find that the emphasis on research has increased considerably. In terms of career prospects, there may be a temptation to see teaching as a diversion from the main task: research.

Without wishing to decry the importance of research and publication, it may be useful to explore some of the possibly undesirable side-effects of this form of competition. It is commonplace to talk about the explosion of knowledge. But this may often mean no more than – to follow Jacques Barzun again – the explosion of publications. The entrepreneurial academic has every incentive to serve up the same meal with different sauces: to re-use his material, slightly reworked perhaps, in a variety of contexts. It is depressingly frequent – as one reads through the various learned journals – to find slightly revamped versions of the same article popping up again and again. The strategy seems to be: if you have got nothing new to say, then say it in a new journal – hoping that you will also be addressing a new audience. The growth in the number of learned journals may thus be as much an index of the expanding need to multiply publications for career advancement as of expanding knowledge.

Again, the emphasis on research in the academic market tends to reinforce the tendency to specialize. It is, after all, easier to make a new contribution in a restricted field than (say) to reconceptualize the major issues in your discipline – although the latter may be intellectually more important as well as more difficult. In turn, specialization may affect teaching: all of us like to ride our own hobby horse. This tendency was already noted by the Robbins Report 15 years ago: 'In a period of rapidly

---

[4] A. M. Halsey and M. Trow, *The British Academics*, 1971.

changing knowledge there is undeniably a tendency to add new knowledge year by year to an already full curriculum. It is easier to add than to take away.'[5] For knowledge, read specialization – and the danger is apparent. It is that universities may increasingly turn out what the Robbins reported called 'mere specialists', instead of 'cultivated men and women' by concentrating on imparting knowledge or techniques rather than on enhancing the capacity to think.

In a world of scarce resources, where the universities collectively are competing with other institutions of higher education, the pressure to produce trained specialists rather than educated graduates may be considerable: trained specialists are far too often confused with 'relevance'. But if universities give in to such market forces, the long-term effect may well be to weaken their competitive position – since they will no longer be able to claim that they are making a unique contribution in terms of a unique product.

The Competition Between University Departments

The competition for resources between departments in the same university is very much like the competition between government departments. Anyone familiar with the battles over public expenditure allocations will find himself in familiar ground on looking at university budgeting. Any Vice-Chancellor reading, for example, Lord Diamond's book on public expenditure[6] – reflecting his experiences as Chief Secretary to the Treasury – would find his own dilemmas mirrored there; the main difference being that he has to deal with insistent professors rather than insistent Ministers. For in both cases, there are no 'rational', self-evidently objective, criteria for deciding to spend more on education rather than health (in the case of public expenditure), physics rather than chemistry (in the case of university budgets). In both cases we are talking about values, attitudes and therefore politics. It is extraordinarily difficult, perhaps impossible, to measure need, efficiency or output.

Still, decisions have to be made – and rationalized. They are all the more difficult since the choice is (nearly always) not between the deserving and the undeserving but between various worthy, and much cherished, schemes. Moreover, just as Ministers are assessed by their civil servants in terms of their success in extracting money from the Treasury, so professors are assessed by their colleagues in terms of their success in extracting resources from the University funds.

---

[5]Committee on Higher Education, *Report*, p. 89, HMSO, 1973. Cmnd. 2.54.
[6]Lord Diamond, *Public Expenditure in Practice*, 1975.

How, in these difficult circumstances, can decisions about priorities be taken? How can the relative 'needs' of different departments be measured? What is the equivalent of the annual 'profit' for an academic firm – i.e. the department? Here there would appear to be a number of what might be called pseudo-currencies: market prestige (as measured by the capacity to attract research funds), productivity (as measured by the number of publications) and consumer demand (as measured by the attractiveness to students). The use of such pseudo-currencies of assessment is probably inevitable – and perhaps preferable to the use of some other possible criteria (e.g. will Professor X resign and decamp to the United States if he isn't given an extra post) – but there are obvious difficulties and dangers about their use.

Market prestige. The standing of business firms is largely measured by their appeal to the capital market. How sensible is it to measure the standing of academic firms by their appeal to the research market? Here there are a number of problems. The amount of money attracted may measure (a) the fact that particular kinds of research are very expensive, or (b) the fact that a particular research field is currently fashionable and so can draw on ample sources of funds, rather than the fact that a department has an exceptionally high standing in the market. The point can be simply illustrated. In the current financial year[7] the Science Research Council has a budget of £146 million, while the Social Science Research Council has a budget of £16 million. This reflects both Governmental priorities as between science and social science research, and the differences in the cost of carrying out these two activities. Fair enough. But it does mean that, in measuring the relative 'market prestige' of science and social science departments, universities should perhaps multiply the income of the latter by a factor of nine.

There is a further complication, however, which stems from the difficulty of balancing measures of quantity against measures of quality. The theoretical economist or physicist may need no more than a blackboard by way of equipment, while carrying out a survey or an experiment will be expensive. So obviously competition in terms of the size of research funds obtained could have undesirable, distorting effects. Hence the need to have other invitations to foreign universities (an exercise which, again, may be somewhat problematic; how does one weight one invitation to lecture at Harvard, say, against six lectures at Mid-Western Liberal Arts Colleges?).

Productivity. The danger of assessing individual performance by totting up the number of publications has already been discussed. The same

---

[7]*The Government's Expenditure Plans 1979–80 to 1982–83*, p. 134, HMSO, 1979. Cmnd. 7439.

point applies in the case of departments, only more so. For qualitative judgments are that much more difficult to make across disciplines. I am perfectly capable of counting the number of publications by my colleagues in, say, engineering or pharmacy. Unfortunately, I am totally incapable of making any sort of informed assessment of their quality. And the same applies, of course, in reverse. The effects of competition by numbers can have ludicrous consequences. For example, one academic institution includes obituaries among the list of the publications by its staff. The moral of that seems to be that if you want to enhance your productivity, choose a field of research where there is a high mortality rate among your peers.

Consumer demand. This, on the face of it, might seem to be the easiest – and most sensible – criterion to apply. If there is a falling student demand for places in the courses offered by department A, while demand for places in department B is clearly buoyant, then it would be eminently reasonable to allocate resources accordingly. But this again raises problems.

If student demand is measured simply in numbers – e.g. the numbers putting a particular department first in their list of choices – this raises the problem of how sensible it is to extrapolate from what may be a short-term trend. Fashions in student preferences may change rapidly. Lecturers, once appointed, tend to remain for ever. The co-existence of volatile consumer preferences and the comparative immobility of the academic profession creates a very real difficulty for future planning. Imagine a fashion industry where some of the producers insisted that they had been trained to make crinolines, that their exclusive skill lay in making crinolines and that they would go on making crinolines. One way of trying to resolve this dilemma is by putting the emphasis on the quality, rather than the quantity, of the students applying for places. But again there are reasons for scepticism – particularly about our capacity to assess the various dimensions of ability adequately on the basis of the information available. 'A' level results certainly measure achievement; but to what extent do they also measure potential? So a competition whose currency is 'A' level scores may ultimately have distorting effects.

The Competition Between Universities

The competition between universities largely takes the shape of competition for students: the number of first-choice applications per place becomes a kind of indicator of popularity, to be deployed in the battle for resources. Once more the metaphor of the market seems appropriate, since this appears to suggest a trend towards consumer sovereignty – perhaps the single most important development of the 'seventies.

What I mean by invoking the phrase of 'consumer sovereignty' is that – at the risk of some exaggeration and to an extent anticipating events – there has been a remarkable change in the relative power of universities and students. This shift has nothing to do with student participation in the administration of universities. It is not the product of student militancy, either. But it does reflect a change in the market situation. It is not the right of students to be represented in Senate, but their position in the market which matters. The relationship between the supply and demand for university places is altering for a variety of complex reasons, some of which have already been touched on: the availability of other, alternative institutions of higher education, the increasing scepticism of the young about the usefulness of a university degree as a passport to well-paid employment, and so on. The changes are by no means uniform across university disciplines or courses. The underlying trends may, quite possibly, be affected by future social and economic development. Still, it does not seem unreasonable to assert that the balance between producers and consumers has shifted decisively and permanently to the latter – and that the movement may well be accentuated in the 'eighties when the size of the relevant age cohort shrinks. Even if the universities do not as yet have to compete to fill their places, they certainly have to compete already to attract the ablest students (however defined).

Clearly in such a competition, universities will vary a great deal in the strategies they adopt. Some, able to draw on an accumulated capital of prestige and exceptional physical resources, may not feel any need to compete overtly at all. Perhaps Oxford and Cambridge fall into this category. History has distributed its favours both capriciously and arbitrarily – and so, it is tempting to add, has the UGC which has tended to perpetuate inequalities. (Indeed there seems to be a surprising contrast between the National Health Service and other social services, where there has been such a strong emphasis on redistributing resources more equitably on clearly defined principles, and the opaque situation in the university world where it is far from clear on what principles funds are shared out). Universities inevitably vary a great deal in their market appeal, and in what they can hope to offer to the consumer.

But there does seem to be one general trend, and a welcome one at that. The dawning realization that universities are in a competitive market situation for students is leading to a far greater degree of diffusion of information. In another context, it would indeed be tempting to talk about advertising. Universities are beginning – if only very diffidently – to see the importance of producing information about their products to potential students, by way of brochures and so on. It is, so far, only a very tentative start. Universities appear to know surprisingly little about the precise processes by which students choose their universities; the relative importance of information diffused by the institutions themselves, the advice of careers masters and feed-back from other students. Yet the logic of present developments is, surely, to carry out market research about the consumers, their sources of information and the factors that influence their choices. This may seem like vulgar commercialism, but since the universities are already competing it would seem more sensible to do so on the basic of well-researched studies rather than on the basis of hunch and guesswork. Consumerism is here to stay: witness the development of the academic equivalent of the Consumers' Association and its magazine *Which* – the anti-prospectuses produced by the students themselves which some universities are now distributing alongside their own, official prospectus.

On balance this is probably a welcome development. It is, after all, in everybody's interest that students should make an informed choice of university rather than complaining subsequently that they didn't really know what goods they were buying. However, there are also obvious dangers. Again, there is the recurring question of the currency of the competition. In theory, everyone would probably claim that the competition should be in terms of the quality of the education offered. In practice, things could turn out rather differently. Again, leaning on the model of the market, it is possible to suggest alternative – and much less acceptable – strategies. Competition could be in terms of product differentiation: the equivalent of producing toasters which also play a tune – i.e. offering new kinds of degrees which combine a variety of different features (which may, of course, sometimes be perfectly sensible). Similarly, competition could be in terms of offering special inducements: the equivalent of offering free rail passes with corn flake packages – i.e. universities might concentrate on advertising various amenities which are not directly relevant to the quality of the education offered. Perhaps most ominously, competition might take the form of price cutting. By this I do not mean competitive fee cutting but rather lowering the price required from students – in terms of their investment of time and energy – in acquiring their degrees.

Lastly, there is the possibility that increased competition between the universities, in a situation of declining student numbers and perhaps declining resources also, may lead to a greater differentiation both in products and in their roles. At present, the assumption is that all universities have the same status and the same role. But, returning to the metaphor of the market, this is like arguing that British Leyland and Rolls-Royce are no different since they both produce cars. In other words, increased competition might force some universities to try to appeal to a particular sector of the market. If their appeal is not high enough (for whatever reason) to attract sufficient students in competition with more prestigious or better-endowed universities, it might still be sufficient to attract students in competition with nonuniversity institutions of higher education. So, as in America, there might be a differentiation between large civic universities and liberal arts colleges with no pretensions about doing research or post-graduate programmes.

All this may, at present, seem rather unlikely. Universities, it may be argued, are not commercial firms. Their behaviour follows different norms. The metaphor of the market leads to implausible conclusions. However, the point of my analysis has been to suggest that there may be tensions between the traditional norms of universities and the market situation in which they increasingly find themselves. The academic as entrepreneur may be tempted to forget his role as the guardian of standards, whose responsibility is not to please but to educate consumers. If in the past this role was too often associated with an arrogant indifference to the needs of society, perhaps now the time has come to recognize explicitly the dangers of an over-anxious responsiveness to volatile market forces.

In any case, an analysis of the universities as a market system must take account of the institutional rigidities: of the factors which inhibit adjustment in the face of competitive pressures. Some of these have already been mentioned: in particular, the fact that universities (in contrast to commercial firms) do not go into liquidation. But there is a further, perhaps more important, source of rigidity. For the paradox is that precisely the same forces that make the competition more fierce may also make it more difficult for the universities to react flexibly. Given a stagnant future, in terms of total resources, the temptation is for everyone to entrench themselves. Promotion may be difficult to get; the incentives to move sideways to another job may be negative (particularly since British universities have so far, in contrast to their American counterparts, resisted the full logic of competition and do not on the whole compete in terms of the salaries they offer). The danger of institutional sclerosis may therefore be no less real than the danger of over-responsiveness to market forces.

Once again, the issue needs to be placed within a wide societal context. Just as the reasons why the universities face a future of increased competition for resources and students largely derive from the overall performance of the economy, so any attempt to tackle the problem of institutional sclerosis must range beyond the world of academia. From time to time, the case for encouraging greater mobility among university staff is argued. Why should lecturers be appointed to permanent posts in their early or mid-twenties? Why, come to that, should appointment to a university professorship be considered a life sentence? So far such arguments, persuasive though they are, have had little practical effect.

The reason is obvious enough: in a society where the trend is towards less mobility, where more and more occupations have effectively achieved security of tenure, it is unreasonable to expect any one profession to carry the risks of moving in the opposite direction.

This would suggest that the universities should be strongly pressing the case for greater flexibility throughout British society. Indeed their problems of institutional rigidity, and occupational immobility, are a paradigm of the larger problems faced by Britain. And they are only likely to be solved if there is an acceptance of the need to introduce more opportunities for movement and exchange of staff in the civil service, in the health and social services and in industry, as well as in the universities. Given a general acceptance of the need to promote such movement – as a substitute for the opportunities created by economic growth – it would then be possible not only for academics to move into other occupations, but for the universities to recruit more widely; to have a fluid mixture of part-time, short-term and permanent staff.

Such a development would at least be a positive reaction to the economic and social trends which are at the root of the difficulties faced by the universities. The emergence of the academic entrepreneur, acting in a competitive market situation, has its problems and dangers, some of which this paper has sought to analyse. But ironically the fact that the universities are, in a sense, the last refuge of the Protestant work ethic may mean that they have a greater contribution to make to British society at large whose poor economic performance may, in part at least, mirror the decline of competitive individualism and the rise of institutional rigidity.

41

The Welfare State:
A Self-Inflicted Crisis?

POLITICAL QUARTERLY
January–March 1980

If I had sat down to write this article 20 or even 10 years ago, and taken as my theme the development of Britain's Welfare State, the result would almost certainly have been the celebration of a national achievement. Naturally I would have qualified my enthusiasm with a few criticisms, but I do not think that I would have had any fundamental doubts about the appropriateness of the underlying structure and policies. Today, it seems mildly eccentric to suggest even two cheers for the Welfare State. Its natural allies on the Left have made an industry of analysing its shortcomings: in particular, there is disillusion because poverty, far from having been eradicated, appears to be as prevalent as ever. Its natural critics on the Right are in the ascendant: there is widespread acceptance of the argument that welfare spending is parasitic on the economy, threatening the prospects of resumed growth. This assumption is not only embodied in the public expenditure policies of the present Conservative Administration but was already reflected in those of the previous Labour Government.

One possible reaction to both the disillusionment and the criticism is to point out that much of it is exaggerated or misplaced. The National Health Service may indeed be shabby and threadbare by the standards of many advanced industrial countries. But, then, Britain is a poor nation by the standards of these same countries, and it is hardly surprising that her public services mirror this fact; additionally, it can be argued that the NHS remains the best instrument yet devised for rationing inadequate resources equitably. Poverty, as it was defined in absolute terms when the Welfare State was created in the post-war era, has virtually disappeared.[1] When people lament the persistence of poverty, they are mostly talking about the persistence of inequalities in incomes – an equally important, but very different, issue. Moreover, Britain devotes a smaller proportion of her national income to welfare expenditure than such successful and virtuous economies as Germany, Sweden and the Netherlands.[2] So there is clearly no simple, causal link between high welfare spending and poor economic performance.

The case for the defence is therefore strong. But proclaiming the very real achievements of the Welfare State is not necessarily enlightening in trying to think about the future evolution of policy. Nor does it really help, in the present climate of opinion, to produce a shopping list of things that ought to be done to remedy the gaps in welfare provision. My purpose in this article is therefore to try to tease out the reasons for the disillusion and criticism: to identify the likely constraints on social policy in the coming decade. In doing so, I shall suggest that the disillusion of the Left is largely self-inflicted: it rests on an inadequate analysis of the political and economic framework of social policy. Similarly, I will try to show that the criticisms of the Right, while based on a more realistic assessment of the political and economic framework, contain some wrong-headed assumptions.

The Politics of Social Policy

Social policy is about coercion. Its very essence lies in compelling people to do what they would otherwise not do, either for their own good or for what is conceived to be the good of society as a whole. Thus people may be compelled to go to prison or to mental hospital. More centrally to my argument, social policy involves parting people from their money through the tax system. If we are interested in the Welfare State, we are therefore necessarily concerned about the political and economic factors which either facilitate or hinder the use of coercion by the State.

In the context of a debate about the role of the State, this might seem a fairly trite remark. In the context of the British debate about social policy over the past decades, however, it is likely to raise some eyebrows. For the British tradition of social policy has been conspicuously strong on prescription but short on any theory of power: significantly one of

[1]G. C. Fiegehen, P. S. Lansley and A. D. Smith, *Poverty and Progress in Britain 1953–1973* (Cambridge University Press, Cambridge, 1977).
[2]OECD, *Public Expenditure Trends* (OECD, Paris, 1978).

Richard Titmuss's most popular books[3] was devoted to the central role of altruism in social policy. Yet a framework of State coercion may well be a necessary condition for encouraging altruism: even if we are altruistically inclined, even if we are ready to see a part of our income transferred to the elderly, the disabled and the sick, we are more likely to do so if we know that others will not be "free riders" – exploiting our good impulses by not contributing. In other words, altruism may grease the wheels of social policy but it is no substitute for a machinery of coercion.

It is the failure to appreciate this simple but central point which explains, I think, the widespread disillusion with the achievements of the Welfare State. Let me illustrate this by looking at the debate about poverty. As already pointed out, this is a debate essentially about inequalities of income (and opportunity). But as soon as we define it in these terms, it becomes apparent that when we ask why inequalities have persisted so stubbornly, we are asking why it is politically so difficult to re-distribute income: a question not about the design of specific social policies but about the political feasibility of achieving certain policy aims.

In defining the problem in this way, I am of course echoing the Marxists.[4] Their analysis is simple: given the inequalities in the distribution of power within a capitalist society, it follows that inequalities of income will be perpetuated. But while I share their "political economy" approach to the analysis of the Welfare State, I draw very different conclusions. The paradox of the modern Welfare State, I would argue, is that it has become more difficult to make any further progress in achieving a more equal distribution of income precisely because both power and income have become more diffused: indeed if Britain were still a classic "capitalist" society, the task would be very much easier. Putting the same point more forcibly still, I would argue that the successful redistribution of power and income in itself creates the strongest impediment to further progress; and that it is precisely this fact which explains why not only Britain but other advanced industrial societies (Communist as well as capitalist) have found it so difficult to change the pattern in recent decades.

For, looking at the long-term evolution of income distribution, a seemingly odd phenomenon is noticeable. This is that the major shifts in income distribution took place *before* the major expansion of the Welfare

---

[3]Richard M. Titmuss, *The Gift Relationship* (George Allen & Unwin, London, 1970). For a highly relevant discussion, see also David Collard, *Altruism and Economy* (Martin Robertson, London, 1978).

[4]For the best Marxist analysis, see Ian Gough, *The Political Economy of the Welfare State* (Macmillan, London, 1979).

State in Britain and elsewhere: over the past two decades rising welfare expenditure has failed to make much of a dent on the pattern of income inequalities. But this seemingly puzzling and perverse phenomenon makes a great deal of sense if we examine the politics of income distribution.

The distribution of incomes is, as is well known, diamond shaped. That is the bulk of incomes is concentrated around the middle. The implication of this is that, as Welfare States expand, it becomes progressively difficult to finance extra expenditure by soaking the rich. It is easy enough to finance the first steps towards the Welfare State by increasing taxes on the well-to-do (however defined). But such a policy becomes progressively less feasible in a mature Welfare State. Similarly, in the early days of a Welfare State the benefits of spending tend to be concentrated selectively on the very poorest at the bottom of the diamond: a considerable income distribution impact can thus be achieved at a relatively low cost. But as the Welfare State becomes more universalised, so the cost of changing the distribution of income becomes higher. The paradox of the mature Welfare State is therefore that more people have to be coerced into paying higher taxes in order to make what will be inevitably less of an impact on the distribution of incomes. Hence the well-known downward creep of taxation: as public expenditure rises as a proportion of national income, so increasingly average and even below average wage-earners are drawn into the tax network.

At the same time, the task of coercion becomes more difficult. For when public expenditure starts to nudge up towards 50 per cent. of the national income (and when a high proportion of that expenditure is devoted to welfare policies in their widest sense), it is inevitable that Governments will come face to face with those organised interests in society whose members have to foot the bill: the trade unions. If income redistribution is difficult, it is not so much because we live in a capitalist society but because we live in a society with powerful trade unions – precisely because, to return to my earlier assertion, power is diffused.

The Collapse of the Social Contract

The point is illustrated by the experience of the Labour Government between 1974 and 1979. The Labour Government came to office committed to expanding the Welfare State and in fact did so by increasing pensions and taking other measures designed to change the redistribution of income in favour of the least-favoured sections of the population. The concept of the "social wage" (or "social contract") was invented to justify such an approach: the idea that trade unionists would restrain their wage demands in return for improved welfare benefits and social services.

The policy, as we all know, collapsed in ruins – as did attempts to introduce similar policies in Norway, Sweden and the Netherlands. The unions insisted on maintaining their net-of-tax take-home-pay. The Government was forced to reverse its policies, and to offer tax *cuts* (which, in turn, implied expenditure reductions) in return for wage restraint. The "social wage" was not, in other words, perceived by union members as equivalent to money in their own pockets: they voted, in their wage bargaining, against a policy of redistribution to the elderly and others via the State. Further, they also voted, by their tactics, against the redistribution of income within the trade union ranks themselves: they fought to maintain traditional relativities as between different occupations, as had the miners in 1974. Attempts to change the distribution of income are, it seems, seen as threatening by a majority of the people – and, most importantly, by the best organised sections of the population. The rhetoric of soaking the rich does not persuade those who would really have to finance the expansion of the Welfare State, *i.e.* the unions, to pay up their inevitable share. As the results of the 1979 General Election showed, the backlash phenomenon is not limited to the middle classes.

One long-term implication of this is that those who are concerned about the future of the Welfare State should also be concerned about Britain's trade union movement. For there would appear to be two necessary conditions for even attempting to pursue a "social wage" strategy. First, there has to be a central trade union body capable of getting the agreement of all the member organisations. Secondly, within each union, the leadership must be able to carry its rank and file within it. In other words, there has to be both the organisational capacity and the leadership ability required to translate official commitment to such an approach into the bargaining arena. In the years after 1974, the Trades Union Congress made the commitment – but was unable to deliver the goods. And the Labour Government, consequently, came unstuck. Unless there are fundamental changes in the nature of Britain's trade-union movement, there would seem to be little point in repeating the experiment of trying to solve the problem of financing higher welfare spending with the help of the TUC.

There is a further reason why those concerned about the problems of the mature Welfare State ought to be preoccupied with the role of the trade unions. The Welfare State is more than a metaphor. It is a set of institutions employing a large number of people: the NHS alone employs some 1,000,000 men and women. The Welfare State provides welfare not only for its nominal beneficiaries but also for those who work for it. Increasing expenditure on the Welfare State cannot therefore automatically be equated with increasing the amount of welfare provided to society: the distinction between Welfare State and Welfare Society is crucial.[5] Rising spending may in part at least reflect the fact that, given the constituencies for the *status quo* represented by organised labour (whether the BMA or NUPE) it is extraordinarily difficult to liquidate existing, perhaps no longer relevant, commitments in order to meet new demands: that there is a built-in inertia, which means that all change tends to be additive. In short, organisational impediments to redistributing resources (whether geographically or by population groups) are built into the structure of the Welfare State.

All this underlines, I think, the inadequacy of what might be called the "moral" tradition of British social policy writing and thinking over the past few decades: it is a tradition which, by ignoring the political context of social policy, invites disillusion and a sense of betrayal. More dangerously, perhaps, the sense of betrayal can all too easily lead to a feeling that unless society as a whole is transformed, it will never be possible to pursue the ideal social policy. This, of course, is perfectly true in the trivial sense that in utopia it is possible to pursue utopian policy. But in practice the demands for fundamental change in the political and economic structure are often another way of saying that if the State's coercive powers were to be strengthened it would be easier to compel people (whether trade unionists or capitalists) to do what the moralists believe ought to be done. In thinking about the future evolution of social policy, it may therefore be more sensible to analyse further what might be called the "enabling conditions" which have allowed the Welfare State to expand over the past 30 years.

Dividends of Economic Growth

The Welfare State is the residual beneficiary of the Growth State.[6] If there has been a steady expansion in both services and cash benefits, until recently, the reason is simple. Economic growth made it possible to finance improvements in the Welfare State while also permitting private consumption to increase: the dividends of economic growth could be shared out among various competing societal aims in an exercise from which everyone emerged as a winner – so easing the problem of coercion. The most successful Welfare States – such as Sweden's and Germany's

---

[5]William A. Robson, *Welfare State and Welfare Society* (George Allen & Unwin, London, 1976).

[6]For an earlier elaboration of this point, see Rudolf Klein, *Inflation and Priorities* (Centre for Studies in Social Policy, London, 1975), p. 1.

– tended to develop precisely in those countries with the best growth record, while Britain predictably began to discover that her social services and provision were falling behind those of other nations, in line with her economic performance. It is only in the last few years of worldwide stagflation that financing the Welfare State has become, particularly in no-growth economies like Britain's, a zero sum game. The need for political coercion, through the tax system, inevitably rises as economic growth declines.

Again, all this is reasonably self-evident.[7] Yet this very obvious insight has been massively neglected in the debate about social policy, except by the Right-wing critics of the Welfare State. Caricaturing only slightly, the industrial system has been seen as parasitical on the Welfare State by the Left while the Welfare State has been seen as parasitical on the industrial system by the Right. Specifically, the Left – and the central tradition of social policy thinking which found its inspiration in the works of Titmuss – tended to stress the damaging side-effects of economic growth: the fact that the Welfare State had to cope with the social disloca-tion, ill-health and the casualties generated by the industrial system. The Right, in contrast, tended to see the Welfare State as a burden on the industrial system: undermining incentives (whether directly through high social benefits or indirectly through taxation), weakening the work ethos and discouraging self-help.

It is difficult to avoid the conclusion that, in this debate, the Right at least asked the right questions – although, as I shall argue, it reached the wrong conclusions. Of course, the process of economic growth imposes considerable costs on society, for which the Welfare State often has to pick up the bill. This is why an increase in the GNP does not necessarily indicate an equivalent increase in national well-being: ironically, the costs of dealing with the disbenefits of economic growth may themselves help to swell the total national income. But assuming that economic growth has made at least some real improvements in welfare possible – such as higher living standards for old-age pensioners – it follows that those concerned about the Welfare State should also be concerned about its relationship with the industrial system in a positive sense: that they should be asking themselves to what extent social policies can contribute to economic growth.

In practice, social policies are largely and inevitably shaped by eco-nomic considerations. The principle of lesser eligibility – *i.e.* that those

---

[7]For a cross-national discussion of the relationship between public expenditure and taxation, see Richard Rose and Guy Peters, *Can Government Go Bankrupt?* (Macmillan, London, 1978).

receiving public support should be treated less generously than those in work – remains central to social policy, even though the 1834 Poor Law report is held out as an example of the heartless excesses of *laissez-faire* principles in most textbooks. The preoccupation with maintaining work incentives still dominates thinking about social policy, even though we have realised that the level of taxes may be as crucial as the level of benefits. Much of Welfare State expenditure also reflects direct economic priorities: for example, spending on education is often explicitly justified on the ground that Britain needs a well-trained labour force.

Unfortunately, those who perceive the Welfare State as an instrument of social justice above everything else find it difficult to proclaim the case for investment in social policy on grounds of economic and political expediency. The field therefore tends to be left wide open to those on the Right who argue that Welfare State spending is parasitical on the economy: a case which appears to have been largely accepted by the present Conservative Government.

Central to the case against Welfare State spending is the argument – put forward by Robert Bacon and Walter Eltis in one of the most influential books published in the last decade[8] – that the social services suck up the labour which would otherwise swell Britain's productive capacity. If Britain's economic performance has been poor, so runs the argument, it is because too many workers have been drawn into the "unproductive" public sector. This line of reasoning is based on some questionable figures and dubious assumptions. It is perfectly true that the numbers employed in the public sector have shot up sharply: but the figures usually given do not allow for the fact that many of those working in the public sector are part-time women – for whom the choice is often not between employment in the public sector and in the "productive" sector, but between employment in the public sector and staying at home. More crucially, perhaps, the assertion that the social services are "unproductive" needs to be challenged: as already argued, much of social expenditure can and should be seen as a necessary condition for maintaining the performance of the economy.

Further, the Bacon and Eltis type of reasoning confuses two quite different arguments. There is the argument that particular *kinds* of service are unproductive: in which case, they represent a waste of national resources, whether provided in the public or the private sector – yet those who support this line of reasoning rarely criticise the provision of social services (*e.g.* health) in the private sector. Alternatively, the services

---

[8]Robert Bacon and Walter Eltis, *Britain's Economic Problem: Too Few Producers* (Macmillan, London, 1976).

may be viewed as desirable in themselves, but it can be argued that problems of economic management may be caused by the difficulties of financing them in the public sector through taxation: a point which has more substance but which leads to the conclusion that such "unproductive" services actually ought to be encouraged, but within the private sector.

Lastly, it is worth stressing that the growth of the Welfare State manpower can – rather more plausibly – be seen as an attempt to fill the vacuum left by the failure of British industry. British industry is in trouble not because the State taxes away its profits in order to finance the Welfare State but because of its failure to make enough profits in the first place.[9] The Welfare State can therefore be seen as an essential instrument for making the consequences of economic decline socially and politically acceptable. The paradox would seem to be that it is the development of the Welfare State which has made it possible for successive Governments – Labour as well as Conservative – to pursue economic policies which, until recently, would have been seen as threatening to the entire social and political order.

A two-fold conclusion would seem to follow if this analysis is accepted. First, the role of the Welfare State in promoting economic growth should be recognised more explicitly when discussing specific policies: which might, for instance, suggest that more emphasis requires to be placed on encouraging mobility in housing policy (particularly local authority housing) and that the possibility of using NHS resources to give priority to active members of the labour force should be considered (which might be more sensible than protesting about the growth of the private sector, which fulfils precisely this function). Secondly, and more generally, it should not be left to the Right to stress the relationship between social and economic policies: here there would surely seem to be a case for stealing the clothes of the Right, but wearing them with a difference – and using their arguments to make out the case *for* the Welfare State.

Implications of Stagnation

So far my analysis has implied that economic growth is still possible, and that renewed growth will once again be the solvent of conflicts about the distribution of incomes and national resources. This may, however, turn out to be a wildly optimistic assumption – and certainly would seem

---

[9]Mervyn A. King, "The United Kingdom Profits Crisis: Myth or Reality", *Economic Journal* (March 1975), p. 33.

to be inappropriate in the present economic climate. In thinking about the future of the Welfare State it is therefore essential to contemplate the possibility that the age of economic growth may be over. If I am right in my assertion that the Welfare State was largely the product of the Growth State, what would be the implications of the No-Growth State for the Welfare State?

One answer, in such circumstances, might be to see the Welfare State as a system for job-creation in a no-growth society: as I have suggested, it is this function which may already help to explain some recent developments. If there is permanent unemployment – fluctuating between one and two millions – the cost of creating jobs in the public sector diminishes: it effectively becomes the difference between the cost of unemployment benefits and the wages or salaries paid. But such an approach raises a crucial question. If the expansion of public sector jobs is not to create problems of finance (and, by definition, the problems of raising extra funds through the tax system become more acute in a no-growth economy), then it means that those jobs will have to be designed to employ unskilled, low-paid workers – i.e. those where the margin of income as between being in or out of work is lowest. In turn, this would mean a deliberate policy of designing social services which can be delivered by a large force of unskilled workers – a process of deskilling, thus reversing the trend of the past decades towards greater professionalisation.

This point illustrates what I take to be the main conclusion to be drawn from assuming that the era of economic growth is over. This is that we can no longer sensibly think about the future of the Welfare State by simply extrapolating from the past. If there is a crisis of the Welfare State it is self-inflicted to the extent that the reaction to a new situation has been to assume that we must demand more of what we have had in the past. The Welfare State should be seen not as an historic monument – to be defended at all costs – but as a set of institutions and policies which have to be adapted to changed circumstances. To conclude, let me therefore suggest three areas where we could be exploring the scope for change.

First, the conventional definition of Welfare State policies is far too rigid. As Titmuss pointed out a long time ago, a great deal of welfare is supplied by the market sector of the economy, e.g. through occupational pension schemes. But the tendency has been to see such developments as somehow second-best to State provision. This proposition is, to put it mildly, not self-evident – if (to pursue the example of occupational pensions) such problems as transferability and inflation-proofing can be dealt with. More neglected still, most analyses of the Welfare State leave out of account those governmental decisions whose costs are carried by the private sector: yet, looking to the future, it may be that the aims of public policy should be to internalise the social costs now generated by the private sector – by regulatory policies designed to improve health and safety at work or to reduce the amount of atmospheric pollution. Such measures are obviously not costless, but they do not have to be financed out of taxation. If we cannot manage politically to increase the budget of the NHS, we might yet be able to limit the demands on the service if only at the margins.

Secondly, and following on from this point, the demarcation line between the public and the private sectors is much too firm in another respect as well. One of the most interesting developments in the field of social care has been the growth of the "grey sector"[10]: smudging the usual distinction between paid and voluntary work, there has been the development of paid volunteers, such as child minders and foster parents. In future, welfare support could increasingly be provided by expanding this sector, rather than by a policy of simply extending the public services we have already got.

Thirdly, we should recognise that some of the existing institutions of the Welfare State may be becoming disfunctional in terms of organisational complexity and resistance to change. The task of administrative co-ordination – as the experience of the NHS shows – may be generating more costs than benefits. This might suggest experiments with new institutional patterns: for example, with the Yugoslav model (echoes of G. D. H. Cole) of services run by co-operatives of producers who negotiate both the financial costs and the level of provision with co-operatives of consumers – the creation of a kind of social market, as it were.

Any movement in these directions would mean abandoning some of the aims of the founding fathers of the Welfare State. It would imply a less tidy system, with more diversity and variation. It would mean less emphasis on national planning and national priorities. But, as I have tried to suggest, the costs of such adaptive changes might be less than the costs of insisting on travelling along the same rail track, even though we know that the bridges have broken down.

---

[10]I am indebted for this point to Roy Parker's paper on "The future of the personal social services", given at the Seminar at the University of Bath to mark the 10th anniversary of the Seebohm report, September 1978.

42

The Social Policy Man: Priest or Pragmatist?

THE TIMES HIGHER EDUCATION
SUPPLEMENT
15 February 1980

Until recently, I suppose it would have been fair to say that the study of social policy could largely be equated with the study of the Welfare State: of its gradual evolution over the past century or so and of the specific bundle of institutions and programmes which we now call the Welfare State. In other words, the study of social policy has tended to revolve around those institutions and programmes whereby society takes collective decisions about the allocation of resources according to non-market criteria.

The study of social policy also tends to have two other characteristics. First, implicit in much of the academic literature is an optimistically evolutionary view of history. The Welfare State is seen as the child of progress. The gradual, faltering steps which lead to its creation – the battles fought to bring about change, the long campaigns of persuasion – tend to be regarded as landmarks in mankind's advance towards a more civilized form of society.

Second, the academic institutionalization of the study of social policy is largely the creation of the Welfare State. By this I mean that the rise and spread of departments of social administration and policy in universities up and down the country has coincided with the growth of the Welfare State.

All this might suggest a rather cosy, symbiotic relationship between the academic activity known as the study of social policy and the institutions of the Welfare State. It might indicate that our prime function is to train our students in the skills necessary to administer and deliver the social services: to produce, as it were, social engineers who can keep the machinery of the Welfare State running, while adapting the technology to meet changing circumstances or perhaps on occasion inventing new tools for policy makers.

This, however, is at best only a partial description of our role. The reason why the study of social policy is now at what I believe to be at a critical stage of its development is that those involved are increasingly being forced to question their own assumptions. Specifically, we are being forced to ask whether the Welfare State – in the institutional form that it has developed in Britain – is an evolutionary dead-end rather than the final, triumphant end-product of mankind's advance towards a more humanitarian form of social organization.

Let me try to justify this rather large claim – with which many of my colleagues will disagree. In doing so, I would like to draw our attention to two crises. The first is what I shall call the *internal* crisis of the subject area: the uncomfortable discrepancies between ideals and realities uncovered by the advance of knowledge about the operations of the Welfare State. The second is what I shall call the *external* crisis of the subject area: the new economic climate within which the Welfare State has operated since the mid-1970s.

The internal crisis of the subject area reflects its own institutional growth. The study of social policy, it is tempting to argue, is an industry whose output is social problems. Multiply the number engaged in it, and you will multiply the number of social problems. So, starting from the early 1960s, we have had an increasing number of studies drawing attention to the shortcomings, failures and gaps in our system of social provision.

The external crisis of the subject stems from the contrast between this expanding programme of aspirations generated by the study of social policy and the contracting economic environment in which these activities are taking place. The paradox of the present situation is that economic stagnation generates extra demands at the same time as it erodes the financial basis of the social services.

Public consumption can only increase at the expense of private consumption, and the evidence is that people get less generous, less altruistic in their attitudes as their economic circumstances get worse. As a result, those engaged in the activity of social policy analysis have had to take on board an entirely new set of issues.

The first item on our new agenda ought to be the relationship between social and economic policies. Social services ought not to be viewed as parasitical on the economy by definition. But if we assume (as I do) that the resumption of economic growth is the most effective social policy that we have got, then can the social policies strictly defined make more of a contribution to this end? It seems to me that they can. One of the causes of Britain's decline, it is generally agreed, are the rigidities of both the industrial structure and the social system. If we are to make the most of new technologies, then we must be able to redeploy our labour force from declining industries to new industries. This, in turn, means that we have got to cut the social costs to the men and women concerned – for otherwise, they will quite rationally and reasonably resist changes.

The second main item on our new agenda should be the future of the Welfare State itself. We should be asking ourselves to what extent the machinery of the Welfare State has become an *end* in itself, as distinct from being an effective *means* towards the achievement of certain policy objectives. In the case of the social services, we have no satisfactory means of measuring their outputs. We assume that if we increase the inputs – if we employ more doctors, nurses, social workers or teachers – then this implies an increase in output (whether in terms of quantity or quality).

But is this really so? We do not really know, though we may suspect that the main beneficiaries may as often by the service producers as the service consumers. Added to this, we can be reasonably certain that as services grow in size and complexity, so the costs of co-ordination increase.

I would therefore suggest that we have got to think seriously about dismantling the Welfare State. By this, I do not want to imply that we abandon the policy aims which lead to its creation, but that we question its specific organizational form. Let me illustrate my point. Last year, when I was working as a specialist adviser to the House of Commons expenditure committee, we looked at the cost of old people's homes. Specifically, we compared the costs in homes run by local authorities and in those run by voluntary agencies.

The cost in local authority homes was 78 per cent higher than in the other homes, and rising much faster. Now there may be a variety of explanations for this amazing difference: local authority homes may have higher standards, the old people in them may be more infirm, and there may be differences in accountancy practices. But another possible explanation may be that small organizations are more efficient – if only because they are less circumscribed by trade-union rules – in delivering social services. If that is so, then perhaps we should be thinking much more about the creation of a social market in the provision of social care.

The third item on our agenda, I would suggest, should be the relationship between publicly and privately provided social welfare. One of the most neglected areas in social policy studies is that of State regulation. Let me illustrate that point. Industry, as we all know, produces ill-health (among other things). There are industrial accidents and industrial diseases. If society is collectively concerned about this, it can react in one of two ways. It can assume responsibility directly, by providing health services and sickness absence payments. Or it can legislate to compel industry to improve health and safety at work, and to assume financial responsibility for the consequences of accidents and disease.

So, if we assume that social policy currently and for the foreseeable future constrained by the inability or unwillingness of governments to raise extra finance through the tax system, one way forward might be to proceed by legislative regulation. And this raises a further issue: what might be called the "internationalization of social policy". Social policy, whether financed through taxation or through regulation, affects the competitive position of industry. Indeed, one of the original aims of the European Community was to harmonize the social policies of its member countries, precisely on the grounds that these affect the competitive position of industry. What Britain can do is therefore affected by what other countries do.

Reading all this, you may conclude that social policy is a very odd form of academic activity. It is clearly not a discipline in the traditional sense, with a clearly defined body of knowledge and theory.

It has rightly been called a magpie subject, in that it steals and borrows theories and techniques from other disciplines. Its areas of activity are not clearly demarcated. Indeed, the implication of what I have said is that social policy ought not be defined as a discrete, clearly delineated area – its boundaries set by the Welfare State – but that it should be seen as affected by, and in turn affecting, the political and economic structure of society.

Inevitably, therefore, we not only borrow from other disciplines but intrude on their territory. Traditionally, the study of social policy has been closely associated with sociology: indeed, historically, the development of sociology in Britain can be seen as an off-shoot of concern with social policy issues. Now we are increasingly, and rightly, drawing on philosophy, political theory and political science, economics and organization theory.

Is there, then, no single organizing principle – no central intellectual paradigm – which defines the activity known as the study of social policy? If there is an answer to this question, then it is to be found – I would suggest – not so much in the area of activity, as in the way in which students of social policy approach their subject. Most of those involved in the activity tend to be committed to improving or changing the world – not just to studying it. Indeed one distinguished professor of social policy defined the subject as being about "doing good to people".

This is an obviously unsatisfactory definition: social policy often involves doing "harm" to people, when we lock them up in prisons or mental hospitals, or when we take away their money to finance welfare programmes. But, however inadequate, the definition does underline that the study of social policy involves a vision of the just society. If we define something as a social problem, it is because we believe that there is a gap between what *is* and what *ought* to be the case.

The study of social policy, I would therefore suggest, is first and foremost a study of the concept of the "just society": of the criteria which we should use when we come to our day-to-day work of analysing the actual workings of the social services or of labelling a specific social situation as a "problem". The British tradition of social policy tends to equate the achievement of social justice with the achievement of equality. But this begs a lot of questions. Are we concerned about equality of opportunities? Or about equality of outcomes? Is equality an absolute value – or are we, for example, prepared to accept some inequality in return for greater economic efficiency?

So our first responsibility is to worry about the meaning of words: to avoid the slipshod use of language which tends to creep into the debates about social policy. Indeed, this is all the more important since issues of social policy are the subject of day-to-day discussion in the media and Parliament: the line between academic discourse and public debate is difficult to draw in the case of social policy precisely because we do not (fortunately) tend to use an esoteric language incomprehensible to the layman.

Our second responsibility, I would suggest, is to analyse the nature of the choices available in decisions about social policy issues. The difficulty about any concept of the "just society" is that it is multidimensional. For example, most discussions of social policy put a high premium on the value of democracy, as well as on the value of equality. But what if there is a collision between the two? In the case of the NHS and other social services, for example, we tend to *assume* that the objective of policy should be to achieve an equitable distribution of resources geographically according to the needs of the population. This implies strict central control over the rationing process. So we inevitably limit the scope for local decisions, and in doing so, the incentives for people to take participation in the decision-making process.

Lastly, I would argue that our responsibility is to avoid the temptation of imposing our own values. Like every other citizen, students of social policy are entitled to have their own values or political preferences, and to take part in political activities designed to bring their achievement about. But if we are concerned with the academic study of social policy, then clearly we should be equally concerned with finding out about the values of other citizens.

We know remarkably little about popular perceptions of the "just society", as distinct from prescriptive academic theories about what the "just society" ought to be. We are abysmally ignorant about what different people consider to be "fair" or "unfair" – and it may well be that the disillusionment of many academics with the achievements of the Welfare State stems from the fact that their prescriptions of fairness are at odds with popular perceptions.

This underlines a central dilemma for those involved in the academic study of social policy. Should they see themselves as social theologians upholding certain absolute values or as pragmatic tinkerers concerned with social engineering? Should they accept the limitations imposed on social policy by the economic or political structure of their society, or do they insist that there can be no compromise with their vision of the just society? Should they settle for moving towards an acceptable society, or do they campaign for the transformation of society?

These questions are now more acute than at any time in the history of social policy as an academic activity. Given the economic and political constraints I have described, it has become clear that society is not going to be transformed by means of social policy: hence the widespread disillusion. So the temptation for the social theologians is to call for the political and economic transformation of society in order to create the environment in which social policy can be based on justice and equality.

As an impenitently pragmatic tinkerer, I do not share this view. I share neither the optimism of the theologians that the political and economic transformation of society will bring us into the promised land of social justice, nor their pessimism about the lack of scope for creating an acceptable society even within current constraints. The activity of studying social policy will always remain a messy business. It will always involve considerations of political and economic feasibility, of choices among many competing (and all desirable) aims of policy. Therein, I would argue, lies its fascination. For it is an activity which calls for both imagination and self-discipline – which requires us to be novelists as well as scholars, extending society's ideas about what is desirable, as well as testing those ideas against reality.

This article is based on Rudolf Klein's inaugural lecture.

43

Edwin Chadwick 1800–90

FROM: FOUNDERS OF THE WELFARE STATE,
PAUL BARKER (ED), HEINEMANN
1984

If any warning against using stereotypes in analysing the development of social policy is needed, it is offered by the career of Sir Edwin Chadwick: the hero-villain of social reform in the first half of the 19th century. As the author of 1842 *Report on the Sanitary Condition of the Labour Population of Great Britain,* Chadwick secured a prominent place in the pantheon of social reform: the first of the great social engineers, who saw the transformation of the environment through state action as the key to both health and prosperity. As the main author of the 1834 *Poor Law Report,* however, Chadwick secured an equally prominent place in the gallery of social oppressors: the archetype of the ruthless ideologue who justified the horrors of the workhouse in the name of promoting individual responsibility.

Through the history books there still stalks the caricature Chadwick, the ruthless and heartless individualist: as in E.P. Thompson's *The Making of the English Working Class.* But among his contemporaries he was pilloried and abused because of his reforming zeal, inspired by – in the words of Sir John Simon, the great health reformer – his "indignation . . . at the spectacle of so much needless human suffering."

Chadwick's life almost spanned the 19th century. Born in 1800, he died in 1890. The son of a failed businessman turned successful journalist who was an admirer of Tom Paine and a life-long radical, Edwin was educated by his father and private tutors: a fact which reflected not the family's wealth but its position in the social fringe of the radical intellectuals.

If Chadwick was never accepted by the Whig or Tory political establishments, he was fully accepted by the intellectual establishment of philosophic radicals who dominated the world of ideas during the first half of the 19th century: the world of the political economists like James and John Stuart Mill, Ricardo and (Chadwick's special patron) Nassau Senior. Trained as a lawyer, Chadwick never practised (although he always tended to interrogate facts rather like a prosecuting barrister). Instead, he became a freelance journalist and, most important, Jeremy Bentham's assistant.

It was the influence of Bentham's system of ideas – in particular, his iconoclastic insistence on testing all legislation and all institutions against the "greatest happiness" principle – which, together with the principles of the classical economists, shaped Chadwick's approach to social reform throughout his life. It was an approach which stressed that policy should be determined by the application of clear-cut principles, not by the operations of special interest groups. It saw individual self-interest as the mainspring of social action, while yet recognising the state's role in creating the legislative and institutional framework required if individual self-interest were to work to the benefit of society as a whole. (The doctrine of pure laissez-faire, as Lionel Robbins pointed out a long time ago, is not to be found in the writings of the classical utilitarians and economists and is largely the retrospective creation of Dicey in his attempt to show that the drift towards collectivism represented a betrayal of the principles of the founding fathers.)

On Bentham's death in 1832, Chadwick became a member of that curious and influential band of philosophic radicals who combined involvement in public administration, journalistic polemics and academic inquiry: a freedom which, eventually, was to be circumscribed by their own success in creating a professional bureaucracy and so drawing a demarcation line between administration and politics. For Chadwick, as for Mill, Macaulay and others, there was nothing inconsistent in holding administrative offices and engaging in the mobilisation of public opinion in support of their views. No pressure group – not even the Child Poverty Action Group – has ever been more assiduous in using the media and its network of contacts to promote its ideas.

First drawn into public administration as an investigator for the Royal Commission of Inquiry into the Poor Law in 1832, Chadwick was to become the main drafter of its report and then secretary of the commission set up to administer the new legislation. Subsequently, in 1848, he became a member of yet another Victorian quango – the General Board of Health – until he was hounded out of office in the mid-1850s. This marked the effective end of his career as a public servant although, until the end of his life, he remained active as an indefatigable pamphleteer and speaker at such bodies as the National Association for the Promotion of Social Science or the British Association for the Advancement of Science.

In the course of his career in public administration, Chadwick was also at various times involved in the farming of factory legislation and the reform of the police. But it is his part in the reform of the Poor Law and in the sanitary revolution that represents his major contributions to the shaping of social policy, and which best demonstrates the futility of trying to capture the nature of his role (and that of philosophic radicalism) in terms of simple stereotypes.

The pressures which led to the appointment of the Poor Law Commission, and the subsequent legislation implementing its recommendations, were long-standing, multiple and varied. There was the concern about the cost of support for the poor. There was the worry that outdoor relief – and especially the Speenhamland system, an early version of the Family Income Supplement, which subsidised the working poor – was undermining labour discipline. There was the Malthusian argument that subsidising the poor would only encourage them to breed, and thus accelerate the trend towards increasing "immiseration." This view led to the conclusion that there should be no support whatsoever for the pauper population (a view which was finally to triumph in article twelve of the Soviet constitution of 1936, which enunciated the principle that "he who does not work, neither shall he eat").

In short, the pressures driving the campaign for reform had little to do with Benthamism or philosophic radicalism, but largely reflected the desire of the landed classes to re-assert social control over "an increasingly numerous, truculent, and workshy peasantry who sent poor rates spiralling at a time of agricultural depression," to quote Anthony Brundage's analysis of the making of the New Poor Law.

However, the way in which the problem of pauperism was re-defined in the 1834 report, and the subsequent legislation, did reflect the influence of Benthamite principles as transmitted through Chadwick who, while no great intellectual innovator, had a rare gift for synthesising and systematising the ideas of others. Crucially, Chadwick rejected Malthusian pessimism, and with it the argument for ending all support for paupers. The real evil, as he saw it, of the existing Poor Laws was not that they encouraged the growth of population, but that they undermined incentives to work. If only the pauper could be forced back into the labour market – instead of being attracted from it by the allowance system – the problem would be solved.

From this definition of the problem, the solutions followed almost automatically. If the real problem stemmed from the system of allowances, then the solution was to abolish all forms of outdoor relief: to concentrate all support in the workhouse. If the real need was to force paupers into the labour market, and by so doing give them an incentive to seek work instead of relief, then it was essential to set support at a level below that which anyone could hope to earn in employment.

The logic of this solution led directly to the workhouse test and to the principle of "less eligibility" – the twin pillars of the New Poor Law. In future, there was to be only one test of need: whether the able-bodied pauper was prepared to enter a workhouse. This would be a "self-acting test of the claim of the applicant," in the words of the 1834 report.

Those administering the Poor Law would no longer have to distinguish "the really destitute from the crowd of indolent imposters." Relief would be automatic: "the able-bodied claimant should be entitled to immediate relief on the terms prescribed, wherever he might happen to be; and should be received without objection or inquiry; the fact of his compliance with the prescribed discipline constituting his title to a sufficient, though simple diet." This would get rid, at a stroke, of the "cumbrous and expensive barriers of investigations and appeals" in a discretionary system.

But, of course, the new system of automatic entitlement to relief could only work if it also reflected the principle of "less eligibility" – adapted by Chadwick from Bentham's *Panopticon*, the latter's vision of an ideal prison (an ominous and significant way of perceiving the role of the workhouse). "Every penny bestowed that tends to render the condition of the pauper more eligible than that of the independent labourer is a bounty on indolence and vice," the 1834 report argued. It was therefore essential that conditions in the workhouse should be less attractive – less eligible – than "the situation of the independent labourer of the lowest class." Only thus could paupers be encouraged to de-pauperise themselves: only thus could the right to relief be reconciled with the need to maintain the incentives and discipline of the labour market. The principles of the New Poor Law can thus be seen as an attempt to combine the requirements of all industrialising societies (whether capitalist or not) for labour discipline with the acceptance of collective responsibility for maintaining standards of subsistence for the whole population. The 1834 report was emphatic that its aim was not to deal with poverty, which it regarded as inevitable, but simply to prevent indigence – ie, starvation.

The new system led not only to literary denunciations from writers like Carlyle but also to political protest and riots. These were the natural reactions to what, in practice, often turned out to be a ruthlessly mean and dehumanising system. So it is not surprising that Chadwick himself came to be portrayed as a dogmatic, insensitive ideologue who created a machine for crushing people in the new bastiles. But it is important to analyse in some detail just why the New Poor Law turned out to be such a disaster. For only so can we solve the puzzle of why Chadwick – the dedicated enemy of "needless human suffering" – came to be associated with a reform which systematically generated humiliation: why a reform which introduced the principle that society should "ensure every individual belonging to it against the extreme of want," in John Stuart Mill's words, came to be perceived as an example of social tyranny.

One answer is that there was a fundamental flaw in Chadwick's analysis of the problem: a flaw which stemmed from the assumptions of the classical economists. Like Mrs Thatcher, they believed unemployment to be largely, if not wholly, self-induced. If the individual worker did not have a job, he had only himself to blame: it was either because he was indolent or because he was pricing himself out of the labour market (which is why the Speenhamland system was denounced with such fervour; it was seen as distorting the natural operations of the labour market).

But this is only part of the explanation. The New Poor Law not only represented the introduction of new principles in social policy. It also represented an attempt at an administrative revolution. It created, for the first time, a national body – the Poor Law Commission – in an attempt to enforce national standards. Parishes were to be amalgamated to form effective units of administration, where "efficient permanent officers" would be in charge. "We deem uniformity essential," the 1834 report argued, while recognising it might take time to achieve.

In the event, Chadwick – like so many social reformers since – found that his intentions were betrayed in their implementation. In a paper read to the Social Science Congress at Edinburgh in 1863, he reflected – with the benefit of hindsight – on the failure of the New Poor Law to achieve its full aims. Basically, he argued, the intentions of the reformers had been defeated by the power of local lobbies: the "sinister interests which operate most powerfully in narrow areas."

"Farmer guardians," he pointed out, "could still give, though indirectly, outdoor relief, which in effect was frequently relief in aid of the wages of their own employees ... The owners of small tenements in towns could still, as guardians, give outdoor partial relief, much of which was in payment of high rents paid by their own tenants."

Here is the voice of the true radical reformer. Like so many social engineers, Chadwick was convinced that if only his ideas had been carried out ruthlessly and comprehensively enough, they would have succeeded. Once Chadwick had made up his mind – once his ideas were developed into a full-blown system where abstract principles were translated into a precise administrative machinery – nothing would shift him.

Indeed it is this which, perhaps, helps to explain his failure as an administrator. His career as secretary to the Poor Law Commission, from 1834 to 1842, was marked by a series of increasingly bitter and public rows with the commissioners, who finally relegated their domineering servant to an administrative limbo, virtually ignoring his existence. As Sir John Simon wrote, Chadwick lacked the quality of "judicial patience": he did not recognise sufficiently that social reform had to be based on the mobilisation of consent.

Simon was writing here about Chadwick in his role as the prophet of the sanitary revolution. But Chadwick's contribution in this role was remarkably similar to the part he played in the creation of the New Poor Law. Once again, he launched a crusade with a report – the 1842 *Report on the Sanitary Condition of the Labouring Population of Great Britain* – published in a large edition with carefully orchestrated publicity. Again, he succeeded in having legislation, based on his report's principles, enacted – if only in a watered-down version. Again, however, he stumbled when it came to implementing the legislation: the General Board of Health failed to overcome local resistance to its policies, and Chadwick himself became the main victim of this failure.

In turning his attention to sanitary reform, almost as a form of occupational therapy for his frustrations at the Poor Law Commission, Chadwick's starting point was the financial burden of disease on the poor rates. But the scope of his inquiry soon widened out. The outcome was a magisterial, comprehensive and horrendous indictment of social conditions in Britain, which makes chilling reading even today.

In the event, the ideas underlying the *Sanitary Report* were very different from those that had shaped the *Poor Law Report*. In it, Chadwick embraced wholeheartedly the environmental theory of disease prevention, brushing aside the claims of curative medicine. It was squalor, dirt and – above all – excrement which caused disease: "All smell is, if it be intense, immediate acute disease," he wrote. The so-called miasmatic theory of disease was soon to be discredited, but Chadwick's recipe for action was not: a good example of how bad theories can actually lead to successful social policies. Further, Chadwick concluded that it was poor social conditions, rather than indolence or lack of moral fibre, which caused poverty. Disease caused destitution; destitution did not cause disease.

In this emphasis on the crucial importance of transforming the environment in order to transform individual lives lay the key to social policy progress for the rest of the 19th century, and beyond. For if Chadwick's particular concern was with drainage and sewerage, precisely the same logic applied to improving housing and working conditions. In this lay the most enduring contribution of the *Sanitary Report*.

Equally important was the way in which Chadwick reached this conclusion: the methodology of analysis which shaped his report, and which has continued to influence social policy ever since. Page after page of the report is devoted to analysing variations in life expectancy by social class and place of residence, in an endeavour to identify the causes of disease. In Manchester, for example, the average age of death of "professional persons and gentry, and their families" was 38, while that of "mechanics, labourers, and their families" was 17; in rural Rutlandshire the equivalent figures were respectively 52 and 38. In this respect, the analysis was not so very different from that of the Black report, published in 1980.

In the event, the sanitary revolution turned out to be a long-drawn-out war of attrition with local vestries and local water companies, of which Chadwick was the first casualty. But although then effectively barred from active administration and politics – his attempts to become an MP failed abysmally – Chadwick continued the battle with words for another 35 years.

In a sense, most of his addresses and articles are a prolonged, and sometimes crotchety, self-justification. He adopted new enthusiasms, such as educational reform, but essentially his aim was to defend his two great reforms: the New Poor Law and the sanitary revolution. However, it is his language of justification which gives these later writings their fascination. For them, he developed what was largely to be the language of social policy analysis for the next 100 years: asserting the claim of dispassionate reason – of scientific methods and bureaucratic rationality – as against the power of vested interests: the "baleful money interests" represented in parliament and the "jobocracies" of public companies, as well as the "imbecility, or the sinister interests of ignorant local administrators."

Facts and figures, as always, continued to be Chadwick's main weapon. Already in the *Sanitary Report*, he had begun to develop a cost-benefit approach to the analysis of social problems. Preventive measures, he had argued with a wealth of statistical evidence, could pay for themselves. It was a point to which he returned, again and again. "When the sentimentalist and the moralist fails, he will have as a last resource to call in the aid of the economist, who has in some instances proved the power of his art to draw iron tears from the cheeks of a city Plutus," he told the British Association in his presidential address in 1862.

Not only was waste sinful, but waste itself could become the source of sin: "it is my deep conviction that whilst waste is sinful, sin by the infliction of animal and human suffering is wasteful," Chadwick wrote (in an essay devoted to the regulation of the cab trade). People represented capital investment – he argued, in an early version of human capital theory – and maximising their welfare would also maximise national wealth. Poor social conditions not only lowered the productivity of labour but also generated social problems: "insanitary conditions are attended with moral as well as physical deterioration; crime following most closely those conditions where there is a perception of the short duration of life, and where the appetites for immediate enjoyment amongst the ill-educated and ill-trained are strong and reckless" – a contention backed up by a statistical table showing the relationship between crime rates and health indicators. In sharp contrast to the assumptions which had shaped the New Poor Law, Chadwick had come to see the poor as the victims of their circumstances: a conclusion which demanded collective social action rather than individual moral rehabilitation.

One of Chadwick's main concerns, therefore, remained the principles and practice of social regulation. "It will not do, however, to base legislation on beneficence, or on the heroic virtues, and the great problem is to unite interest with duty," he stressed. The challenge was to create a framework of state regulation and intervention which would give individuals incentives to behave in the public interest. It was a principle which led him to advocate more and more intervention: in particular, public control of water authorities and railways. Unregulated competition between small firms – whether for the cab horse trade or for funerals – was inefficient: far better have one, publicly regulated, monopoly enterprise (a long cry, this, from the classical free market doctrine).

In turn, this required improved methods of legislation and more professional administration. Chadwick's contempt for democratic politics – whether national or local – grew with age. Instead of starting with an inquiry into facts, legislation reflected the prejudices of public men. Instead of the "close and secret" cabinet procedure for preparing legislation, there should be open inquiries: "In legislation, as in other things, gross ignorance sees no difficulties, imperfect knowledge descries them, perfect knowledge overcomes them." In local government, matters were worse still, since it was the self-interested who had the greatest incentive to participate, with the result that "the performance of honorary municipal duties, instead of devolving upon the highest class of citizens, is sinking into the hands of the lowest grade of persons of the middle classes." From this followed the need for a more professionalised bureaucracy.

In all this, Chadwick anticipated most of the themes that were to occupy social reformers for the next century. He was a pioneer not only in developing methods of social inquiry for analysing problems but also in realising that devising solutions meant designing new instruments of administration. Like so many social reformers since, he was a man dominated by a "strain after perfection which necessarily becomes one-sided in a world of many mixed considerations," in the words of one politician sympathetic to him. This "strain after perfection" helps to explain both his immediate failure to achieve his aims and his long-term influence. An opinionated optimist, sustained by his conviction that social engineering exploiting the knowledge of the social sciences could transform the world, Chadwick may often seem naive and over-simple in the present age of disillusion and pessimism. But it is difficult not to be impressed by his intrepid, single-minded conviction that rational analysis could defeat the forces of ignorance, prejudice and self-interest, and create a better society.

44

O'Goffe's Tale, Or, What Can We Learn From the Success of the Capitalist Welfare States?

NEW PERSPECTIVES ON THE WELFARE STATE IN EUROPE. CATHERINE JONES (ED), 1993

This paper starts with a puzzle. Looking back on the literature on the welfare state published in the 1970s and the early 1980s (Moran, 1988), there is a striking asymmetry. On the one hand, there are the grim prophecies of crisis – if not worse – threatening the welfare state in capitalist societies. On the other hand, there is the almost total silence about the likely fate of the welfare state in communist societies. Yet if we look around us now, there is a very simple observation to be made. On the one hand, the welfare state in capitalist societies has survived the crisis in remarkably good health. On the other hand, the welfare state in communist societies is going through precisely the same paroxysms of reconstruction as the regimes that created it. It is a contrast which, as I shall argue in this paper, has some important implications for both the practice and theory of comparative social policy studies.

The best starting point for exploring this puzzle is perhaps O'Goffe's tale. In constructing O'Goffe's tale, I have taken the three leading exponents of the neo-Marxist thesis (O'Connor, 1973; Gough, 1979; Offe, 1984) and conflated the main features of their accounts. The result may not be fully fair to any individual member of the trio – and is not intended to be so – but it gives a sense of the logic of their argument. For what distinguished O'Goffe from the myriad of other scholars wringing their hands about the plight of the welfare state at a time of economic turmoil was that he sought to explain these troubles by invoking the nature of *capitalist* states. In O'Goffe's view this was not just a crisis. It was something much more serious: a contradiction. In other words, the difficulties of the welfare state did not just reflect contemporary or evanescent problems of capitalist societies but were inherent in their nature. They were inherent because of the in-built, inescapable conflict between the needs of legitimation, consumption and the demands of capital accumulation. To maintain political legitimacy, the capitalist state had to spend on welfare services and programmes; to maintain the machinery of capitalism, however, it had to promote capital accumulation and ensure profits. And all this was in addition to freeing enough resources for consumption. The development of the welfare state threatened the process of capital accumulation. While the Keynesian Welfare State had for 30 years created the illusion that both objectives of policy could be reconciled in an ever-more prosperous world, the loss of belief both in Keynesian theories of economic management and in the compound arithmetic of growth meant that conflict was inevitable. The conflict could be resolved and the welfare state saved, O'Goffe concluded, only in a new kind of socialist society.

There were important insights in this approach. It was a much-needed antidote to the kind of bland, historicist accounts of the welfare state typical of the hitherto dominant Marmuss school.[1] This tended to present the rise of the welfare state everywhere as an inevitable process: a milestone in the progress of mankind. O'Goffe rightly argued that welfare policies involved conflict about resources, and therefore raised questions about the distribution of power in society. Equally important, he pointed out that welfare policies could not be separated from economic policies, and that both are inevitably shaped by political institutions. In short, O'Goffe concluded, the welfare state could be understood only as the product of economic and political forces: as part of the total social environment.

The impact of O'Goffe's critique was all the greater because it echoed, and in many respects overlapped with, that of Hayman.[2] The New Right

---

[1]Otherwise known as T.H. Marshall and Richard M. Titmuss.
[2]Otherwise known as Friedrich A. Hayek and Milton Friedman.

also argued that the welfare state would destroy capitalism. The growth of social spending, so the case ran, was undermining work incentives, sapping the ability to invest, creating self-serving welfare bureaucracies and fuelling inflation. Worse still, it was a threat to liberty: the political system was being corrupted (as well as being overloaded) by having to take decisions about the distribution of resources that should be left to the market. Not the least important common element between O'Goffe and Hayman was their shared distrust for the capacity of Western political systems. For very different reasons, they had little faith in politics – seen as a dialogue between groups with different interests but a common concern to solve societal problems – as a way of tackling the difficulties posed by rising social expenditures in times of economic stringency. Indeed, rising social expenditure was seen as a symptom of political failure: democratic politics, it was often argued (Brittan, 1977), generated extravagant public expectations which in turn led to excessive expenditure.

O'Goffe had nothing to say, however, about the welfare state in communist states. Indeed, on his own premises, there was no need to say anything about this. For was not the whole point of his argument that the crisis – indeed contradictions – of the welfare state derived from the very nature of capitalist societies? There was no need to test the premises, even though some of us suggested at the time that it might be a good idea to do so (Klein, 1979): that communist societies might well have the same dilemmas – such as the conflict between meeting needs and maintaining work incentives and between the demands of capital accumulation and social spending – as capitalist ones. O'Goffe clearly took the premises to be self-evidently true. In fact, the events of the past few years suggest that they were self-evidently wrong: that the same conflicts, contradictions or crises afflicted the communist Welfare States (CWS) as the Keynesian Welfare States (KWS). The real difference lay in the fact that while the capitalist societies of the West were able to cope with the supposedly irreconcilable contradictions, the communist societies of the East collapsed under their weight. While the KWS has emerged virtually intact from the 1980s almost everywhere – a point to which we return below – the CWS is crumbling in the wake of the collapse of the regimes that created it.

A number of implications can be drawn out from O'Goffe's tale. The first is about the logic of political analysis. Before we can make a statement about cause-and-effect in a particular society – or class of societies – we surely have to be able to test it against a counter-factual. Otherwise, we are operating in a solipsistic universe. The point is as obvious as it is frequently neglected. The comparative method is not just a luxury add-on to the study of social policy but an essential component if we are to avoid repeating O'Goffe's blunder in over-predicting the crisis of the welfare state in the West while under-predicting its collapse in the East.

The point can be simply illustrated. Take O'Goffe's assertion about the conflict between the competing claims of political legitimation, capital accumulation and consumption. What evidence is there to support the assumption that this is somehow peculiar or unique to capitalism? None. But if O'Goffe had chosen to search for evidence that such conflict was also apparent in communist regimes, he might well have found it; certainly there are hints that communist regimes used welfare spending as a means of buying legitimacy and popularity (Ferge, 1986) when they failed to deliver the goods of economic prosperity or political acceptability. Indeed, it might quite plausibly be argued (using the O'Goffe line of reasoning) that, in doing so, they damaged their capacity for capital accumulation and further undermined their legitimacy, so creating what proved to be a fatal downward cycle.

But of course it may be argued in O'Goffe's defence that information about social policy in the communist bloc was remarkably scant at the time (as it still is). Therein, however, lies the second implication which can be drawn out from O'Goffe's tale. It suggests the need for self-examination in the social policy community. Why was there so little information in the 1970s and 1980s? And why, as anyone trying to teach comparative social policy soon found, were most of the available studies unsatisfactory in quality? Part of the answer lies, obviously, in the fact that communist regimes did not release accurate data or encourage research; even now it is extraordinarily difficult to establish with precision, for example, what percentage of the national income is spent on health care (or education and the social services) for purposes of comparison. But this is an incomplete answer. Even when there was evidence of the failure of the communist regimes in the welfare field – notably that provided by rising mortality (Wnuk-Lipinsky and Illsley, 1990) – it tended to be neglected in comparative social policy studies.

Similarly, the evidence of parallelisms between capitalist and communist welfare states tended to be overlooked: for example, Wilensky's conclusion (1975) that much the same (non-ideological) factors explained the growth of welfare state spending in capitalist and communist countries. It is therefore difficult to resist the conclusion that the under-prediction of crisis reflected both the linguistic incompetence and ideological predispositions of most of the scholars in the field. There has always been, and continues to be, a serious shortage of scholars in the field equipped with the languages required for the serious study of East European welfare systems. And there is a lingering tendency to use comparative studies as a search for ammunition in domestic political battles: to be able to cite examples of how much better things are done in other (preferably non-capitalist or left-wing) countries.

This is not to imply that O'Goffe was necessarily or invariably uncritical of the welfare state in communist societies. Indeed, some Marxists (Deacon, 1983) argued that the social policies of the Eastern bloc countries were, in themselves, evidence that these countries could not be considered to be fully communist or socialist societies. Despite the limitations of their analysis, dependent as they were on English-language sources, they were able to see the multiple inadequacies of the CWS. The analysis also conceded that, to establish a fully socialist welfare state, there would have to be a 'class struggle' against the political leadership in Eastern Europe. But it crucially stopped short of considering whether a form of economic organisation that rested on the collective ownership of the means of production was compatible with a fully socialist welfare state. Might not the capture of the welfare state by the self-interest of the party bureaucracy represent an inherent, unavoidable contradiction in communist societies? Rather than conceding this point, the Marxist literature sought to argue that some communist regimes had demonstrated that truly socialist social policies were feasible. In Deacon's case, the examples cited were China, Cuba and (incredibly) Mozambique.

In short, the Marxist literature represents the search for a social policy Utopia, i.e. a society where there is no conflict between the self-interest of the welfare state producers and consumers or between competing claims on national resources. The quest for the 'Eldorado banal de tous les vieux marxistes', to adapt Baudelaire, goes on – undiscouraged by the fact that infatuation inevitably leads to disillusion, as successive candidates for the 'Eldorado' turn out to be flawed. While the failures or problems of capitalist societies are seen as being inherent in their very nature, the failures or problems of communist societies are seen only as evidence that they are not truly communist. In the first case, the system is showing its true face; in the second, it is a betrayal of what the system should be like – and therefore no conclusions can be drawn about the model's viability. It is a line of argument which, of course, can never be proved wrong by mere empirical evidence.

To summarise the argument so far, then, the paradox is that the neo-Marxist analysts of the welfare state developed an analytical tool-kit which might well have been quite useful in predicting the impending disintegration of the CWS – but chose not to use it. Instead, they applied their explanatory drill to the KWS, and it broke in their hands. And it broke in their hands precisely because of their assertion that the dilemma of choice was unique to capitalist societies. In doing so, they overlooked the possibility that these societies might have the *political* institutions and resources required to cope with the reconciliation of competing claims and the so-called 'crisis of the welfare state': a rather overblown way of describing the problems of adaptation to new circumstances which faced Western societies in the wake of the global economic crisis of the mid-1970s. In contrast, the communist societies lacked these institutions and resources, which is, of course, why O'Goffe under-predicted the turmoil in the East and over-predicted the crisis in the West. In the next section, we therefore discuss in rather more detail what can be learnt from comparative studies of this success story for the capitalist societies of the West.

From Crisis to Success

Although the 1970s spawned a formidable body of literature on the 'crisis of the welfare state' – a phrase which also haunted the early 1980s – the actual story turned out to be one of successful adaptation (Jobert, 1991). The welfare state, on balance, turns out to have discomfited those who were writing its obituary (Ringen, 1987). The contradictions, it turned out, could be managed if not eliminated. If choice between competing claims on increasingly scarce resources could not be avoided – and where, except in Utopia, can it be avoided? – at least Western societies turned out to have the political capacity for dealing with the challenge.

Most important, perhaps, is what has not happened. There has been no crisis of legitimacy in the Western capitalist societies, in sharp contrast to the communist nations of the East. The existing political order has not been challenged. There is little evidence of massive disillusion with the political system. If one of the purposes of social spending is to legitimate the state, as O'Goffe would put it, then it appears to have been achieved. Bismarck's invention, 'conceived of as an essay in practical politics' (King, 1983), has turned out to be a success. The welfare state has helped to maintain the political stability – and probably also the social cohesion – of the Western world.

The achievement is all the more remarkable if we consider that the period of the 'crisis of the welfare state' was also the era of quite exceptional social change and dislocation in Britain and other countries of the West. The nature of the transformation is well known: the move from traditional industry to the service economy (Gershuny, 1978). So is the fact that it was accompanied everywhere by unemployment on a scale which, until the mid-1970s, would have been considered a threat to political stability: no government, so ran the conventional political wisdom of post-1945 Britain, could survive unemployment figures above 500,000 – let alone 1 or 2 million. If the welfare state is conceived of as an instrument for insuring against the risks of change, or as a way of compensating those who bear the social costs (Baldwin, 1990), then again it seems to have earned its keep during these critical years. This is not to assert that the social costs of change were necessarily equitably or fully compensated everywhere; the level of unemployment benefits was one of the casualties of public expenditure retrenchment in many OECD countries (OECD, 1985). It is to argue, however, that – whatever its weaknesses or inequities – the welfare state did succeed in helping to smooth the social and political pains of a dramatic economic transformation.

Nor is there much evidence that social spending was at the expense – as both O'Goffe and the New Right argued – of capital accumulation (Cameron, 1985). The real conflict was between social spending and consumption; hence the famous tax back-lash of the late 1970s. It was this that seemed to vindicate O'Goffe's prophecy. If the accelerating expansion of social spending characteristic of the 1960s and the early 1970s had been maintained, then clearly personal disposable income would have been severely squeezed: public consumption would effectively have replaced private consumption. Extrapolation could easily produce a doom scenario of government bankruptcy and falling personal incomes (Rose and Peters, 1978). In the event, governments did not go bankrupt and, on the whole, personal incomes continued to rise; one of the few countries in which the incomes of the 'middle mass' have failed to rise substantially over the past decade is the United States, a notoriously low welfare spender. For what the predictions of crisis and collapse had overlooked was the institutional resilience of the welfare state and the effect over time of marginal, incremental changes. Nowhere was total welfare state expenditure reduced; everywhere, however, governments sought ways of reducing the inherited rate of increase.

On the one hand, the welfare state therefore emerged from the 1980s everywhere looking much as it had at the start of the decade. There were no dramatic changes in its institutions, policies and programmes. The welfare state, it turned out, had created a powerful political constituency for its own survival even in countries, like Britain (Hills, 1990) and the United States (Marmor, Mashaw and Harvey, 1990), which had governments ideologically committed to cutting it back. On the other hand, there turned out to be unexpected scope for decelerating the rate of growth in spending. In part, this was achieved by disguising retrenchment as technical change in the method of calculating benefits over time (for example, by decoupling them from movements in earnings); in part, it was done by concentrating economies on those groups with least political power (for example, welfare beneficiaries and the unemployed). On balance, the beneficiaries of the welfare state concentrated in strong, permanent constituencies – like the elderly and the service providers –

seem to have emerged remarkably unscathed, while the shifting populations of those at the margins or outside the labour force appear to have
done rather worse. The outcome, in fact, is what might be predicted if
one sees the welfare state not as an instrument for 'doing good' – let
alone for achieving equality – but as both the product and the producer
of coalitions of self-interest.

The welfare state also demonstrated, in the 1980s, its capacity for
organisational adaptation. In response to economic stringency, it moved
to meet some of the criticisms once again common to O'Goffe and the
New Right: notably, the criticisms of a self-serving welfare bureaucracy
imposing their own preferences on captive consumers. The current
reforms of Britain's National Health Service (Day and Klein, 1991) are a
case in point, as are the changes in the education system designed to tilt
power towards parents, which in part at least inspired the health policies.
The NHS changes are more likely to change the balance of power between
managers and providers, rather than that between consumers and professionals. But, interestingly, Sweden is currently experimenting with a rather
similar set of ideas (Saltman, 1990, and Gould in this volume), if within
a totally different ideological framework: there the intention appears to
be to see how far it is possible to create choice for health care consumers
by forcing public providers to compete for customers. There is, of course,
a standard O'Goffe response to such changes. These are seen not as
demonstrating a capacity for flexibility or innovation but as evidence that
capitalism is trying to re-build the welfare state in its own image; that
the welfare state has been saved only at the cost of distorting its real
essence by introducing the values of the market place: by commodifying
welfare. In short, the prediction of disaster has turned out to be correct,
only the nature of the disaster was mis-specified. The contradictions of
capitalism have been resolved – if only temporarily – by invoking managerial efficiency. O'Goffe's capacity for salvaging predictions of impending
doom from apparent success stories should not be underestimated.

But, of course, there are varieties of adaptive strategies and degrees
of success. So far the discussion has been in terms of the 'welfare state'.
It is useful shorthand, but a dangerous abstraction. The welfare state is
a bundle of institutions, policies and programmes which varies in its
composition from country to country (and some of its most important
components, like labour market policies, may even be excluded under
conventional definitions). As Figure 1.1 shows, countries reacted to the
economic crisis of the 1970s in very different ways. Some, like the USA,
'over-reacted' to the crisis, perhaps predictably: that is, the rate of increase
in spending declined by much more than would be predicted from the
fall in the rate of economic growth. Others, like Sweden, 'under-reacted',
again unsurprisingly: that is, the momentum of social spending continued

	Pensions	Health	Education
Canada	△	▲	▲
France	○	▲	NA
Germany	▲	▲	▲
Italy	▲	▲	△
Japan	○	▲	△
UK	△	△	▲
USA	▲▲	▲▲	▲▲
Ireland	▲	▲	▲
Netherlands	▲	▲	▲
Norway	▲▲	▲▲	▲▲
Sweden	△	▲	△
Finland	▲	▲	△
Australia	▲	▲	▲
New Zealand	○	△	▲

△ 'Under-reactors': spending rate declines by less than the fall in GDP rate.
▲ 'Over-reactors': spending declines by more than the fall in GDP rate.
○ 'Non-reactors': spending rate increases even though GDP rate falls.
▲▲ 'Heavy over-reactors': spending declines by much more than the fall in GDP rate.

FIGURE 1.1   A summary of reaction ratios for programme expenditure in 14 OECD countries (1960–75: 1975–81).

relatively unaffected by economic problems. Similarly, these are significant variations in the pattern of retrenchment/continued expansion as between different programmes: pensions, health and education.

The pattern was much the same in the 1980s: common themes of concern about rising social spending, but many variations in the national solutions adopted. A recent analysis of developments – by a research group that included contributors to the original O'Goffe thesis (Pfaller, Gough and Therborn, 1991) – demonstrates considerable variations in both the nature of the policy debates and policy outcomes in a range of capitalist societies: Germany, France, the United States, Britain and Sweden. If there are conflicts between different interest groups in capitalist societies – as in all societies – then, quite clearly, they are mediated by specific national factors: the nature of the political culture and the political system. The point is obvious enough, and needs stressing only because of past attempts to anchor all analysis and explanation in the nature of that mystical entity, capitalism.

Generalised theories – whether of the O'Goffe or Hayman variety – are not helpful in explaining such particular patterns, however ingenious the *post hoc* rationalisations offered when predictions fail. The history of the 1980s offers a special opportunity for comparative social policy studies precisely because it allows us to look at the way in which common economic problems were translated into policy change by very different political systems, and the relative weight given by these different political systems to equity and efficiency. It gives us an opportunity to explore different strategies of adaptation and to ask what kinds of social policies and welfare institutions provide most scope for flexibility. For not the least important reason why the crisis of the Western welfare state was over-predicted, while that of the communist welfare state was under-predicted, was that far too little attention was paid to the respective learning capacity of the two systems (Deutsch, 1966). And if it is indeed the case that an effective learning system, plus a well-developed capacity to adapt, is the necessary condition for the welfare state's survival, then perhaps we should be using the 1980s to draw some conclusions about the kind of conditions and institutions that best promote both learning and adaptation.

There is perhaps a further conclusion that we can draw from O'Goffe's tale, both for social policy discourse in general and for comparative analysis. We have noted throughout the surprising fact – given their ideological opposition to each other – that O'Goffe and Hayman agreed on so many issues. Why should that be? Fifteen or even ten years ago, one might have been tempted to answer the question by saying that they had intellectual insights denied to those of us in the soggy middle who rejected both approaches. Events since then suggest that this is not a plausible explanation. More recently Hirschman (1991) has provided a more persuasive explanation, which is that both O'Goffe and Hayman use the same type of rhetoric or style of argument. They tend to make apocalyptic prophecies based on the contention that, given the nation of mankind or of a particular class of society, change will inevitably be either futile or have perverse consequences. What this would suggest is that social policy needs a very different kind of theorising: one that is based not on large and often vacuous generalisations about the nature of capitalist or any other kind of society but on a rigorous analysis of the policy conflicts in particular societies and of the criteria used to justify specific choices (Weale, 1991). Diagnosing 'contradictions', i.e. conflicts, in societies does not get us far. Investigating how different societies tackle those conflicts – their institutional capacity for so doing, the structure of power and the arguments used in the process – is likely to provide far more illumination.

Acknowledgements

I am grateful for the comments of all the participants at the conference which gave birth to this book, and for the specific suggestions from Bob Deacon, Nicholas Deakin and Richard Rose.

References

Baldwin, Peter (1990) *The Politics of Social Solidarity*, Cambridge: Cambridge University Press.

Brittan, Samuel (1977) *The Economic Consequences of Democracy*, London: Temple Smith.

Cameron, David R. (1985) 'Public expenditure and economic performance in international perspective' in Rudolf Klein and Michael O'Higgins (eds) *The Future of Welfare*, Oxford: Basil Blackwell.

Day, Patricia and Klein, Rudolf (1991) 'The British health care experiment', *Health Affairs*.

Deacon, Bob (1983) *Social Policy and Socialism*, London: Pluto Press.

Deutsch, Karl W. (1966) *The Nerves of Government*, New York: The Free Press.

Ferge, Zsuzsa (1986) 'The changing Hungarian social policy' in Else Oyen (ed.) *Comparing Welfare States and their Future*, Aldershot: Gower.

Gershuny, Jonathan (1978) *After Industrial Society?* London: Macmillan.

Gough, Ian (1979) *The Political Economy of the Welfare State*, London: Macmillan.

Hills, John (ed.)(1990) *The State of Welfare*, Oxford: Clarendon Press.

Hirschman, Albert O. (1991) *The Rhetoric of Reaction*, Cambridge, Mass.: The Belknap Press.

Jobert, Bruno (1991) 'La Réstructuration des États Européens', Mimeo, University of Grenoble.

King, Anthony (1983) 'The political consequences of the welfare state' in *Evaluating the Welfare State: Social and Political Perspectives*, London: Academic Press.

Klein, Rudolf (1979) 'Welfare as power', a review of Gough op. cit, *New Society*, 20 September, 632–3.

Marmor, Theodore R., Mashaw, Terry L. and Harvey, Philip L. (1990) *America's misunderstood welfare state*, New York: Basic Books.

Moran, Michael (1988) 'Crises of the welfare state', *British Journal of Political Science* 18 (3) 397–414.

O'Connor, James (1973) *The Fiscal Crisis of the State*, New York: St Martin's Press.

Offe, Claus (1984) *The Contradictions of the Welfare State*, London: Hutchinson.

Organisation for Economic Co-operation and Development (1985) *Social Expenditure, 1960–1990*, Paris: OECD.

Pfaller, Alfred, Gough, Ian and Therborn, Goran (1991) *Can the welfare state Compete?* London: Macmillan.

Ringen, Stein (1987) *The Possibility of Politics*, Oxford: Clarendon Press.

Rose, Richard and Peters, Guy (1978) *Can Governments Go Bankrupt?* London: Macmillan.

Saltman, Richard B. (1990) 'Competition and reform in the Swedish health system' *The Milbank Quarterly* 68(4), 597–618.

Weale, Albert (1991) 'Principles, process and policy' in Thomas and Dorothy Wilson (eds) *The State and Social Welfare*, London: Longman.

Wilensky, Harold L. (1975) *The Welfare State and Equality*, Berkeley: University of California Press.

Wnuk-Lipinsky, E. and Illsley, Raymond (1990) 'International comparative analysis: main findings and conclusions' *Social Science and Medicine* 31 (8), 878–89.

Part 4

The Politics of Health Care

The health policy and politics area probably contains the work for which Rudolf Klein is best known, although there is ample evidence in the previous sections of this volume that health research was only one of his special interests; it is certainly true that health care and the British National Health Service provided him with a rich source of research and analysis. But although this last section is dedicated exclusively to Rudolf's health policy work, this should not be taken to imply that health care has provided his final intellectual resting place. Rudolf was writing about the politics of the NHS before he became Professor of Social Policy at Bath University in 1978 and, conversely, he has continued to contribute to the wider policy literature in the 1980s and 1990s, as is evident from the previous section.

On the face of it, it appears that Rudolf is juggling with different academic interests and certainly with different policy fields. To an extent this is true and is a source of admiration among his colleagues. However, a closer examination of this collection reveals a more complex picture: it shows that his work has common conceptual themes which provide links across apparently different areas. What Rudolf has actually managed to do is to turn the British health services into one case among several different public policy study areas which, studied alongside each other, provide a greater depth of understanding of the policy process; a policy analysis whole which is greater than the sum of the parts. No doubt he will find this description of him as an intellectual juggler a compliment rather than a criticism: he has always seen his strength as working between disciplines rather than within any one of them.

45

N.H.S. Reorganisation: the Politics of the Second Best

THE LANCET
26 August 1972

First reactions to the white-paper on the reorganisation of the National Health Service[1] have, rightly, been concerned with the actual proposals. The other way of analysing the document is to examine it as an output of the policy-making process and as an example of how decisions are made. Such an approach has advantages. It puts the whole issue of N.H.S. reform in the context of the Government system as a whole, so avoiding the dangers of an exclusively medicocentric view of the Health Service. It also, as I shall try to show, leads to a more realistic judgment than criticism which ignores many of the factors involved in evolving policy on such a complex issue as the future shape of the N.H.S. There are also some disadvantages: many of the key decisions are taken in secret, and it will not be possible to describe the actual process until the Government files are opened in another thirty years, if then.

There are two basic models of the decision-making process. The first – expounded in its most sophisticated form by Dror[2] – is what may be called the optimising, rational model. In this the decision-maker first analyses the objectives he wants to achieve in tackling a given problem, then looks at all the possible ways of achieving them, weighs up the disadvantages and advantages of each policy option, and finally chooses the policy which best fulfils his aims. The second model assumes that the administrator or policy-maker "satisfices"[3] – i.e., he looks for a course of action that may not be ideal but that is satisfactory or good enough. This, it has been argued,[4] is not only a more accurate description of what

319

happens but also a more rational way of going about things, since it leads to a cautious, incremental approach to change informed by the realisation that most decisions have to be based on inadequate information, without the time needed to explore all the options.

These two very basic models do not by any means exhaust the literature on policy-making.[5,6] Of particular relevance to the Health Service may be the "garbage-can model of organisational choice".[7] However, using the two over-simplified models – the optimising and the satisficing – provides a helpful starting-point for considering the reorganisation of the N.H.S.

Muddling Through?

It immediately becomes clear that reorganising the N.H.S. is an example of the satisficing approach: indeed it has been argued[8] that the N.H.S. as a whole is an example of the "muddling-through" approach in policy-making. The optimising model simply does not apply. Thus, most conspicuously, the optimum solution of putting health and personal social services under the same administration has been excluded from consideration. This is not a political issue in a party sense. Mr. Richard Crossman has argued that "there is, in reason, no case for saying that the new great local authorities should not take over the health service", but this was after leaving office.[9] As long ago as 1924 a distinguished Conservative Minister of Health, Neville Chamberlain, argued in a private memorandum[10] for "the creation of a single health authority in each local area". But since the medical profession is opposed to local authority control, and the local authorities are opposed to losing control of the social services, and no Government wishes to take on either of these interest groups, any reorganisation of the N.H.S. has to settle for the second best. Similarly, the present Government, like its predecessors, has ducked a confrontation with general practitioners, who remain, in effect, a self-governed enclave within the N.H.S.

To emphasise these points is to direct attention to the constraints within which the white-paper, like its green-paper predecessors of 1968[11] and 1970,[12] has been produced, and the reasons why at best it can only hope to offer a "satisficing" solution. The first constraint is that all the actors involved in its production have multiple roles. Any Minister trying to reorganise the N.H.S. is also trying to extract more funds from the Treasury. In the latter role he may need allies in the Cabinet who might be alienated if, for example, he were to seek to expand the N.H.S. at the expense of local government. The Civil Servants at the Department of Health and Social Security, besides seeking to improve the Health Service organisation, must meet the representatives of the health professions across the negotiating-table for years to come in pay and other talks: they cannot afford to invest too much of their resources of energy and prestige in one particular battle. As one ex-Minister has written,[13] many Civil Servants feel that "it is good to be right but it is better not to be defeated". The representatives of the professions, similarly, have to take a long-term view, and to reconcile their own private preferences with the demands of the more militant members: at the same time as they are bargaining, they are also trying to educate. Thus in 1911, when the Government and the medical profession were engaged in a fierce fight, the B.M.A.'s Medical Secretary, Dr. Smith Whitaker, was saying in private conversation: "If the Association throws itself at once on the side of the new régime then it will dominate it, if it opposes its development the new scheme will organise itself as a rival"[14] – a classic exposition of the "insider" approach of the professional negotiator.

There are other constraints as well. The quest for efficiency is only one of the dimensions of decision-making.[15] The other dimensions are those of political practicability and administrative feasibility. Thus all policies have political costs[16]: that is, they will alienate some people and enlist the support of others. This is a crucial consideration (again not in a party sense), since the costs of pushing a policy through may be such that a Government or Minister may exhaust their credit before the stage of implementation: trade-union legislation is a case in point. Again, a policy which may appear to be the most "rational" in the abstract may be irrational in practice if it demands non-existent administrative resources for its execution: one of the chief constraints on the reorganisation of the N.H.S. is that – with very few exceptions – exactly the same people, with the same talents, will be running it after 1974 as before, both at the Department of Health and Social Security (D.H.S.S.) itself and in the rest of the country.

Interacting Forces

In short, the white-paper only makes any kind of sense if it is considered as the product of a complex bargaining process involving forces partly exogenous to the N.H.S. itself and partly indigenous. This is perhaps not so very different from the bargaining process by which decisions are reached in individual hospitals.[17] The interest in analysing it from this point of view is to see where the different parties have been prepared to compromise (and why) and what their "sticking-points" have been.

Here one of the most illuminating as well as controversial issues to examine is the membership of the new health authorities. The Consultative Document[18] proposed that the main criterion for selecting members of the new area health authorities should be "management ability". This proposal crystallised both professional and political opposition to the document. It was seen by the profession as an attempt to impose an unacceptable degree of managerial control, and led the B.M.A. to reiterate its call for "elected representation on the health authorities for the professions and the community at all levels of the N.H.S."[19] It also provided the main theme for the Labour Party's criticism in the House of Commons, echoed once again on the publication of the white-paper.[20]

One interesting aspect of this debate is that it has very little to do with political ideology. Although "good management" may appear to be a very Conservative slogan, it was the 1968 green-paper which emphasised the need for "strongly staffed management authorities". In short, the pressure for a more managerial approach has been persistent because it has come from the Whitehall machine.

In turn this pressure can only be understood if the N.H.S. is seen in the context of the trend towards a more managerial style of public administration. In 1967 the Maud Report on the Management of Local Government[21] criticised the involvement of amateur councillors in detailed decision-making; and it suggested a small, more professional management board, with a clerk chosen for his "managerial ability". In 1968 the Fulton Report on the Civil Service[22] criticised the amateurism of Civil Servants ill-equipped "to use new techniques of analysis, management and co-ordination". Far from being selected for any sort of special treatment, the N.H.S. is one of the last services to be given a managerial face-lift.

Power

However, in the case of the N.H.S. the argument is as much about power as about methods. The reason why Sir Keith Joseph wants a new structure of authorities is much the same as Mr. Richard Crossman's, though the former's instrument is nominated members while the latter's would be elected members.[23] Both are concerned to break the mould of existing patterns – notably in the allocation of resources – as established by the existing members, professional and lay, both at the regional-board and at the management-committee level. A new structure is seen as a way of preparing the way for a new set of priorities – with first priority, as Sir Keith Joseph's foreword to the white-paper emphasises, going to the non-acute services.

The main point of a managerially neat structure and hierarchy – running from the D.H.S.S. to the regional health authorities to the area health authorities to the districts – is therefore to create a machinery for the introduction of a new set of priorities and (hopefully) to monitor their adoption. The structure is not as neat as it might be. Partly this is because of exogenous constraints: local-government boundaries have not been drawn with the health services primarily in mind, with the result that the areas have in turn to be divided into districts which do not correspond to any local authorities. Partly, too, this is because of administrative problems: one of the reasons why the regions have steadily gained in power, as green-paper has succeeded green-paper, and the white-paper has succeeded the Consultative Document, is the sheer administrative problem of monitoring the activities of 72 area health authorities (excluding London) and finding suitably high-powered members. This task is obviously much simplified if limited to 14 regions.

Concessions

This interpretation helps to explain Sir Keith Joseph's pattern of concessions and non-concessions in his white-paper. He has made very few concessions which would weaken the ability of the centre to determine priorities in the allocation of resources. The various authorities will be appointed, not elected, though members will be chosen, in the revised version, "for their personal qualities", as distinct from their "management ability" (a diplomatic touch). 4 out of 15 members of the area health authorities will be appointed by the corresponding local authority. This is only one less than proposed in the 1970 green-paper, though this was criticised by the then Conservative spokesman on health – Lord Balniel – who said: "Personally I would prefer strengthening the professional representation and diminishing still further the Ministerial appointments."[24] However, unlike the Crossman green-paper but in line with the Robinson green-paper, there will be no quota of representatives of the authority's professional staff.

A possible explanation of this emphasis on a ministerially appointed majority could be that it represents a victory for the Treasury. The Treasury has always taken the view that since the N.H.S. spends the taxpayer's money, "a hundred per cent ministerial appointments were needed to get full financial control", as Harold Wilson records[25] in his account of the Crossman reform proposals. Hence the Crossman plans "had not been easy to get through". It may be that Sir Keith Joseph has made a concession to the Treasury point of view here. If so, he may in exchange have got both extra funds for the N.H.S.[26] and some significant concessions recorded in the white-paper. Thus "authorities will have freedom, within limits, to use funds allocated for capital expenditure to meet revenue expenditure and vice versa. Arrangements will also be worked out to enable unspent revenue allocations to be carried over from one year to the next."

A complementary explanation could be that Sir Keith Joseph himself wants to prevent the health professions from controlling the allocation of resources. The built-in tendency of all organisations is to perpetuate and accentuate existing patterns.[27] In the N.H.S. the powerful, established specialties tend to attract resources at the expense of the less prestigious or weaker ones: for example, the latest report of the Hospital Advisory Service[28] records that "It is still usual to find that new hospitals are being planned with far too few geriatric beds, on the assumption that the geriatrician and other staff will be content to take over old and inconvenient premises vacated by other specialties." To the extent that the policy of the D.H.S.S. is to divert resources to these less prestigious and weaker specialties, so it must resist pressure to allow the health professions themselves to control the allocation. However – and here again one can see the makings of a bargain – it is clear that in return the profession need have little fear about managerial interference with the *use* of resources once they have been allocated and even less about public pressure, given the shadowy role of the community health councils.

Quality of the Final Decision

To analyse policy-making as the product of bargaining, compromises, and deals does not, in itself, tell us anything about the quality of the final decision. It does, however, tell us something about the priorities of the policy-makers, and it suggests that it is a mistake to assess the products of policy-making – like the white-paper – on a once-and-for-all basis. The constellations of power which produce the policies – the interplay of forces between Government departments, professional pressure groups,[29] local authorities, and all the rest – survive individual decisions, and continue to affect their outcome. Specifically, most of the factors which have shaped the white-paper and which will shape the legislation will also affect the way in which the policy is implemented after 1974.

This analysis, if accepted, suggests that one of the chief tests which should be applied to the white-paper is not so much whether it has produced anything like an ideal solution – it patently has not – but whether it has produced what is an implementable solution capable of improvement on an on-going basis. Looking at the evolution of policy, it is clear that it is the product of conflicts of view and sometimes conflicts of interest: notably on the crucial point as to who allocates resources. To the extent that there are such differences and conflicts, a policy of gradualism is enforced on the policy-makers. There will always be some frictional costs in carrying out any change. The problem for policy-makers – and those who try to assess the outcome of the process – is to know whether the right balance has been struck between overestimating the frictional costs, and thus missing an opportunity for improvement, and underestimating the frictional costs, and thus creating a situation of opposition to evolving change.

I thank Prof. J. N. Morris and Dr. J. S. A. Ashley for their constructive criticism.

References

1. Department of Health and Social Security. National Health Service Reorganisation: England. Cmnd. 5055. H.M. Stationery Office, 1972.

2. Dror, Y. Public Policymaking Reexamined. San Francisco, 1968.

3. Simon, H. A. Administrative Behaviour. New York, 1965.

4. Lindblom, C. E. The Policy-Making Process. New Jersey, 1968.

5. Heclo, H. H. Br. J. polit. Sci. January 1972, 2, part 1, p. 83.

6. Rose, R. (editor) Policy-Making in Britain. London, 1969.

7. Cohen, M. D., March, J. G., Olsen, J. P. Admin. Sci. Q. March, 1972, 17, no. 1, p. 1.

8. Maddox, G. L. Med. Care, September/October, 1971, 9, no. 5, p. 439.

9. Parliamentary Debates, July 1, 1971, 820, no. 170.

10. Feiling, K. The Life of Neville Chamberlain. London, 1946.

11. Ministry of Health. The Administrative Structure of the Medical and Related Services in England and Wales. H.M. Stationery Office, 1968.

12. Department of Health and Social Security. The Future Structure of the National Health Service. H.M. Stationery Office, 1970.

13. Bray, J. Decision in Government. London, 1970.

14. Webb, B. Our Partnership. London, 1948.

15. Levin, P. H. Publ. Admin. Spring, 1972, 50.

16. Wildavsky, A. Publ. Admin. Rev. December, 1966, 26, no. 4, p. 292.

17. Strauss, A., et al. in The Hospital and its Negotiated Order in Decisions, Organisations and Society (edited by F. G. Castles, D. J. Murray, and D. C. Potter). Harmondsworth, 1971.

18. Department of Health and Social Security. National Health Service Reorganisation: Consultative Document. May, 1971.

19. Report by council to the Special Representative Meeting, Br. med. J. 1971, iii, suppl. p. 1.

20. Parliamentary Debates. Aug. 1, 1972, 842, no. 1168.

21. Committee on the Management of Local Government. Vol. I: Report. H.M. Stationery Office, 1967.

22. Committee on the Civil Service. Vol. I: Report. H.M. Stationery Office, 1968.

23. Crossman, R. *Times*, Aug. 9, 1972.

24. Parliamentary Debates. March 23, 1970, **798,** no. 85.

25. Wilson, H. The Labour Government 1964–1970. London, 1971.

26. Klein, R. *Lancet*, 1971, ii, 1306.

27. Downs, A. Inside Bureaucracy. Boston, 1967.

28. Hospital Advisory Service. Annual Report for the Year 1971. H.M. Stationery Office, 1972.

29. Eckstein, H. H. Pressure Group Politics. London, 1960.

46

Ideology, Class and the National Health Service

JOURNAL OF HEALTH POLITICS, POLICY
AND LAW
Fall 1979

For most of the thirty-odd years of its existence, the history of Britain's National Health Service (NHS) has been one of conflict within consensus.[1] There have been a number of issues which have provoked sharp differences either between the Labour and Conservative Parties or, more usually, between the medical profession and the government of the day. But, despite party clashes on such issues as prescription charges and despite periodic threats of mass resignations by the doctors over pay claims, the consensus about the basic structure and principles of the NHS has constrained and limited conflict.

There has, however, been one notable exception. This is the conflict, between 1974 and 1976, over the issue of pay beds in the NHS: i.e., the beds set aside in NHS hospitals for the treatment of the private, fee-paying patients of consultants. For this was a conflict which called into question – and indeed revolved around – the basic concordat on which the NHS was built. It was ideological in character, in that much of the argument reflected clashing perceptions about the moral and social basis of the health service. It brought into opposition, furthermore, the Labour Party and the trade-unions on the one hand, and the Conservative Party and the medical profession, on the other: a seemingly neat and symmetrical illustration of a conflict where disagreement about a specific health issue reflected a clash of class interests.

The two-year political battle over the pay beds issue is therefore of greater interest than the intrinsic importance of private practice within the NHS might suggest. Indeed, as this paper will seek to show, the pay beds issue became important not because it could be shown to have much impact on the day-to-day effectiveness, efficiency or even fairness of the service, but because it was linked to – and symbolic of – a number of more fundamental concerns involving the principles on which the NHS is built. The reason for analyzing the battle in detail is, therefore, that it is an opportunity to test theories about the nature of policy change in health services: the relative importance of exogenous, socio-structural factors and of factors endogenous to health care systems.[2] Further, the episode illustrates, in the British context, the emergence of a new set of policy actors, the trade-unions, in the health arena.[3] Lastly, the question of private practice and the NHS draws attention to some of the political problems created by the existence of a near-State monopoly of health care in a pluralistic, liberal democracy.

For ease of presentation, the first section of this paper will set out the basic facts about private practice and the NHS and the second section will give a brief account of the events in 1974 and 1976. Following sections will then examine the conceptual problems of analysis, the roles of the Labour Party, of the trade-unions and of the medical profession, while the conclusion will discuss the implications for the study of the politics of health.

Private Practice in the National Health Service

Private practice in British health care takes a number of forms. There are some doctors, insignificant in numbers, who are totally outside the NHS. There are other doctors, however, who have the right to engage in private practice once they have fulfilled their contractual obligations to the NHS. This category includes virtually all general practitioners and about half the hospital consultants. In turn, these may treat their private patients either in their own offices or in privately-owned hospitals or use the facilities specifically set aside in NHS hospitals. These are the so-called pay beds, established by the 1946 Act setting up the NHS.[4]

Determining the scale, and nature, of private practice is far from easy. There are no routinely collected statistics and hardly any special studies,[5] a fact that, in itself, suggests both low salience and small scale. But there are a number of sources from which it is possible to stitch together a general, if somewhat rough and ready, impression. Taking, first of all, the number of people covered by private insurance schemes, there was a fourfold increase in the 20 years between 1955 and 1975, largely because of the rise in group schemes organized by employers for their white-collar workers (from 585,000 to 2,315,000),[6] most of it in the period before 1970. In other words, one out of every 25 people in the population is covered by such a scheme and they paid out £52 million for private medical care in 1975, the equivalent of just over one percent of the national expenditure on the NHS. Additionally, of course, patients outside these schemes may have paid for private care out of their own pockets, but no satisfactory information is available about the extent of such transactions. The only available source, the Family Expenditure Survey,[7] suggests that the scale of such private spending on health care is insignificant in total (though, of course, it may be quite large in particular cases).

Turning to the other side of this equation, information about medical incomes from private practice is equally scarce and unsatisfactory – although crucially relevant when trying to assess the economic importance of this issue to the medical profession. Twenty years ago, in 1955/6, the Royal Commission on Doctors' and Dentists' Remuneration[8] carried out what still remains the most comprehensive survey of medical earnings. This showed that the average net income of part-time consultants with private practice was 20 percent higher than that of full-time consultants without this additional source of income – an excess that, however, rose to 43 percent for the highest decile. This differential does not appear to have changed greatly over time. In 1969/70, the average income of part-timers was 23 percent higher than that of full-timers,[9] while in 1971/2 the difference was 18 percent.[10] Given the problems involved in collecting and interpreting such data, it would be a mistake to try to make anything of the fluctuations over time; the safest conclusion would seem to be that, taking all consultants and ignoring differences between specialties, private practice adds roughly a fifth to the incomes of those engaged in it. For general practitioners, earnings from private practice and other fee-earning activities outside the NHS is more marginal still: in the early nineteen seventies, it added less than ten percent to their average income.[11] Even allowing for the possibility that some fees may not be declared (and the advantage of being able to offset earnings against tax-exempt expenses) the picture is consistent with the figures of fee payments from patients. The sums involved are only a very small proportion of all spending on health care in Britain.

Similarly, the pay beds themselves form only a small proportion of all NHS resources. In 1949, there were 6,647 pay beds in England (the numbers in Wales and Scotland are, relative to population served, smaller still and can therefore be ignored). Thereafter, the numbers declined steadily, if slowly, and in 1974, at the beginning of the pay bed crisis, there were 4,500.[12] However, the number of patients treated in these beds moved in the opposite direction. As a result of the general acceleration of turnover, it increased from 86,064 to 111,400, having reached a peak of 118,000 in 1972. Thus in 1974, pay beds represented just over one percent of all NHS beds, and the private patients treated in them represented two percent of all non-psychiatric cases handled in the NHS. No analysis is available of the patients by diagnosis or form of treatment, but the fact that the average length of stay in pay beds is shorter than that in either general medical or general surgical beds (7.4 days, as against 13.1 and 8.8 days respectively in 1974)[13] confirms the accepted view that private patients tend to use these facilities for routine procedures, rather than for long-stay conditions or major operations.

In all this, one of the most significant facts, in view of the political crisis which broke in 1974 and which is described in the following section, is precisely the paucity of information. This suggests that private practice was not only marginal to the NHS in its scale of operations and finance (as indicated by the available data) but was also marginal administratively and politically. And while it could be argued that the lack of information was in the interests of those who benefit from private practice (the doctors) or from not stirring up the issue (the administrators), the same cannot be said about the opponents of private practice. In other words, lack of information would seem to suggest lack of political salience in the years before 1974, a point which will be analyzed further when the reasons for the sudden eruption of this issue are discussed.

The Political Battle, 1974–1976

In February 1974 the Labour Party fought and won, albeit on a minority vote, a national election. Its manifesto[14] included the following short paragraph: "A Labour Government will revise and expand the National Health Service; abolish prescription charges; introduce free family planning; phase out private practice from the hospital service and transform the area health authorities into democratic bodies." In the subsequent October election of the same year, which confirmed Labour in office, the commitment became more specific still: the Labour Government, the manifesto declared, "has started its attack on queue-jumping by increasing the charge for private pay beds in National Health Service hospitals and is now working out a scheme for phasing private beds out of these hospitals."[15]

In between these two manifestos, the political climate within the NHS had changed dramatically. Starting at one of the London Teaching Hospitals, Charing Cross, rank and file members of the National Union of Public Employees (representing mainly the semi-skilled and unskilled workers in the NHS) took industrial action against pay beds. NUPE members refused to serve meals for, or otherwise help in the care of, private patients. Other unions, notably the Confederation of Health Service Employees, and staff at other hospitals followed suit. Although it was never quite clear just how much industrial action was being taken at how many different hospitals, the issue of private beds was overnight put on the front pages of the newspapers and onto the television bulletins – helped by the fact, perhaps, that Charing Cross Hospital happened to be conveniently accessible to Fleet Street and the television company headquarters. In reply, the British Medical Association's Central Committee for Hospital Medical Services, representing the consultants, threatened a work-to-rule unless the Secretary of State for Social Services, Mrs. Barbara Castle, took immediate action to restore normal working and to rescind the union ban on admission to private beds.[16]

So, in the summer of 1974, the battle lines were drawn. And perhaps the most important outcome was to force Mrs. Castle to take a public stand and to declare her position on the issue. After long negotiations between the Secretary and the representatives of the medical profession and of the unions (probably the first occasion when all three had met around the negotiating table) an agreement of sorts was worked out. The unions agreed to call off their industrial action and the consultants withdrew their threat. The question of pay beds was referred to a working party already appointed to negotiate the details of a new contract for hospital consultants. The Secretary of State condemned the use of industrial action to compel policy change in the NHS but endorsed the aims being pursued by the trade-unions. Indeed, in doing so she explicitly stressed the ideological aspects of the debate: "The issue before us is whether the facilities of the NHS, which are supposed to be available only on the principle of medical priority, should contain facilities that are available on the different principle of ability to pay. We say that those two principles are incompatible in the NHS."[17] So, in effect, the trade-union protesters had asserted their right to take part in the policy debate, raised the emotional temperature of the dispute, and persuaded the Secretary of State to define the issue in terms which made it central to the Labour Party's vision of itself as a crusader for social justice. The religious metaphor is apt, as Mrs. Castle was to point out on a subsequent occasion: "Intrinsically the National Health Service is a church. It is the nearest thing to the embodiment of the Good Samaritan that we have in any aspect of our public policy. What would we say of a person who argued that he could only serve God properly if he had pay pews in his church?"[18]

The next major step in the battle came with the publication, in August 1975, of a consultative document by the Government outlining proposals for the separation of private practice from NHS hospitals.[19] This proposed a dual strategy. First, legislation was to be introduced to revoke the authorization of pay bed facilities in the NHS and set a specific date for completing the process of separation. Second, legislation was to be introduced to establish a licensing system for the private sector designed to ensure "that the total provision for private medical care after pay beds are phased out shall not materially exceed . . . that which obtained within and outside the NHS in March 1974." In short, the total size of the private hospital sector was to be permanently frozen.

The consultative paper appeared at a time when the medical profession was already in conflict with the government over other issues, in particular, the negotiations over a new contract for consultants. The threat to pay beds also produced a specific reaction from the medical profession. By the beginning of December 1975 The Secretary of State faced a militant profession; the Council of the British Medical Association had recommended that senior hospital doctors should limit their work by caring for emergencies and existing patients only, and was collecting undated resignations.[20] This coincided with an on-going pay dispute with the junior hospital doctors, who had already introduced an emergencies-only rule, and produced a counter-threat from NUPE to blockade pay beds in retaliation against any consultants who obeyed the BMA call. On the assumption that all those involved in the battle actually meant what they said, the NHS appeared to be on the point of total collapse. So, not surprisingly, there followed an intervention by Prime Minister Harold Wilson and a series of meetings at No. 10 Downing Street with the medical profession. Lord Goodman, who had previously acted both as the Prime Minister's solicitor and as legal adviser to the medical profession, was called in as a mediator, reputedly to the dismay of Mrs. Castle, and produced an acceptable compromise formula which became the basis of the subsequent legislation embodying the new concordat between the government and the medical profession on private practice.

The Goodman compromise,[21] like the subsequent legislation, was based on the explicit recognition of two principles: first, that private beds and facilities should be separated from the NHS; second, that the government made a formal commitment to the principle that private practice should be maintained in Britain, and that doctors should be entitled to work both privately and in NHS establishments. The second principle was no more than a reiteration of the Government's acceptance of private practice as a fact of life. Indeed, the Secretary of State had maintained throughout the crisis that it was no part of her intentions to try to abolish private practice, as distinct from separating it from the NHS. The medical profession, however, was skeptical on this point and its doubts had been further reinforced by the Labour Party conference in the autumn of 1975. This had carried a NUPE resolution calling for the eventual abolition of all private practice and the prohibition of all private insurance schemes, against the advice of Mrs. Barbara Castle.[22]

More specifically, the Goodman compromise showed a number of important changes in the proposals put forward in Mrs. Castle's consultative document, all designed to provide concessions and reassurance to the medical profession. Only 1,000 (under a quarter) of the private beds were to be phased out immediately. Decisions about phasing out the rest were to be taken not by the Secretary of State but by an independent Board with half its four members drawn from the medical profession and the other half appointed after consultations with the trade-unions and other interested parties, and the casting vote held by an independent chairman. The Board, to quote the Secretary of State, would be guided by the following criteria in phasing out the pay beds: "that there should be a reasonable demand for private medicine in the area of the country served by a particular hospital; that sufficient accommodation or facilities existed in the area for the reasonable operation of private medicine, and that all reasonable steps had been, or were being taken to provide those alternative beds and facilities." No limit was set on the future size of the private sector. No date was set for the completion of the phasing out operation.

In the event, the Government's legislative proposals followed the Goodman concordat almost to the letter. The Parliamentary Bill, published in April 1976, filled out some of the details left open by the Goodman agreement but did not touch any of the principles: for example, it gave the Board power to license the construction of all new private hospitals with more than 100 beds in London and more than 75 beds in the rest of the country, but did not specify any maximum. The medical profession took the view that, while it was still opposed to the principle of the Bill and felt free to campaign against it, the legislation represented the most acceptable form of rape. The Government took the view that, while it would have preferred the more radical approach of its consultative document, it was committed to the Goodman compromise and was not prepared to make any further concessions either to the doctors or to the trade-unions.

The final Act of Parliament showed few changes from the initial Bill, and none affecting the main architecture of its provisions. This was despite the prolonged and well-orchestrated rearguard action fought by the Conservative Party on behalf of the medical interests. The Conservatives opposed the Bill both in principle and in detail, both in the Commons and in the Lords. No sooner had it been introduced than a body of advisers representing the BMA and other professional organisations was set up to brief the Conservative spokesmen, who tabled 400 amendments and a number of new clauses during its passage through Parliament. A rota of advisers organised by a member of the BMA Secretariat was "in constant attendance at all the Parliamentary sittings."[23] But only a few, minor concessions were wrung out of Mr. David Ennals who, by this time, had succeeded Mrs. Castle as Secretary of State, following the change of Prime Minister from Mr. Harold Wilson to Mr. James Callaghan. At one stage it seemed possible that the Conservatives might succeed in killing the measure by exhausting the available parliamentary time. However, Ministers – their backs stiffened by threats of industrial action from the trade-unions, should the Bill be abandoned –[24] insisted on pushing their measure through, cutting short the parliamentary discussion by means of the guillotine (a procedural measure for time-tabling the debate).

The Government's insistence on sticking to the Goodman compromise was reflected also in its attitude towards its own supporters. Ministers resisted the repeated attempts of the Labour Left – backed by the unions – to give the measure more bite: in particular, to fix a date by which all pay beds would have had to be phased out. So, in the end, the Government could rightly claim to have stuck to the Goodman compromise and to have been totally faithful to the concordat reached with the medical profession. And the medical profession – though frustrated in its desire to defeat the principle embodied in the Government's legislation – could reflect that, in practice, it could look forward to the continuance of private practice within the NHS for the indefinite future, if on a reduced and perhaps slowly contracting scale.

The Problems of Analysis

The above account of the 1974 to 1976 crisis is by no means a comprehensive history of events; it simply presents the context of analysis in order to define the questions which require further investigation. Some of these are general in kind, and applicable to all fields of policy study. How, for example, do we identify the precipitating factors which convert a dormant political issue into an active one? Others are more specific to the study of health services. How, for instance, do we account for the emergent influence of the trade-unions during the crisis, and does this mark a shift in the balance of power within the health care system to the disadvantage of the medical profession? In turn, does such a shift (assuming that there was one) reflect a more general structural shift in society?

In addition to such *political process* questions, Britain's 1974 to 1976 crisis also raises some puzzles about *policy substance*. So far little attention has been paid to the arguments used in the debate about private practice and pay beds. But, as we shall see when we turn to them in detail in the following sections, the debate was not exclusively ideological in character. It cannot be reduced to the simple symmetry of a clash between those who were opposed to private practice out of a general dislike of the market economy (reinforced by a specific dislike of the commercial element in medicine) and those who saw private enterprise as desirable, whether in health care or elsewhere. That, of course, was an important element in the conflict and certainly helps to explain the vocabulary of the consequent rhetorical babble. But equally, some more practical policy considerations were also involved, in particular, the question of the extent to which comprehensive health care planning is feasible while there is a private sector outside governmental control.

To analyze these questions further, it is perhaps useful to think of the policy drama in terms of the inter-action between three groups of actors: the Labour Government, the trade-unions and the medical profession. Each of these groups has its own stage or arena, where its internal differences are acted out. But there is also a large stage where the three groups confront each other, and act out their differences. That dialogue, however, can only be interpreted in the knowledge both of the strains and tensions within each group and of the audience for whose sympathy they are competing.

The Labour Government

In the 1974 to 1976 debates, Labour ministers tended to take it for granted that opposition to private practice within the NHS had always been an article of faith for the party. The 1946 decision of Aneurin Bevan to permit pay beds and part-time private practice was seen as a tactical concession, a necessary sacrifice of principle to expediency without which it might not have been possible to launch the NHS.[25] It was this which had helped Bevan to split the medical profession, by buying the support of the hospital specialists and thus isolating the general practitioners.[26] But Bevan's tactics should not be confused with Bevan's aims, it was argued in the nineteen seventies, and therefore Labour Ministers were only carrying out the original intentions of the architect of the NHS. The 1976 legislation, seen in this light, simply represented the delayed implementation of what had always been the Labour Party's aims. Immanent policy had simply become explicit action.

In fact, the history of the emergence of private practice as an active political commitment by the Labour Party is more complex and more puzzling. Effectively, it submerged for more than 20 years after 1946. Bevan's compromise was criticized by a number of Labour backbench MPs during the 1946 debates, and the issue was subsequently kept alive (if only symbolically) by the Socialist Medical Association. The SMA periodically moved motions at the annual Labour Party conference directed against private practice. But these produced little more than vague pledges, on behalf of the leadership, to take "steps to combat queue jumping for hospital beds," in the words of the 1964 Manifesto.[27] In 1967 the Labour Minister of Health, Mr. Kenneth Robinson, reduced the number of pay beds (which had been much under-utilized) in agreement with the medical profession, in return for lifting the limit on the fees charged by consultants. Even this, however, was not seen as an ideological move – either by the Labour Party or by the medical profession – and only produced mild dissenting noises from some Conservative MPs.[28]

The puzzle of the emergence of private practice as an issue is compounded when the history of pay beds is compared with that of prescription charges. Ideologically, the latter was far more highly charged. It was undoubtedly one of the Labour Party's articles of faith that health services should be free at the point of delivery. This, after all, was one of the issues over which Aneurin Bevan had resigned from the Labour Government of 1951. Prescription charges were thus anathema, and the 1964 Labour Government duly abolished them soon after taking office. Two years later, however, they were reintroduced in the wake of an economic crisis. This, in turn, provoked a strong reaction from the Party activists. Of the 30 resolutions submitted about the NHS to the 1969 Labour Party Conference, 20 called for the abolition of prescription charges. Only six called for the abolition of private practice or beds in the NHS.[29] Moreover, this pattern was by no means exceptional,[30] throughout the nineteen fifties and 'sixties, prescription charges were a much more salient and emotive issue for the Labour Party's rank and file activists than private practice and pay beds. Yet when another Labour Government was returned to office in 1974, it was the phasing out of private beds – not the abolition of prescription charges – which was put on the political agenda and carried into execution, although both commitments had appeared in the election manifesto.

Then why was priority given to the issue of private practice? One answer might be that, in the nineteen seventies, private practice within the NHS had grown in scale and therefore importance. But to judge from the evidence already presented about the growth of private practice, this does not appear to have been the case; if there was any increase, it was incremental and marginal. Alternatively, of course, the explanation might be that although private practice had not increased to any extent, knowledge about its impact had – thus transforming perceptions of the problem, if not the configuration of the problem itself.

There is at least some evidence in support of this latter interpretation. In 1971/2, the Employment and Social Services Sub-Committee of the

Parliamentary Expenditure Committee carried out an inquiry into NHS facilities for private patients.[31] And the Labour majority on this Sub-Committee used the opportunity to direct attention to the abuses (as they saw it) of private practice within the NHS – although their conclusions were overturned by the Conservative majority on the main Public Expenditure Committee. The findings of the Sub-Committee are interesting in that they both encapsulated past criticisms of private practice and anticipated the main themes of Labour spokesmen during the 1974 to 1976 debates.

Private practice in the NHS was indicted on a number of counts. In the Sub-Committee's view, it permitted "queue-jumping for non-medical reasons, allowing patients to by-pass the waiting-lists for reasons that have nothing to do with their medical conditions." It was unfair on junior hospital doctors, nurses and technicians "used for private practice purposes and without willing consent." It led to "dual standards of service" within the NHS. It encouraged the most highly skilled consultants to congregate in those parts of the country – notably London – with the greatest scope for building up a private practice rather than with the most urgent medical needs.

In all this, there was general agreement among the witnesses appearing before the Sub-Committee that there might be *some* abuse. Even the Department of Health officials and the representatives of the medical profession, who resolutely defended the status quo, conceded that some consultants might exploit both patients and staff. The real question, therefore, was whether the scale of such abuses was such as to balance the advantages of private practice and to justify the political costs of change. The advantages, it was argued in evidence to the Committee, were that private pay beds ensured that consultants were on duty in NHS hospitals – instead of dashing off to private clinics – and that private patients introduced a more exigent type of consumer into the NHS, so creating pressure to improve standards.

In practice, the Sub-Committee was never able to draw up a balance sheet. It received a variety of anecdotal evidence about abuse from junior doctors, nurses and trade-unions, but no firm evidence about the scale of the problem. A questionnaire sent out by the Royal College of Nursing, designed to elicit whether consultants deliberately built up their NHS waiting lists in order to persuade their patients to pay for private treatment, produced only five examples of "queue-jumping."[32] Yet, interestingly, this lack of evidence, and the subsequent decision by the Conservative-majority of the Expenditure Committee to repudiate the Sub-Committee's critical comments, did not prevent the report from gaining wide currency: its authority was, for example, frequently invoked by Labour speakers in the 1974 to 1976 debates. Even though there had been no change in the actual situation within the NHS, and even though no extra information had become available, the private practice issue had acquired a new political salience in the context of the Labour Party at any rate.[33]

But salience does not explain action, though it may help to account for the appearance of the issue on the agenda. Once again, there is the already-noted contrast between private practice and prescription charges to point up the puzzle. And the puzzle can only be resolved by placing the issue of private practice in the larger context of the political and economic situation in which the in-coming Labour Government found itself in 1974. It is when policy-making is seen as the product of political pushes and economic constraints that the actions taken by Labour Ministers fall into a coherent pattern. On the one hand, there was the inevitable pressure on any in-coming Government, particularly strong in the case of an activist Administration of the Left, to do something to satisfy the expectations of its supporters. On the other hand, there was the fact that the Government had inherited a distressing economic situation, where both unemployment and inflation were rising against the background of a rapidly increasing balance of payments deficit.

The Secretary of State for Social Services, Mrs. Barbara Castle, and her Minister of State, Dr. David Owen, were therefore in something of a dilemma. Their ability to improve the NHS, in terms of increasing the available resources, was severely constrained by economic circumstances and by their own decision to give priority to raising the wages and salaries of employees, as distinct from improving the scope or scale of service provision.[34] Yet they somehow had to satisfy the expectations of their own followers and, in particular, of the trade-unions: for the foundations of the Labour Government's policies, in the period 1974 to 1976, was the understanding that the unions would accept wage restraint in return for priority being given to spending on the social services – the so-called Social Contract.[35] The tactical problem for Ministers was therefore how best to make the maximum political impact at the minimum expense.

Given this context, the decision to press ahead with the issue of pay beds rather than prescription charges followed logically – if not inevitably. Abolishing prescription charges would have been expensive, and immediately and unmistakably so. Phasing out pay beds had no visible cost consequences. There was much argument in the parliamentary debates about the spending implications of the Government's policies, but no conclusion since the income foregone from private patients had to be offset against the expenditures generated by them, and it was far from clear what the net impact on the NHS's budget would be.[36] In short, the decision to phase out pay beds can be interpreted as an attempt to satisfy the ideological demands on Labour Ministers at the cheapest price (although it must be stressed that a price which may be low in terms of one unit of analysis may be very high when the currency is changed: thus the pay beds was a "cheap" issue in public expenditure terms, but "expensive" in terms of its impact on the government's relations with the medical profession).

Other factors were also involved, some endogenous to the NHS and others exogenous to it. In the former category comes the emphasis placed by Labour Ministers on the need to redistribute resources – both of manpower and of plant – within the NHS,[37] both geographically and as between different sectors of health care. The system of part-time consultants with private practice was seen as an obstacle to policy implementation. It tended to encourage doctors to choose those areas and specialties with the best prospects of private practice. Neither the Government's tactics, nor the medical profession's reaction, therefore make sense unless both are seen in the context of the simultaneous negotiations that were going on between them to devise a new consultant contract. In these negotiations (more fully discussed in the section below dealing with the attitudes and role of the medical profession) the Government's concern was mainly to change the incentives so as to encourage full-time commitment to the NHS and thus discourage private practice. So the concern about pay beds in particular, and private practice in general, can be seen as reflecting both political and managerial considerations. In particular, it reflected the concern to secure the rational allocation of resources within the NHS that had already provided the intellectual justification for the administrative reorganization scheme introduced by the Conservative Government in 1974.[38] In other words, the egalitarian ideology of the Labour Party was married to the planning ideology of DHSS administrators.

One of the most important factors exogenous to the NHS in the pay beds issue was the personal history of the Secretary of State, Mrs. Castle. In the 'fifties she, like Harold Wilson, had been one of the "Bevanites," both a personal and political disciple of Aneurin Bevan. Like her Cabinet colleague, Michael Foote, she owed her influence partly to the personal backing of the Prime Minister[39] and partly to the massive support given to her by the party activists in the elections to the Labour Party's National Executive. Moreover, she had a past to live down. In the last days of the 1964 to 1970 Labour Government, she had been responsible for introducing a bill to regulate industrial relations which had antagonized the trade-unions and split the Labour Party.[40] Politically, it was therefore particularly important for her to avoid another such confrontation if she was to maintain her reputation as a radical.

The history of Mrs. Castle's lost battle with the trade-unions in 1969 is the key to another, and more crucial, factor. This is the role of the trade-unions in influencing government policy generally and shaping the decisions of the 1974 to 1976 Labour Administration specifically. It was the trade-unions, as we have seen, whose rank and file membership started industrial action against pay beds in 1974 and thus precipitated Mrs. Castle's decision to translate the manifesto commitment into immediate policy action. No account of the 1974 to 1976 crisis can thus make sense without considering the transformed role (no less a phrase will do) of the trade-unions in the 'seventies.

The Trade-Unions

The 1974 Labour Government took office after an election largely fought over the issue of a national strike by the miners' union.[41] The election had been called by the previous Conservative Government in an attempt to assert its own authority by invoking the popular mandate as against union power. The failure of the Conservative Government thus opened the way for the Labour Government to design its overall strategy on the principle that government could effectively only be carried out with the cooperation of the trade-unions. The industrial relations legislation introduced by the Conservatives, and bitterly opposed by the unions, was repealed. The Labour Government's economic program hinged on the support of the unions. All in all, therefore, the period 1974 to 1976 was characterised by the increasing incorporation of the unions into the government decision-making process, an explicit acknowledgment of a shift in the balance of social power.

Within the NHS, too, the unions (as distinct from the traditional professional organizations like the BMA or the Royal College of Nursing) were growing in both numbers and influence. In line with trends in the United States and other countries,[42] the proportion of unionized workers in the health industry had increased. It has been estimated that the overall proportion rose from two-fifths in 1948 to three-fifths in 1974,[43] so that by the latter year the NHS was more highly unionized than the British labor force as a whole, only 50 percent of whose members belong to unions. But this estimate conceals the real significance of the rise: its concentration in the late nineteen sixties and early nineteen seventies. This comes out dramatically in Figure 1, which shows the membership trend of the Confederation of Health Service Employees (COHSE). This is the only union whose membership – partly nurses, partly ancillary workers – is concentrated exclusively in the NHS, and is therefore the only reliable source of figures about the unionization of the service.[44] Between 1956 and 1966, the membership of COHSE rose by a mere 16,000 members, a rise of 32 percent. Between 1966 and 1976, the rise was 147 percent. There was a similar explosion in the membership of the National Union of Public Employees (NUPE) over the same period,

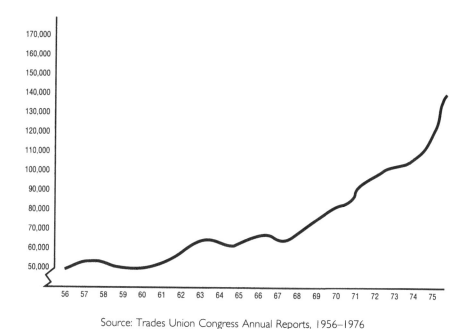

Source: Trades Union Congress Annual Reports, 1956–1976

FIGURE 1.   Membership of the Confederation of Health Service Employees, 1956–1976

thus confirming the trend (although it is impossible to put a precise figure on what happened in the NHS since a high but uncertain proportion of NUPE's membership is in the local government sector).[45]

So here there would appear to be striking evidence of growing militancy in the NHS, particularly among the least skilled workers. The nurses recruited by COHSE, for example, tended to be concentrated among those with the least prestigious professional qualifications and in the least popular sectors of the NHS, such as mental care and long-stay hospitals. It is tempting, therefore, to push the point one step further and to talk about growing self-awareness and militancy among what might be called (somewhat imprecisely) the working-class of the NHS, in contrast to the long-established and organized professionals.

But what might be called the radicalization of the labor force thesis, though it fits in snugly with the rank and file action about pay beds in 1974, requires qualification. If there was any radicalization, the evidence suggests that it was instrumental rather than ideological. In other words, NHS workers were getting more assertive about pay. In 1967 the National Board for Prices and Incomes published a report,[46] which suggested that, in order to improve the traditionally very low rates of pay in the NHS, local productivity schemes should be introduced. Thus the national pay bargaining system was supplemented by a local system of negotiation. One result, therefore, was to give local union officials and shop-stewards a direct incentive to recruit more members, while the members themselves could see direct results from adopting a more assertive stance towards management.[47] A further result was that rates of pay in the NHS, relative to other occupations, began to improve, particularly among manual workers.[48] The process of growing militancy over pay culminated in the 1973 strike of ancillary workers against the then Government's incomes policy: a national demonstration of industrial power, in contrast to the more sporadic and largely verbal protests that had marked earlier disputes. Militancy paid dividends for both union members and union leaders. It brought better pay for the former and more members for the latter. Thus growing union assertiveness was also associated with growing competition between the unions involved in the NHS. The NHS even now is much less highly unionized than the rest of the public sector: its 60 percent unionization rate compares with figures of 90 percent in central and 86 percent in local government. It thus offers an attractive recruiting ground. In particular, there was no clear demarcation line between COHSE and NUPE, and these unions competed not only against each other but also against bodies like the Royal College of Nursing, since one of the aims of the union movement was to exclude professional organizations from wage negotiations.[49] Militancy could thus be seen by the union leaders as a form of advertising – a recruiting campaign, in effect.

The situation in 1974 can therefore be best described as one in which there was scope for action by radical elements in the NHS labor force, rather than one which the labor force as such had been radicalized in any ideological sense. Indeed, given the composition of that labor force, with its high proportion of women and part-timers,[50] this is not surprising. Consistent with this interpretation, the lead in directing attention to the pay beds issue was taken by the National and Local Government Officers' Association – with a relatively small number of members (about 80,000) in the NHS – representing chiefly white-collar administrators. It was NALGO which moved a resolution calling for the "abolition of all part-time posts and the abolition of private pay beds" at the 1973 meeting of the Trades Union Congress.[51] This was the first time that the pay beds issue had been given prominence at a TUC conference – which, like the Labour Party, had previously always concentrated its ideological fire on prescription charges. Subsequently, the extrusion of private practice from the NHS became official TUC policy.[52]

There is a further piece of evidence to support the interpretation that the industrial action taken in 1974 should be seen as reflecting the views of self-selected activists rather than a general groundswell among the union rank and file. Later, in April 1976, the British United Provident Association (representing independent hospitals) commissioned a public opinion survey[53] as part of its campaign against the Government's bill. This indicated that rather more trade-unionists (42 percent) were in favor of keeping pay beds than were in favor of their removal (25 percent). Again, it is clear that the industrial action was concentrated in those hospitals, particularly London teaching hospitals, where the provision of pay beds was particularly visible: where there was, in one way or another, some tangible evidence of private patients being treated differently (if only in terms of accommodation and food) from NHS patients. In short, action may have sprung from a down to earth sense of unfairness (combined perhaps with resentment towards consultants) rather than ideological considerations.

So, in effect, a spontaneous but limited rank and file protest forced the trade-union leaders to activate what had been a long-standing, but dormant, attitude: an implicit policy bias became an explicit policy commitment. Given the competition for members, it was clearly not in the interests of any one leader to resist the growing militancy; rather, each had an incentive to put himself at the head of it. Once again, however, the puzzle remains why the trade-unions pursued this issue rather than that of prescription charges. One explanation could be that the perceived "unfairness" of pay beds was less their effect on patients than their impact on staff: that the system allowed consultants to increase their incomes at the expense of the supporting staff, who contributed their work but did not receive any rewards. In contrast, the deterrent effect of prescription charges, to the extent that it exists, is less visible because it is limited to precisely those patients who (by definition) are kept outside the NHS system as a result. Another explanation, of course, may be that symbolic actions are not the monopoly of governments. To the extent that the trade-unions realized that there was little chance of securing the abolition of prescription charges, there may have been a displacement effect, and the need for a symbolic ideological victory may have been satisfied by taking up the issue of pay beds.

The Medical Profession

So far the recurring theme of this inquiry has been why an issue so marginal in its impact on the operations of the NHS as that of pay beds should have become the cause of so prolonged and so bitter a political conflict. Granting that the Labour Government and the trade-unions had determined to act, it would seem redundant to seek any elaborate explanations for the resistance of the medical profession. Straightforward economic self-interest would appear to be the answer: the medical profession was defending its income in defending pay beds.

But this explanation requires qualification and elaboration. Taking the medical profession as a whole, the evidence already discussed indicates that the income from private practice is marginal (though allowance must be made for the possibility that the official figures under-state the cash flow to doctors). Further, the proportion, though not the numbers, of hospital consultants with part-time contracts entitling them to undertake private practice has been declining: by 1973 it had fallen below the 50 percent mark.[54] For most of the profession, therefore, private practice would seem to be a source of pocket-money, at best, with only a small minority making large incomes.

To understand the battle over pay beds it is therefore once again necessary to put this particular dispute in a wider context. In the first place, it came at a time when the medical profession already felt its standards of living to be threatened, both relatively and absolutely. Rapid inflation was eating away the value of earnings, while the incomes and tax policies of the 1974 Labour Government deliberately discriminated against all higher-income groups. At the same time, the use of the militant tactics by other health service employees was improving their relative position; soon after coming into office in 1974 the Labour Government made generous pay awards to both nurses and ancillary workers. So, as Table 1 shows, medical practitioners – and in particular the top 25 percent of them – were slipping down the earnings hierarchy between 1970 and 1975, an example of relative deprivation in terms of their own expectations. Moreover, absolute incomes were falling: according to the 1977 report of the Review Body on Doctors' and Dentists' Remuneration,[55] the living standards of general practitioners and consultants fell by 20 percent between April 1975 and April 1977.

Second, the battle over pay beds coincided (as already indicated) with the negotiations over a new contract for consultants. These negotiations had been initiated in 1974 by the profession itself. The aim was to create a system of rewards which would relate earnings more closely to effort, either by fee-for-service payments or by basing salaries on a specified working week, with extra payments in return for extra duties performed. The fee-for-service approach was ruled out of court by the Secretary of State from the start of the negotiations. But talks about a "closed contract," with extra payments for extra duties, continued. The Labour Government also saw this as an opportunity to change the bias of the payments system in favor of full-time consultants, and so to create added incentives for them to move into the shortage specialties and deprived parts of the country. It therefore proposed to offer a new form of incentive payments, "career structure supplements," for which only full-timers would be eligi-

TABLE I. Movements in Earnings, 1970–75 (full-time men only).

	Medical practitioners[a]	Nurses	Ancillary staff (NHS)	All manual workers
Lower quartile				
1970	100 (£34.2)	50.6	51.5	60.8
1975	100 (£66.8)	58.2	60.6	66.0
Percent increase				
1970–75	95.3	124.9	130.1	112.0
Median quartile				
1970	100 (£50.0)	42.4	41.2	51.2
1975	100 (£92.0)	56.0	52.4	57.7
Percent increase				
1970–75	84.0	142.9	134.0	107.8
Upper quartile				
1970	100 (£82.3)	29.2	30.7	38.0
1975	100 (£146.9)	43.5	40.0	43.9
Percent increase				
1970–75	78.5	166.3	132.4	106.1

a. The index is based on the gross weekly earnings (=100) of medical practitioners; their actual earnings are shown in parentheses.
Source: New Earnings Survey for 1970 and 1975 (adapted from R. Klein, "Incomes: vive la différence," British Medical Journal, July 10, 1976).

ble.[56] These supplements, it was proposed, would replace distinction awards, criticized on the grounds that they reinforced and preserved the traditional values, structure and distribution of specialists.[57]

In the outcome, these negotiations dragged on for more than a year before being abandoned in the face of the medical profession's opposition: confirmation of the thesis that while the medical profession may not be powerful enough to insist on its favored system of payments, it has veto power over what it regards as threatening changes.[58] But as long as the negotiations continued, they reinforced the medical profession's suspicion that the Government's policy over pay beds was only the beginning of a campaign to make it impossible for NHS consultants to engage in private practice of any kind. And while Labour Ministers denied that they were trying to compel consultants to withdraw from private practice, the contract proposals were self-evidently an attempt to devise a new system of rewards designed to encourage full-time commitment to the NHS. This strengthened the conviction of the medical profession that the Labour Government was repudiating the basis of the 1946 NHS agreement and was moving from a mixed economy towards a State monopoly.

The third element in the situation – mirroring the position among the trade-unions – was competition between different bodies claiming to represent the interests of the NHS consultants. The British Medical Association was under increasing attack throughout the period from the Regional Hospital Consultants and Specialists Association, which argued that the BMA had concentrated on promoting the interests of general practitioners at the expense of hospital doctors. Already at the beginning of 1974, long before the pay bed crisis broke, some 900 consultants had resigned from the BMA to join the RHCSA.[59] So the rival spokesmen for the consultants had a direct interest in competitive militancy: to show their zeal in defense of the medical profession's interests.

Given all these considerations, it is not surprising that the medical profession's reactions to the Government's pay beds policy appears disproportionate to the immediate financial interests involved. The policy was seen as the first step towards turning the medical profession into full-time State employees, precisely the fear which had inspired resistance to Aneurin Bevan's proposals in 1946.[60] As it was, the dependence of doctors on the NHS for most of their income appeared to be leading to a progressive decline in their incomes; moreover, they were clearly doing much worse than their peers in the Common Market countries like Germany or France.[61] But there was also the fear that total dependence on a state monopoly employer, through the gradual elimination of private practice, would lead to a further deterioration in the financial position of the medical profession. In reality, private practice in Britain may be economically insignificant, and certainly does not offer the medical profession an alternative form of financial support. In the profession's mythology, however, it embodied the doctor's traditional image of himself as an independent entrepreneur, rather than a salaried civil servant.[62]

So far all the factors analyzed would seem to be consistent with the mobilization of the medical profession against the Government's pay beds policy, culminating in threats of sanctions. The Government, it would thus seem, had to retreat in the face of a united profession and to make the concessions embodied in the Goodman compromise. But, as in the case of the trade-unions, the picture of ideological commitment and single-mindedness is overly simple. In practice, the Government did not face a homogeneous or united medical profession, as became clear in the wake of the Goodman concordat.

Following the concordat, the BMA's Central Committee for Hospital Medical Services organized a ballot of all consultants,[63] to get their views about the agreement and about the profession's future tactics. This confirmed the results of an earlier ballot, held in 1974,[64] by showing a 73 percent majority of consultants to be opposed to the principle of separation. But only a minority of consultants were willing to fight for the maintenance of this principle to the point of being prepared to resign from the NHS. Sixty-three percent declared themselves ready to accept the Goodman compromise. The replies to the questionnaires showed some interesting differences between the various specialities and parts of the country, indicative of the heterogeneity of views within the medical profession. The proportion of consultants in favor of the Goodman compromise ranged from 60 percent in England to 88 percent in Scotland (where the number of pay beds is negligible), from 83 percent for full-time consultants to less then half for part-timers, from 81 percent for specialists in pathology (where there is virtually no scope for private practice) to 49 percent for surgeons (where there are the greatest opportunities). Altogether only 54 percent of eligible consultants took part in the ballot, a figure which suggests that the issue was less salient for most doctors than the rhetoric of the official leadership might have suggested.

The militants among the consultants saw the results of the ballot as a disaster. In any negotiations with the Government, one of them argues bleakly, doctors "would be like inmates of a concentration camp meeting to discuss their future." This was, another declared, "a black day for the whole of hospital medicine."[65] But although the verbal campaign against the principle of the Government's measure continued, both in and outside Parliament, the threat of sanctions or mass resignations was withdrawn. The government had won its symbolic victory and the profession had won its practical safeguards. The real battle was over, despite the oratorical fireworks that were to follow in parliament.

Politics, Policy and Health Care Systems

One clear conclusion to emerge from this analysis of the 1974 to 1976 crisis over pay beds in Britain is that to study the politics of health care issues in isolation is to risk mystification or misinterpretation. It is to support the conclusion that: "We have political struggles in the arena termed health, but not a politics of health."[66] There are no factors endogenous to the health care system which can explain the sudden emergence of this issue. Nothing in the situation affecting pay beds and private practice had changed in 1974, except for the political environment in which decisions about the NHS were made. The crisis is therefore an example of the importance of politics, in the most old-fashioned and traditional sense of party politics, as against organizational routines or pressure group bargaining.

This, in turn, would suggest that the usefulness of different theoretical perspectives depends on the nature of the puzzle or problem being tackled. In trying to account for the evolution of Welfare State systems over time, and in trying to explain their growth in terms of expenditure, it has been found that ideological factors are largely irrelevant.[67] But ideology may not be irrelevant when it comes to trying to explain *how* different systems operate: their operational assumptions and policy priorities. The fact that the Labour Government had an egalitarian ideology, and a moral commitment to the proposition that health care should be provided irrespective of the ability to pay, was a necessary condition for its actions in the period 1974 to 1976, although it was by no means a sufficient condition.

The ideological commitment of the Labour Party only represents what may be called a predisposing factor. The Labour Party has a variety of ideological commitments on a great many subjects which, in practice, never get translated into policy, or only partially so. And this, of course, is true of all political movements. What, then, activated this latent commitment? In trying to answer this question, the Alford thesis[68] of the importance of societal and structural factors is particularly relevant. The emergence of the pay beds issue depended not just on the election of a Labour Government; previous Labour Administration had, after all, quite happily ignored the whole question of the scope for private practice. It depended quite crucially on the fact that this particular Labour Government was dependent on the support of the trade-unions. In short, there had been a shift in the societal balance of power towards organized labor (which is not to assert that this change must be necessarily permanent).

It was precisely because of this change in the environment of the NHS that the trade-unions within the service were able to exert political pressure on the Secretary of State. One way of viewing the Government's commitment to act on pay beds is, therefore, to see it as the price paid for collective trade-union support on national, as distinct from NHS, issues. In turn, this underlines a more general point of political analysis. Ideological commitments, like all policy commitments, carry a price-tag. Hence an implicit cost-benefit analysis takes place in choosing which ones to carry into execution, an exercise complicated by the fact that different actors in the policy arena use different currencies. For Labour Ministers, the pay beds issue appeared to be a cheap way of obtaining union support: the opportunity costs, as measured in terms of expenditure, appeared to be low. For civil servants in the DHSS, however, the opportunity costs were extremely high, as measured by the effects on long-term relations with the medical profession. As a consequence, Labour Ministers received little support from DHSS officials.

So far the emphasis has been on analyzing the *political* influence of the trade-unions in the NHS. This method of analysis inevitably draws attention to the importance of structural factors, or the role played by organized labor in a particular society. But this is to neglect the possibility that the influence of the trade-unions may also be based on their industrial strength. In other words, the unions in the NHS may derive their power as much from their increasing ability (reflecting an increasing membership) to disrupt the work of the NHS as from any political leverage that they may be able to exercise. In practice, this conceptual distinction may be blurred, since one source of power clearly feeds on the other. But to make this point is to draw attention to the fact that health services are complex organizations. They require the cooperation of a large variety of organized groups, not because they are delivering a commodity called "health," but because they are dependent on a complicated mix of specialized skills. In short, we are dealing not with the politics of health but with the politics of complex public services when discussing the role of organized labor.

This perspective is also helpful in analyzing the role of the medical profession in the 1974 to 1976 crisis. If the medical profession is seen as one example, among many, of organized labor – distinguished mainly by the fact that it organized itself earlier and better than other groups of health workers – then much of what is otherwise puzzling about the whole episode falls neatly into place. For the pay beds battle is destructive of most of the accepted theories for explaining the political role of the medical profession. Elite theory does not help: the fact that the medical profession shared both much of its social background and its values with the leadership of the Conservative Party (and with civil servants) did not prevent the emergence of the pay beds issue. Nor does this approach account for the compromise that ended the confrontation: the political battle fought by the Conservatives on behalf of the doctors did not, as we have seen, effectively make any difference. Again, political culture theories[69] are inadequate. They do not help to explain what is really interesting about the pay beds issue – that it represented a political challenge to the existing order, a discontinuity in the incremental process and organizational style of policy-making in the NHS.

But if the situation is analyzed in terms of industrial power within complex organizations, then both the failure of the medical profession to prevent the Labour Government from taking up the pay beds issue and its ultimate success in compelling a compromise become comprehensible. Moreover, the relationship between factors exogenous and endogenous to the NHS is also clarified. The NHS trade-unions were able to force pay beds onto the political agenda because of structural factors extrinsic to the NHS. So much is grist for the mill of those who argue that change within health services is possible only if the societal environment is also altered. But the medical profession was able to prevent the Government from pushing through its program of change because of industrial factors intrinsic to the NHS as a complex organization. It was because the Government needed the cooperation of the medical profession (in exactly the same way as it needed the cooperation of nurses, technicians and laundry workers) that it had to compromise. To sum up, then, while structural factors may be a necessary precondition for change, organizational factors may explain the problems involved in carrying out new policies.

The events of 1974 to 1976 show that a new set of actors are now involved in the policy arena of the NHS: the trade-unions. This is not to say that the arguments about policy will in the future be carried out along class lines. Although, on the face of it, the dispute over pay beds would seem to fall neatly into such a category, this view is not supported by detailed analysis of what actually happened. There is as much difference in the social class composition within the trade-unions (representing as they do both unskilled workers and highly skilled technicians and administrators) as there is between the medical profession and the unions. Indeed our analysis would seem to underline the need for microanalysis in seeking political explanations, since otherwise it is all too tempting to reify heterogeneous social categories like "the medical profession" and the "trade-unions" as though these have a collective, homogeneous and indivisible identity – which is far from being the case, as we have seen.

It would therefore be premature to conclude that the emergence of this new set of actors will lead to a radicalization of health politics, although it may give greater scope to a radical elite as it did in 1974 to 1976. Structural change, by promoting the growth of organized labor, has created a situation where there may be more pluralistic bargaining. But in the future it will no longer be possible to analyze pressure groups politics in terms exclusively of the relationship between governments and the medical profession. The problem, rather, will be to analyze the interaction of a whole complex of organized interests. In other words, the paradoxical conclusion is that structural and pluralistic theories of policy making are mutually supportive rather than exclusive. It is structure which shapes the universe and provides the value-language of pluralistic bargaining. But it is the interaction of the various interests involved, not the structure, which determines the outcome of any particular policy dispute.

The case of the pay beds issue is, however, interesting not only because of the insights it provides into the problems of explaining political processes, but also because it raises a fundamental question about the political limits to health care systems engineering. The logic of comprehensive health care planning is total state control over the resources required, just as the logic of rationing health care exclusively according to need is the elimination of all payments by patients. In a sense, therefore, the battle over pay beds – and indeed over private practice within the NHS – was a "phoney war." To exclude private practice from the NHS might, even if successful, encourage the growth of the independent sector and thus increase the problems of resource allocation within the public service. To make it impossible for patients to get quicker treatment or more comfortable surroundings within the NHS may simply persuade them to take their business elsewhere. Thus, preserving the ideological purity of NHS, as it were, may in practice do nothing to improve the distribution of services or to prevent the buying of preferential medical care.

Yet, to move beyond this point would mean changing not just the health system but society's entire value system. In other words, the ideal health service may only be achievable at the cost of sacrificing other deeply entrenched values: of strengthening the power of the state bureaucracy by giving it a monopoly control over health services, of limiting the rights of individual citizens either to buy or provide particular services. Thus, when we talk about structural factors limiting the possibilities of change within health services, it would often be more accurate to talk about the social values which constrain state hegemony, and embody a concept of freedom opposed to the abuses of both market and bureaucratic power.

Notes

1. R. Klein, "Conflict Within Consensus: The Case of the British NHS," paper given at conference on "Instrumente der Gesundheitpolitik," June 1977.

2. R. Alford, *Health Care Politics* (Chicago: University of Chicago Press, 1975).

3. R. F. Badgley, "Health Worker Strikes: Social and Economic Bases of Conflict," *International Journal of Health Services, (IJHS)* 5 (1975): 9–17; B. and J. H. Ehrenreich, "Hospital Workers: Class Conflicts in the Making," *IJHS* 5 (1975): 43–51.

4. National Health Service Act, 1946 9 & 10 Geo.6. CH 8 Section 5 Her Majesty's Stationery Office (HMSO), London.

5. The only study to have appeared is now 10 years old: S. Mencher, *Private Practice in Britain* (London: G. Bell & Sons, 1967).

6. *UK Private Medical Care: Provident Schemes Statistics 1975* Lee Donaldson Associates, (London: 1976). For an earlier review of private insurance, see Michael Lee, *Opting out of the NHS* (London: Political and Economic Planning, 1971).

7. Department of Employment, *Family Expenditure Survey: Report for 1975* (London: HMSO, 1976).

8. Royal Commission on Doctors' and Dentists' Remuneration, *Report* (London: HMSO, 1960), p. 62 (Cmnd. 939).

9. Review Body on Doctors' and Dentists' Remuneration, *Report, 1972* (London: HMSO, 1972), p. 52 (Cmnd. 5010).

10. Idem, *Fourth Report, 1974* (London: HMSO, 1974), p. 41 (Cmnd. 5644).

11. Idem, *Report, 1972* (London: HMSO, 1972) (Cmnd. 5010); Idem, *Fourth Report, 1974* (London: HMSO, 1974), p. 40 (Cmnd. 5644).

12. House of Commons, Expenditure Committee, Session 1971–72, Fourth Report, *National Health Service: Facilities for Private Patients* (London: HMSO, 1972), p. 4 (H.C. 172); Department of Health and Social Security, *Health and Personal Social Services Statistics for England* (London: HMSO, 1972 onward).

13. Idem, *Health and Personal Social Services Statistics, 1975* (London: HMSO, 1976), Table 4.8, pp. 74–75.

14. F. W. S. Craig, ed., *British General Election Manifestos, 1900–1974* (London: Macmillan, 1975), p. 404.

15. Ibid., p. 460.

16. "NHS Private Beds: Summary of Events," *British Medical Journal*, July 13, 1974, pp. 127–28.

17. *Hansard*, July 3, 1974, col. 394.

18. *Hansard*, April 27, 1976, cols. 238–39.

19. Department of Health and Social Security. *The Separation of Private Practice from National Health Service Hospitals: A Consultative Document* (London: DHSS, 1975).

20. *Hansard*, December 1, 1975, cols. 1255–61.

21. *Hansard*, December 15, 1975, cols. 971–79; Department of Health and Social Security, "Proposals considered at a meeting on 15 December between the Secretary of State for Social Services and representatives of the medical and dental professions," *Press Release 75/241*, December 15, 1975.

22. *The Times*, October 2, 1975, p. 5.

23. *British Medical Journal*, June 25, 1977, p. 1667.

24. *Health Services: The Newspaper of COHSE*, November 1976, p. 1.

25. M. Ryan, "Hospital Pay Beds: A Study in Ideology and Constraints," *Social and Economic Administration* 9 (1975): 164–83.

26. M. Foot, *Aneurin Bevan: A Biography, Volume 2* (London: Davis-Poynter, 1973), p. 137.

27. Ryan, p. 170.

28. Ryan, pp. 173–74.

29. *Resolutions for the 68th Annual Conference of the Labour Party* (London: The Labour Party, 1969).

30. See, for example, *Resolutions for the 65th Annual Conference of the Labour Party* (London: The Labour Party, 1966).

31. Fourth Report from the Expenditure Committee.

32. Ibid., par. 40, p. xix.

33. *Health Care: A Report of a Working Party* (London: The Labour Party, 1973).

34. R. Klein, "The National Health Service" in *Social Policy and Public Expenditure 1975: Inflation and Priorities,* ed.: R. Klein (London: Centre for Studies in Social Policy, 1975).

35. Trades Union Congress, *The Development of the Social Contract* (London: TUC, 1975).

36. *Hansard,* April 27, 1976, cols. 229 and 325.

37. D. Owen, *In Sickness and in Health* (London: Quartet Books, 1976), pp. 48–60.

38. Department of Health and Social Security, *National Health Service Reorganization: England* (London: HMSO, 1972) (Cmnd. 5055).

39. See, for example, R. Crossman, *Diaries of a Cabinet Minister Volume I* (London: Hamilton and Cape, 1975) p. 378.

40. P. Jenkins, *The Battle of Downing Street* (London: Charles Knight & Co., 1970).

41. D. E. Butler and D. Kavanagh, *British General Election of February 1974* (London: Macmillan, 1974).

42. R. F. Badgley, and B. and J. H. Ehrenreich.

43. Department of Trade, *Report of the Committee of Inquiry into Industrial Democracy* (London: HMSO, 1977), p. 13 (Cmnd. 6706).

44. Trade Union Congress (TUC), *Annual Reports,* 1956–1976 (London: TUC).

45. Ibid. NUPES Membership rose from 175,000 in 1956 to 248,000 in 1966 and 584,000 in 1976.

46. National Board for Prices and Incomes, *The Pay and Conditions of Manual Workers in Local Authorities, the National Health Service, Gas and Water Supply* (London: HMSO, 1967) (Cmnd. 3230).

47. S. J. Dimmock, "Participation or Control? The Workers' Involvement in Management," *Conflicts in the National Health Service,* ed.: K. Barnard and K. Lee (London: Croom Helm, 1977): T. Manson "Management, The Profession and the Unions," *Health and the Division of Labour,* ed.: M. Stacey (London: Croom Helm, 1977).

48. P. B. Beaumont, "Incomes Policy, Productivity and Manual Workers Earnings in the Local Government Sector," *Local Government Studies* (January 1977):

17–29. This finding is very much in line with American trends, as reported by V. R. Fuchs, "The Earnings of Allied Health Personnel," *Explorations in Economic Research* 3 (1976): 408–32.

49. Lord McCarthy, *Making Whitley Work* (London: Department of Health and Social Security, 1976).

50. National Board for Prices and Incomes, *The Pay and Conditions of Service of Ancillary Workers in the National Health Service* (London: HMSO, 1971) (Cmnd. 4644).

51. TUC, *Report 1973* (London: TUC, 1973), p. 602.

52. Idem, *Report 1974* (London: TUC, 1974), p. 114.

53. British United Provident Association, *NOP Survey April 1976* (mimeo.).

54. *Hansard,* December 5, 1974, cols. 625–32.

55. Review Body on Doctors' and Dentists' Remuneration, *Seventh Report, 1977* (London: HMSO, 1977), p. 2 (Cmnd. 6800).

56. "The Consultants' Contract" *The Lancet,* November 23, 1974, pp. 1254–56.

57. S. Bourne and P. Bruggen, "Examination of the Distinction Awards System," *British Medical Journal,* January 18, 1975, pp. 162–65.

58. T. R. Marmor, and D. Thomas, "Doctors, Politics and Pay Disputes: 'Pressure Group Politics' Revisited," *British Journal of Political Science* 2 (1972): 421–42.

59. *BMA News* No. 44, February 1974.

60. H. Eckstein, *The English Health Service* (London: OUP, 1959).

61. D. Deliege, J. Lievens, and C. Zeegers-Dooreman, *Medical Doctors in the Nine Countries of the Common Market: Systems of Payment and Levels of Remuneration* (Louvain: University of Louvain, 1976).

62. "Private Practice and the NHS: Memorandum by Organizations Representing the Medical and Dental Professions and by the Independent Hospital Group," *British Medical Journal,* October 4, 1975, pp. 54–58.

63. *British Medical Journal,* February 21, 1976, pp. 475–76.

64. *British Medical Journal,* December 7, 1974, p. 608.

65. *British Medical Journal,* February 21, 1976, p. 478.

66. T. R. Marmor, A. Bridges, and W. L. Hoffman, "Comparative Politics and Health Policies," October 14, 1976, paper prepared for a conference at Cornell University.

67. H. L. Wilensky, *The Welfare State and Equality* (Los Angeles: University of California Press, 1975).

68. Alford, *Health Care Politics,* pp. 13–21.

69. H. Eckstein, *Pressure Group Politics: The Case of the British Medical Association* (London: Allen & Unwin, 1960).

47

Models of Man and Models of Policy: Reflections on *Exit, Voice, and Loyalty* Ten Years Later

MILBANK MEMORIAL FUND QUARTERLY
1980

Stalking the debate about health policy in the United States are two models of man. The first is that of *homo economicus*: a lonely, self-regarding and rational shopper in the marketplace. The second is that of *homo politicus*: a social animal whose habitat is the world of political activity. In turn, each model of man yields a different policy prescription. Adopting the economic model of man tends to lead to the advocacy of competition in the health care market, unfettered by restrictive professional practices or distorting tax concessions. Adopting the political model of man tends to lead to the advocacy of institutional solutions to the problems of health care delivery: the use of planning and regulatory mechanisms. In the former case, it is competition that ensures responsiveness to consumer preferences. In the latter case, it is institutionalized political activity that guarantees responsiveness to citizen wishes.

Instinctively most of us probably feel somewhat uneasy about this dichotomization of man. Applying either model to the problems of health care policy seems, in many ways, unsatisfactory. The rational shopper model may capture some aspects of the health care consumer, but does not begin to incorporate the very complex patterns of behavior or the relations between providers and consumers in this field. Nor is the political model entirely satisfactory. It assumes that political activity is a natural way of life, when we know that in fact political apathy tends to be the norm. Consequently the assumption of producer responsiveness – implicit in both models – is highly questionable. The economic model, it may be argued, neglects issues of professional dominance. The political model, it may be said, neglects issues of bureaucratic dominance. Moreover, health care has some of the characteristics of both a private and a public good: that is, it affects both those individuals actually receiving it and society at large. Thus a hospital not only benefits the patients (and staff) but also brings contingent reassurance to the surrounding population. The challenge of health care policy is therefore how to combine sensitivity to both consumer preferences (the economic model) and citizen wishes (the political model): what the consumer wants, the citizen may wish to deny him, or vice versa.

It is problems such as these that may help to explain the impact of Hirschman's (1970) *Exit, Voice, and Loyalty* since it was published ten years ago. On the face of it, the subsequent infiltration of this book into the intellectual repertory and footnotes of the health care literature may seem odd: there is no explicit discussion of health care in the book, and Hirschman has made no extended attempt to apply his insights to this particular field in his later reflections on his original work. In practice, however, the importance of his book lies in its pioneering endeavor to bring together the two models of man within the same framework of analysis: to rub together the intellectual sticks provided by two disciplines – economics and politics. If the resulting fire still burns, it is because the debate about health care policies continues to revolve – as I have sought to argue – around competing models of man. This, indeed, is why a discussion of Hirschman's work remains as relevant today as when his book was first published.

Hirschman's book starts with a puzzle. In the economist's paradigm, the response to deteriorating performance by a firm (or public service organization) is exit by the consumers. That is, consumers take their custom elsewhere, so giving the required alarm signals to the firm (or organization) to improve its product or service. If the alarm signals are heeded, then the performance will pick up again. If they are ignored, the firm or organization will go out of business, and its products or services will be provided by others. All will be for the best in the most efficient of all worlds. In reality, as Hirschman (himself an economist) points out, things do not work out so neatly or conveniently. Firms (or organizations) may actually welcome the exit of particularly demanding customers, and may tacitly conspire with each other to shuttle such troublesome customers back and forth between them. Exit may, in other words, inhibit complaints. The signals provided by exit may be ambiguous, in the sense that they may not give a precise message as to what it is that actually disgruntles customers. Such signals may therefore not provide the information required to adjust performance to consumer preferences.

So we come to voice, or what might be called political activity. In Hirschman's analysis, this is an essential complement to exit: the two models of man join hands, and the trick is to find (for any relevant area of policy) the best combination of voice and exit. Voice, in contrast to exit, is rich in information. It denies firms (or organizations) the easy and inviting option of getting rid of the most demanding customers. In turn, decisions by individuals as to whether to employ the exit or the voice option will depend on the degree of loyalty that they feel to the firm or organization in question: a high degree of loyalty is likely to inhibit exit and may encourage voice.

The optimal mix of exit and voice will, naturally, depend on the precise nature of the situation at issue. At one extreme, imagine a highly competitive market in which firms manufacture virtually identical products. In such a situation, exit may well be the response best calculated to convey the appropriate warning signals to the firm whose product is deteriorating in quality. At the other extreme, imagine (to take an example discussed by Hirschman) the public school system. Here, exit, such as switching children from the public to the private school system or moving to the suburbs, may simply reinforce the trend towards deterioration. If the most articulate parents, most sensitive to issues of quality, vote with their feet instead of engaging in voice—that is, traditional pressure group activities – then, Hirschman argues, there will be no incentive to those responsible for the public school system to try to arrest or reverse the process of deterioration. The policy implication is clear. Relying on policy models based on *homo economicus* may bring about perverse results in certain conditions, and it may be necessary to invoke *homo politicus* to redress the balance.

There are a number of problems about Hirschman's conceptual framework (Barry, 1974), and in applying it to specific policy areas. Some of these he has himself identified in subsequent reflections on his book (Hirschman, 1974, 1975). For example, the original argument tended to assume that exit would be costless and that voice would be expensive, and that there would be a consequent asymmetry in the likely reactions to deteriorating performance. But, as he himself has pointed out since, this is an over-simple view. Exit carries costs, such as the search for information or breaking the mold of existing habits (as in the case of divorce, or exit from marriage). Conversely, voice may be valued as an activity in its own right – setting aside any costs – in the sense that

Aristotelian man engages in political activity because this represents his fulfillment as a human being.

More seriously, perhaps, Hirschman's neat antithesis between exit and voice does not – as Barry has pointed out – capture all the available options. It is possible to exit and, having done so, either to complain (i.e., use voice) or to remain silent. Similarly, it is possible to reject the exit option out of loyalty, but to reject voice also and remain silent. Further, Hirschman's analysis is applied to a very specific kind of situation: the *deterioration* in the quality of a product or service. But, as I shall try to argue in discussing the application of his ideas to health, it is important to bear in mind that – especially when it comes to heterogeneous services – discontent may stem from dissatisfaction not with falling quality but with the mix of types of product offered. Again, Hirschman's treatment of loyalty is somewhat sketchy: it is treated as a residual, to explain what otherwise cannot be accounted for in his analysis. Yet, and again this is highly relevant when it comes to health, the deliberate manufacture of feelings of loyalty might well be considered as a defensive strategy by threatened producers: certainly the doctor-patient relationship is highly charged with emotion and is manipulable (indeed, it could be argued that we need a model of *homo sociologicus* to complete the picture convincingly). Many services have symbolic outputs whose function is precisely to reinforce loyalty (Edelman, 1971).

These are important criticisms but, in a sense, they are beside the point when it comes to assessing Hirschman's influence. If, a decade after the publication of his book, his ideas are still bubbling away through the literature, the explanation does not lie in the formal rigor of his analytic method. His influence stems, I would argue, from the style of thought he introduced into the discussion of a wide range of issues, including health policy; he prompts interesting questions rather than providing ready-made solutions, Overall, the significance of his work has been admirably summed up by Young:

> Hirschman's contribution to a dynamic theory of public service organization is several fold. First, he teaches us to combine our consideration of political and economic forces. Second, he isolates the key mechanisms – exit and voice – and, in so doing, puts the focus on the *clients* or *consumers* as the key element for controlling organizational performance. Third, he identifies the essential channels through which organizations receive information about, and incentives to improve, their performance. Fourth, he instructs us that when these channels are not properly structured, organizational behavior can be expected to deteriorate. (Young, 1974: 52)

So it seems eminently worthwhile to make use of the insights provided by Hirschman by applying them to the field of health care policy. Specifically, to return to the point made at the beginning of this essay, what does his analysis imply for the continuing debate over whether a competitive or an institutional model is most appropriate for the organization of health care? Which market – the economic or the political – offers the best deal?

In the first place, asking such questions in the context of Hirschman's conceptual framework compels further analysis of just what we mean when we talk about "consumers" and the "product" in the field of health care. The health care market (Stevens, 1974) is characterized by a high degree of uncertainty about the product, "about which diagnostic and treatment procedures are most apt to prove efficacious." Moreover, the standard consumer strategy of seeking information through a process of trial and error may not always be appropriate in the health care market. Trading in a Ford for a Chevrolet may be a reasonably satisfactory way of obtaining information about the comparative performances of two cars; shopping around from doctor to doctor is somewhat less satisfactory, since the performance of the first physician may actually affect what the second one can do. (To take an extreme case, the freedom to shop around in order to find the most competent physician is hardly relevant to the patient who has not survived the operation by the first surgeon consulted). Lastly, the search for medical care tends to be contingent on something happening to us: so, at least in the case of sudden, acute illness, the incentives to seek information may be greatest at precisely the time in our lives when we are physically least able to shop around.

From this, it follows that – to the extent that we are concerned with exit as a corrective mechanism in the health care market – we should also be concerned to minimize the information costs or, to put it positively, to equip the shopper with the evaluative know-how required to make a sensible choice. This would suggest either more emphasis on "full disclosure" (Stevens, 1974:38) or using proxy consumer groups to generate relevant information (Young, 1974:54).

But there are a number of problems about this approach. For example, the question of how to assess the quality of medical care is notoriously contentious. There is little agreement even among the experts (e.g., McAuliffe, 1979), so that equipping the consumer with adequate information is no easy task. More centrally still, it is not self-evident that exit is necessarily an effective corrective mechanism, because of the heterogeneous, complex character of health care, which consists of delivering not only a number of very different technical procedures, but also of an environmental package (waiting rooms, hospital rooms, etc.). A consumer might well be satisfied with the technical treatment provided, but highly incensed about the quality of the environment in which it has been provided. If, then, he or she chooses to protest by using the exit option, the consequent signal to the producer is ambiguous. Exit, as Hirschman rightly stresses, is poor in information: in complex services, it provides little or no guidance as to the precise nature of the dissatisfaction. Moreover, any system of health care tends to shape the expectations of its own consumers: cross-nationally, there is some evidence (Kohn and White, 1976) that health care consumers tend to be satisfied with what they get, however different the nature of the delivery system. This reinforces the point made earlier about the capacity of health care systems to generate loyalty, and helps to explain why silence is so often the norm.

But it could still be argued that exit plus voice might provide both the incentives and the information required to persuade producers to respond to consumer wishes. Are there any mechanisms, in short, that could allow consumers both to vote with their feet and, having done so, to continue to exert pressure? The classic example of exit followed by voice in the health care market is, perhaps, the malpractice suit. However, this is generally not felt to be a very satisfactory mechanism because of its arbitrary character and its perverse effects on medical practice. For example, one study has shown that there is little correlation between the number of malpractice suits a hospital attracts and such measures of quality as are available (Department of Health, Education, and Welfare, 1973). An alternative approach might therefore be to argue for forms of consumer participation (Stevens, 1974): the deliberate creation of channels of influence through which consumers, having chosen to exit, can transmit information about the precise nature of their dissatisfaction.

The creation of such mechanisms of consumer representation may help to meet some of the difficulties inherent in relying on a strategy of exit followed by voice. But such strategy, it might be said, requires a considerable degree of altruism on the part of the disgruntled consumer: having made his exit, why should he bother to press for improvements that will benefit others? To the extent that representative bodies lower the cost of voice, by acting as proxy political activists, this objection may be weakened. Conversely, however, it could equally well be argued that the mere existence of such bodies will paradoxically weaken the incentive to exert voice because of the well-known free-rider problem inherent in all collective action (Olson, 1965). If we know that others are taking action anyway – and suspect, furthermore, that adding our voice will make little or no difference to the likely outcome – why bother to do anything, particularly when we have already made our exit? Economic man, balancing the costs and benefits, almost certainly would remain silent, though political man, with a regard to the public interest arguments involved, might decide otherwise. Consequently, it does not seem that creating new mechanisms for articulating consumer voice will necessarily solve the problems created by exit followed by silence.

So far, the discussion has been in terms of an atomistic market for health care: the implicit assumption has been that individual consumers deal with individual producers. Now let us complicate this picture (and make it more realistic) by introducing institutional providers. Imagine a city where three health maintenance organizations (HMOs) control the market and are competing for customers. Imagine also a family of three: the husband worried about a possible coronary, the wife expecting a baby, and a three-year-old child suffering from chronic asthma. The first HMO has a high reputation for the quality of its coronary and maternity care, but the pediatrician is notoriously unwilling to turn out at nights in emergencies. The second HMO has excellent maternity services and a responsive pediatrician, but its coronary care facilities are suspect. The third HMO scores high on acute and pediatric services, but low on maternity.

What, then, are the choices for the family faced with such a dilemma? If they exit from one HMO, they will only solve one problem at the price of creating another. In this situation, the consumer has a direct incentive to use voice in order to try to correct a deficiency (not, it must be stressed, necessarily to be equated with a deterioration in service provision). Unfortunately, as Hirschman points out in a different context, it does not follow that producers have an incentive to respond: a circular, and self-balancing, procession of consumers in search of the ideal package may suit all three HMOs very well. In this instance, introducing an element of consumer representation or participation into the governance of each HMO may indeed be the most effective solution: i.e., the implication would seem to be that creating mechanisms for articulating voice may be most important in those situations where exit does not provide a satisfactory option for the consumer. As this example would suggest, the problems of finding an appropriate balance between exit and voice in health care spring from the fact that consumers are not purchasing a product but a complex and heterogeneous package of very different services.

A further peculiarity of the health care market must be noted here, if only as an aside. Most consumers in the United States do not pay directly for the product or package, an obvious fact that raises an intriguing question, in the context of the kind of analysis prompted by Hirschman's approach. The literature generated by *Exit, Voice, and Loyalty* has produced, as noted above, a number of suggestions for strengthening the opportunities for voice by individual consumers. Yet this is to ignore the fact that most consumers are already collectively organized as members of insurance schemes such as Blue Cross. One of the missing elements in the American debate about health insurance, insofar as a transatlantic spectator can judge, is any discussion of the consumer *qua* consumer of insurance policies: why, in fact, insurance schemes are not considered as a mechanism for transmitting voice. If one of the problems of health care is the need for some kind of proxy organization to evaluate services and to articulate consumer voices, why not use existing organizations? The obvious answer may be that membership in insurance schemes tends to follow employment rather than individual choice. Even this answer, however, leaves the puzzle as to why there have been no suggestions, in the American context, for using insurance schemes as mechanisms of voice. Certainly the European experience would suggest that there is some scope for introducing an element of consumer representation in such schemes: for example, in both Germany and France there is a system of elections to the boards of the *kassen* or *caisses* that operate the insurance system.

To return to the main theme, however, there is a third model of health care organization that requires analysis. So far, we have considered an atomistic market of individual consumers and producers and a market with competing institutional providers. But the Hirschman framework of analysis would seem to provide a strong case for creating a monopoly provider of health care, something along the lines of Britain's National Health Service (NHS). This assertion follows from his discussion of the public school system, already cited. If a health care system combining public and private provision permits easy exit, then the result will be (as in the case of schools) to encourage precisely those with the most demanding standards to leave the public domain. Consequently, there may follow a process of self-reinforcing deterioration in the public sector – a prediction, drawn from Hirschman's analysis, that is certainly not falsified by American experience. In short, a pluralistic system will encourage self-regarding economic man to consult only his own interests, with perverse effects for the collectivity at large. In contrast, a monopolistic organization locks consumers into the system, and forces them to engage in voice – to act as political animals – whether they want to or not, pursuing the collective welfare. Moreover, voice provides the information that is essential in such a heterogeneous service as health, where the producers require signals not only about deterioration in quality but also about the appropriateness or adequacy of what is being provided.

Is the inference from this type of analysis that the United States should be moving toward the adoption of something like Britain's NHS? Not quite. For at this stage in the argument we meet again the peculiar paradox of health care: that, by and large, people like what they get, and what they are accustomed to. Despite its obvious shortcomings – poor physical conditions in hospitals, long waiting lists for some conditions – the NHS is extremely popular (Klein, 1979a). As this would indicate, it is possible not only in theory but also in practice to generate loyalty. In the case of the NHS, it could be argued that its most important symbolic output is equity – i.e., perceived fairness in dealing with people, regardless of their financial circumstances – which inhibits both voice and exit.

In turn, this would suggest that when quality deteriorates, one possible reaction is for consumers to rally to their organization. Certainly there was no evidence of an increase in exit from the NHS – i.e., an increased number of subscribers to private insurance – in Britain during the mid-1970s (Klein, 1979b) when there was much talk of a crisis of morale and declining standards (Royal Commission, 1979). Indeed, the prevailing rhetoric of crisis during this period suggests another intriguing application of the Hirschman thesis: it indicates that exit and voice may be options for service providers as well as for service consumers. In particular, a near-monopoly service like the NHS may give a greater incentive to service providers than to service consumers to use voice to articulate their grievances, a strategy frequently pursued by Britain's doctors (Powell, 1966). Such an outcome is even more likely in the circumstances of the 1980s when the choice of exit through emigration seems likely to be increasingly limited, and therefore service providers will increasingly be locked into the system. The point explains why one of the characteristics of all national health services, in all nontotalitarian countries, is a periodic confrontation between public authorities and the medical profession. Voice, in the sense of political or industrial action, becomes the main weapon of service providers.

Of course the NHS is not a total monopoly. There is, in Britain, a small private sector: about one in twenty of the population is covered by private insurance. It could therefore be argued that it is precisely the existence of this safety valve that accounts for the lack of voice from consumers, the conclusion that would be drawn from Hirschman's illustrative example of the public school system. If the most demanding health care consumers can exit, why be surprised that there is so little voice? This indeed is the view taken by the Labour Party, and explains its hostility to private practice. As against this, it has also been argued (Birch, 1975) that the possibility of exit is a necessary condition for the exercise of voice. The more tightly the consumers of any service are locked into the system, the more inhibited they will be in voicing their grievances, for fear of retaliation from the service providers; even if they are dissatisfied with the quality of the service provided, they are likely to take refuge in silence in such circumstances. One conclusion that might be drawn is that the more the health service organizations acquire a monopoly, albeit perhaps only a local monopoly, the more important it becomes to have proxy bodies capable of exercising voice on behalf of consumers who may be afraid of articulating their own grievances.

But the Hirschman thesis helps to explain at least one feature of the British NHS to which American critics (for example, Lindsay, 1980) frequently draw attention: the persistence of queues. Waiting lists are predominantly, though not exclusively, for nonurgent, elective procedures. In contrast, there is no queueing for acute conditions. And this is precisely what would be expected, on the basis of the Hirschman analysis, from the special characteristics of the private sector. The private sector in Britain does not offer a comprehensive alternative to the NHS: it concentrates overwhelmingly on precisely the kind of conditions for which there are waiting lists in the NHS, so giving paying customers a chance to circumvent the queue. It is therefore not surprising that the incentives to the NHS to get rid of waiting lists are blunted: the most exigent consumers have no reason to use voice, since they can buy exit. In contrast, there are fewer opportunities for exit in the case of life-endangering illness, and (predictably therefore) the NHS offers a better service in such cases. Also in conformance with Hirschman's thesis, the NHS is extremely poor in the provision of privacy and comfort within the acute sector; this, again, is what might be expected from the fact that those who put a high value on privacy and comfort can exit to seek them in the private market.

Using this kind of analysis also raises some troublesome questions of equity. The apparent inequity of the exit option is self-evident: it seems to provide a built-in bias toward the better off, who can buy improved services for themselves at the cost of those who cannot afford to leave the system. But the voice option does not guarantee equity, either. As Hirschman has pointed out, the ability (and willingness) to use voice may not be distributed equally among all consumers. Indeed, there is ample evidence to be drawn from the political science literature to show that willingness to engage in political activity, or to participate in civic affairs, tends to be associated with such factors as education, income, and age. So a system designed to encourage voice may have its own built-in biases as well, a conclusion that is of special relevance to health care policy, given the fact that the interests of consumers may often be in competition with each other.

The problem is, essentially, that a given population of consumers is not homogeneous but comprises four groups, with differing potentials for exit and voice:

Group 1: Voice potential high, exit potential high.
Group 2: Voice potential low, exit potential high.
Group 3: Voice potential high, exit potential low.
Group 4: Voice potential low, exit potential low.

This situation suggests that different kinds of institutional arrangements may be appropriate for different sectors of the health care system, depending on the characteristics of the consumers who use them.

Specifically, this very simple scheme shows why there are certain health service clients in group 4 – such as the mentally handicapped or the elderly infirm – who appear to get a rough deal in *all* health care systems, whether the American or the British. Given the low voice and low exit potential of this group, it is inevitable that resources will be directed disproportionately to those consumers who rank high on both counts: hence, no doubt, the international phenomenon of high expenditure on the acute hospital sector and high technology to the neglect of other areas. There is no need to invoke, as so often happens, a medical conspiracy to explain this; the phenomenon is adequately explained by Hirschman's framework of analysis.

The puzzle, rather, is to explain why those in group 4 – the most disadvantaged, those lacking in both market and political power – get any resources at all. To ask this question is to underline a curious gap in Hirschman's approach. The value of *Exit, Voice, and Loyalty*, as I have tried to show in these variations on Hirschman's theme, is that it is enormously stimulating, that it sparks off illuminating questions. But its limitation is that its focus is the behavior of *consumers* within specific organizational settings: economic man dominates even in political behavior (Barry, 1974) – the reconciliation of the two models of man remains somehow incomplete, even though Hirschman has used his approach to analyze the behavior of voters and governments. Yet, as argued earlier, we are interested in health care not only as consumers, actual or potential. We may also be interested as citizens who happen to believe that adequate and comprehensive health services for all sections of the population are a public good. In a sense, therefore, although Hirschman allows us to understand better the politics of the health care arena, he does not help us as much to understand the political market in which decisions about health care are taken. Yet, in many ways, this is the crucial issue. Hirschman's work has sensitized us to the problems involved in designing the mechanisms required within the health care arena, or any other organizational arena. But the introduction of those mechanisms will depend on political decisions taken outside the health care arena. So perhaps we still need another volume from Hirschman: the politics of exit, voice, and loyalty.

References

Barry, B. 1974. Review article: *Exit, Voice, and Loyalty. British Journal of Political Science* 4:79–107.

Birch, A.H. 1975. Economic Models in Political Science: The Case of *Exit, Voice, and Loyalty. British Journal of Political Science* 5:69–92.

Department of Health, Education, and Welfare. 1973. *Medical Malpractice: Report of the Secretary's Commission on Medical Malpractice*. Washington, D.C.: U.S. Government Printing Office.

Edelman, M. 1971. *Politics as Symbolic Action*. New York: Academic Press.

Hirschman, A.O. 1970. *Exit, Voice, and Loyalty*. Cambridge, Mass.: Harvard University Press.

————. 1974. *Exit, Voice, and Loyalty:* Further Reflections and a Survey of Recent Contributions. *Social Science Information* 13(1):7–26.

————. 1975. Exit and Voice: Some Further Distinctions (unpublished). A shortened version appeared as "Discussion," *American Economic Review* 66(2) (May 1976):386–389.

Klein, R. 1979a. Public Opinion and the National Health Service. *British Medical Journal* (12 May):1296–1297.

————. 1979b. Ideology, Class and the National Health Service. *Journal of Health Politics, Policy and Law* 4(3):464–490.

Kohn, R., and White, K.L., eds. 1976. *Health Care: An International Study*. Oxford: Oxford University Press.

Lindsay, C.M. 1980. *National Health Issues: The British Experience*. New York: Hoffmann-La Roche, Inc.

McAuliffe, W.E. 1979. Measuring the Quality of Medical Care. *Milbank Memorial Fund Quarterly/Health and Society* 57 (Winter): 95–117.

Olson, M. 1965. *The Logic of Collective Action*. Cambridge, Mass.: Harvard University Press.

Powell, E. 1966. *Medicine and Politics*. London: Pitman Medical.

Royal Commission on the National Health Service. 1979. *Report*. London: Her Majesty's Stationery Office.

Stevens, C.M. 1974. Voice in Medical-Care Markets: "Consumer Participation." *Social Science Information* 13(3):33–48.

Young, D.R. 1974. Exit and Voice in the Organisation of Public Services. *Social Science Information* 13(3):49–65.

48

Health Care in the Age of Disillusionment

BRITISH MEDICAL JOURNAL
5 July 1982

Over the past decade there has been a profound, if gradual, change in the way we think about health services and the role of medicine. It is a change which mirrors wider and deeper shifts in our intellectual, social, and economic environment. The ideology of optimism has given way to an ideology of disillusion. The assumption that the future would inevitably be better than the past – that the combination of economic growth, technological change, and rational planning would transform our society for the better – has begun to look increasingly moth-eaten. In Britain at least, economic growth can no longer be taken for granted. Technological change appears to create as many problems, such as nuclear waste, as it solves. In the new conventional wisdom rational planning is seen as a recipe for bureaucratic meddling. The three sustaining assumptions of the ideology of optimism are crumbling.

The pessimistic assumptions supporting the new ideology of disillusionment may well turn out to be as friable as those they have displaced. We simply do not know. If this article had been written in 1832, at the time of the BMA's foundation, it would no doubt have been based on a very constrained view of the scope for public policy, citing the classical economists in support of the view (now associated with the name of Milton Friedman) that there is little that governments can usefully do to create a wealthier or healthier society. But if we cannot predict what will happen we can explore the implications of the changes in our collective view of the world – our new perceptual lenses – for the ways in which we define problems and for health services and the medical profession. Precisely because health services and the medical profession represent a microcosm of the wider world (although they may have some unique characteristics) they cannot expect to be immune from the effects of the larger societal shifts.

No More Economic Growth?

Consider first the implications of no longer being able to take economic growth for granted. The problems are symbolised by the hospitals designed in the '60s and built on the assumption that future generations could afford much higher standards. They opened in the late '70s or early '80s to the financial embarrassment of all those concerned. In short, if we cannot take economic growth for granted, can we take improving standards for granted? And if we cannot what does this imply for the medical profession and other healthcare providers?

The medical imperative is to maximise the quality (and quantity) of care to the individual patient. In a sense, that is the doctor's ethical responsibility. If the scope for medical intervention continues to grow while resources remain limited then the dilemma always inherent in the organisation of a national health service is going to grow much sharper: the dilemma of balancing the doctor's responsibility to the individual patient and his responsibility to the community of potential patients. The former would indicate giving the individual patient the best treatment, regardless of the resource consequences. The latter might indicate giving the patient less than the (medically) optimum treatment if this were to make more resources available for others. In short, we should be debating whether medical audit should be about the standards of care provided for individual patients or for the community being served.

If accepted, this argument would in turn indicate that we should have to become increasingly concerned with the management of tragic choices: "the conflicts society confronts in the allocation of tragically scarce resources."[1] Who should carry the responsibility, and according to what criteria, for turning people away to die? The question is neither rhetorical nor new. The case of renal dialysis underlines that it is all too real and may also indicate the answer. For what is so puzzling about renal dialysis is that the NHS has actually managed to make a policy of rationing acceptable to the public, even though the consequences are so tragic. In this respect the NHS appears to be far more ruthless than most other

---

[1]Calabresi G, Bobbitt P. *Tragic choices*. New York: Norton and Co, 1978.

Western health care systems.[2] The reason would seem to be twofold. Firstly, the NHS is perceived to be equitable: it does not ration by money. Secondly, it disguises a national decision about resources as a series of discrete medical judgments: in individual cases medical criteria are used to determine who is going to be treated.

Clearly this gives the medical profession great power: hence the argument that members of the public should be involved in devising the criteria to be used in tragic choices.[3] But this argument may miss the real point, which is that the social acceptability of such decisions depends crucially on their being diffused and invisible – and that to have explicit criteria (whether derived from moral philosophy or cost-benefit analyses) would impose intolerable strains. What may be acceptable as a seemingly technical decision about an individual patient may be unacceptable as an explicit, collective decision about the distribution of the rights to treatment. The illusion of equal rights may be all important. To adapt the famous description of professionals as the people we hire to make our mistakes for us,[4] doctors are the people we hire to make our tragic choices for us. And the real question for the future may well be whether the medical profession is prepared to accept responsibility for what may be increasingly difficult decisions as a tolerable price for preserving its clinical autonomy. The price of guarding its patch, of repelling all attemtps by the outside world to penetrate the secret garden of clinical practice, may rise sharply. If resource contraints compel the medical profession to perform at what they consider to be less than acceptable standards, or to make too many tragic decisions, then ironically it may be in their interests to accept a system of accountability which clearly allocates responsibility between them and those who make the decisions about resources.

Disillusion with Technology

The proliferation of tragic choices links our first theme, the new agnosticism about economic growth, to our second theme, the new mood of disillusion with technology. For, to some extent, developments in medical technology often create the need for such choices. Indeed, it is precisely ths characteristic of medical technology which helps to explain the current disillusionment, though much rhetoric about excessive investment in "high" technology (never clearly defined) reflects a wider disen-

[2]Anonymous. Audit in renal failure: the wrong target? *Br Med J* 1981;**283**:261–2.
[3]Kennedy I. *The unmasking of medicine*. London: Allen and Unwin, 1981.
[4]Hughes E. *Men and their work*. London: Collier-Macmillan, 1958.

chantment: witness the demonstrations against nuclear power stations. If at the time of the creation of the NHS medical science was seen as a powerful instrument of progress, a way of actually creating a healthier society, this is no longer the case. Not only have its claims been challenged[5]; even when accepted, medical science is recognised as creating as many problems as it solves. With only slight exaggeration, the NHS may be seen as a machine for generating social problems, particularly among the elderly suffering from chronic degenerative diseases.

Indeed, the irony here is that the medical profession can effectively rebut its critics only by rejecting the criteria which it has itself tended to use in measuring its own achievements. If the critics argue that the capacity of medical science to extend life has been exaggerated – that social factors largely determine life expectancy – then, surely, the right response is to concede the point. If further investment in medical intervention can be justified it is in terms of improving the quality of the lives that have (for a variety of reasons) been so successfully extended over the past century.[6] Once again, this argument has profound implications for the future of health services and the medical profession. For it implies a reversal of the medical profession's own hierarchy of prestige: it suggests that priority should be given to applying technology to those procedures, perhaps boringly routine ones, which improve the quality of life for the many – cataracts, hip replacements, hernias, and so on – rather than to virtuoso innovations which may help the few. The distinction may often be difficult to draw: today's virtuoso innovation may turn out to be tommorrow's routine procedure. But it does offer at least a rough and ready benchmark for decision making.

More fundamentally, the new mood of agnosticism about technology in our societies – the awareness of its double-edged nature, and its capacity to destroy as well as to create – can only reinforce the tensions within the medical profession: between the humanist and the technological traditions of medicine. The point is familiar; the implications for the future are, however, unclear. Over the past few decades subspecialisations within medicine have proliferated in line with growing technological sophistication, and if we extrapolate these developments into the future what then is left of the doctor's traditional all-embracing role? The overcrowded medical curriculum, desperately stretched as it tries to accommodate demands for both a more rigorous scientific training and a return to a more social orientation, symbolises this tension. Is the caring

---

[5]McKeown T. *The role of medicine*. London: Nuffield Provincial Hospitals Trust, 1976.

[6]Morris JN. Are health services important to the people's health? *Br Med J* 1980;**280**: 167–8.

role to be relegated to nurses and social workers? Is the technological role to be devolved, increasingly, to non-medical technicians and scientists? The fashionable answer to these problems has been to emphasise the doctor's role as the co-ordinator of a team, the manager of a medical supermarket. But this redefines the nature of the tensions, rather than resolving them. It begs the question of why doctors should be the managers, a question which has come increasingly to the fore in recent years and will certainly not go away.

Just as economic stagnation creates conflict about resources, so the increasing use of technology in health services creates conflict about roles. If health care is about the application of technology, what is so different about doctors? The nurses have their own technology of care; laboratory technicians too have their own technology. If medicine is the first health-care occupation to have established itself as a profession, the others have followed suit: health care is a rampant example of the "professionalisation of everyone."[7] And the characteristic of a profession, as defined by the medical profession itself, is the fierce assertion of autonomy – a "hands off" syndrome. Furthermore, the medical profession has over the past decade undermined its own claim to a unique status. While health-service providers as a group have moved towards greater professionalisation, the medical profession itself has moved in the opposite direction in one crucial respect by adopting a trade-union strategy of industrial action.

If medical domination crumbles over the next few decades it will result from pressures within the health-care system – the competition between rival, professionalised technologists – rather than an assault by laymen asserting consumer rights. If it survives it will be because the medical profession manages to show that medicine is more than applied technology: paradoxically, perhaps, because it manages to show consumers that doctors are their best allies in coping with the organisational complexities of the health-care system – in providing them with the information required to make real choices.

Scepticism About Planning

To discuss the organisational complexities of health care systems is to introduce the third theme of our argument: the growing scepticism about rational planning. Again, this is not unique to the NHS, which is why

[7]Wilensky HL. The professionalization of everyone? *American Journal of Sociology* 1964;**70**:137–58.

tinkering with its structure is unlikely to make this issue disappear. Large-scale organisations are increasingly seen as out-of-date monuments to the optimistic belief in rational planning which dominated the '60s and early '70s. Left and Right alike indulge in the rhetoric of antibureaucracy. The technology of social engineering is under much the same sort of cloud as other forms of technology. The change is epitomised in the difference between the 1974 and 1982 reorganisations of the NHS. In 1974 the emphasis was on the centralisation of planning; in 1982 it has switched to the decentralisation of responsibility. The change is, of course, related to the transformation of the economic climate: in 1974 it was reasonable to assume that the centre could claim credit for the dividends of growth, while by the '80s it had become apparent that governments were well advised to diffuse the blame for bad news.[8]

Once more, the NHS can usefully be seen as a microcosm of its social and political environment. Its problems are particularly acute because it has an especially florid form of complexity. Technological complexity also means organisational complexity, and the proliferation of professional groups multiplies the power to veto change. The snaffle is more in evidence than the horse. And here, of course, the argument comes full circle. If economic stagnation means that change cannot be achieved by distributing the dividends of growth – if changing the priorities of the NHS between different client groups or redistributing resources geographically becomes a zero-sum game – then the built-in inertia of the organisation presents real problems.

We can therefore assume that the pressure for breaking up the NHS will grow in intensity. The attractions of a smaller scale and the promise of organisational flexibility can be expected to grow. Against this, however, two factors seem to argue against a fundamental transformation of Britain's health-care system. Firstly, the 1,000,000 people now employed in the NHS represent a powerful coalition for the status quo. Secondly, if the aim of public policy remains the achievement of equity in distributing scarce resources, it is difficult to see an alternative to a national health service.

Squaring the Circle

Conceivably technology may help to square this particular circle. In the long run the development of microtechnology may permit the creation

[8]Klein R. The strategy behind the Jenkin non-strategy. *Br Med J* 1981;**282**: 1089–91.

of information systems which permit the individual units within the NHS to operate as independent entrepreneurs in a kind of social market, buying services from each other (and perhaps the private sector as well). Equally, technology may help to transform the relationship between providers and consumers of health services. At present the former have a monopoly of information. In future consumers may be able to have direct access to information which allows them to cope better and more confidently with organisational complexity. The emergence of the new technology may also encourage the development of a "self-service economy" in health.[9] The potential for self-treatment might be greatly increased by access to information. Self-diagnosis will become a real possibility, with very considerable implications for the role of the general practitioner, and the do-it-yourself movement could well spread to health care.

To speculate about such developments is, however, to embark on a reckless trip down the Cresta run of futurology. In discussing the future of health services and the role of the medical profession the best guide remains the past – the strains and stresses which are already visible in the healthcare system and which will be accentuated by changes in the social, political, and economic environment. The only prediction that can be made with reasonable confidence is that the implications of adapting to the new situation are likely to be less painful than the implications of reacting to the new environment by defending the status quo, in terms of the distribution of resources, power, and status. If the future is simply like the past, only poorer, it will be very bleak indeed.

---

[9]Gershuny J. *After industrial society.* London: Macmillan, 1978.

49

The NHS and the Theatre of Inadequacy

UNIVERSITIES QUARTERLY
1983

Since its creation 35 years ago, the National Health Service has been in a permanent state of crisis. In the 1950s, there was the drama of over-spending, culminating in Bevan's resignation. In the 1960s, there was the drama of confrontation with the general practitioners. In the 1970s, there was the drama of confrontation with just about everybody: nurses, ward orderlies and consultants. In the 1980s, there is the drama of impending collapse, with large numbers of the health care professions abandoning the wards and operating rooms to take to the television studios to prophecy that the day of reckoning is fast approaching. The longest death bed scene in British institutional history appears to be nearing its climax: the next instalment of the series may – who knows? – even be the last.

To apply the language of the theatre – or the metaphor of soap opera – to the NHS may appear irresponsibly frivolous. Yet we cannot even begin to analyse the real problem of the NHS if we do not first grasp the extent to which the politics of health care are a branch of dramaturgy. The NHS *is* a political theatre, with a permanent cast of 1,000,000 and as such it generates drama as well as producing health care. It is an institution with a built-in incentive to dramatise its own difficulties, to exaggerate shortcomings and to shock its audience: the theatre of inadequacy.

The reason for this is self-evident. In Britain, the NHS has a near-monopoly of health care. Private spending on health care (about which more later) accounts for only five per cent or so of total expenditure.

For doctors and others with specialised skills which they cannot easily apply in other areas, there is little alternative employment outside the NHS – particularly now that the traditional escape routes to North America and elsewhere are being closed down. If, therefore, those working in the NHS want to improve conditions for themselves – if they want higher pay or more resources – they have a direct incentive to dramatise short-comings and inadequacies. Since they cannot exit, they must use voice. Or, as Enoch Powell was the first to point out almost 20 years ago[1], those working in the NHS have a vested interest in denigrating it. To improve conditions for themselves they have to point out how awful conditions are for patients.

The theatre of inadequacy takes many forms. At the local level, there is Grand Guignol: the surgeon pressing his case for a new piece of equipment will make blood-curdling statements about the danger of patients dying ('shroud-waving', as this is known in the trade) if he doesn't get what he wants. At the national level, the various professional interest groups – ranging from the British Medical Association (BMA) to the Confederation of Health Service Employees (COHSE) – will regularly issue warnings about the NHS's inadequate funding and the dire, if unspecified, consequences that will follow if governments do not find more money.

But granting that the chorus of self-denigration is part of a long NHS tradition, we are still left with a number of puzzles. Why, in recent years, should the chorus have become both louder and shriller? Why, furthermore, should there be – to judge from the explosion of media coverage – such an upsurge of audience interest in medical horror stories? Why, finally, is the political consensus which has for so long cocooned the NHS breaking up?

In trying to answer these questions, there are various possible lines of explanations. Throughout the 'seventies, the NHS became steadily more highly unionised, with competition between both professional bodies and trade-unions intensifying. The incentives to advertise through mili-tancy, and other public displays of indignation, have thus been reinforced. Moreover, the NHS is bound to reflect the growing rhetorical polarisation of politics. But, of course, all this is to ignore what may be the glaringly obvious explanation: that people are getting more indignant about the state of the NHS because the service itself is becoming more inadequate. The next section therefore addresses itself directly to this issue.

How Adequate is the NHS?

Like so many deceptively simple questions, this one is strictly unanswer-able. To ask about the adequacy of the NHS – and to inquire about changes over time – is rather like asking whether a train is on time, when there is no Bradshaw. Not only do we lack a time-table, but we do not even know the destination of the train. Indeed, the 1979 Royal Commission on the National Health Service[2] noted the 'absence of detailed and publicly declared principles and objectives', and was forced to produce a shopping list of its own. The objectives of the NHS should be – in the Royal Commission's view – to provide 'a broad range of services of a high standard', ensure equality of entitlements and access and satisfy 'the reasonable expectations of its users', among other things. But as the Royal Commission was forced to concede, some of these objectives lack precision, while others may actually conflict with each other. So we are still left looking for benchmarks against which to assess the performance of the NHS in our attempt to establish whether or not services are deteriorating.

The most obvious way of assessing the NHS's performance would seem to be, of course, to ask about its impact on the people's health. Are we getting healthier as a result of the NHS's activities? Unfortunately the statistics we have got don't tell us much about the impact of the NHS on the nation's health, while the statistics which we would need do not exist[3]. While we know everything about the quantity of deaths, we know remarkably little about the quality of life. That is, there is a vast literature about the causes of declining mortality over the past century, and a fair consensus among the experts that the reasons for this have to be sought in rising standards of living rather than improvements in medical technology[4]. If the only objective of health services were to extend life, there would be little point in spending much money on them. But, of course, the real justification for spending money on health services is to improve the quality of life: to prevent the birth of handicapped babies, to cure crippling disabilities or, when this is not possible, to minimise the suffering of those who cannot be cured. And, incredibly enough, we simply lack the information required to come to *any* conclusion about the impact of the NHS on the quality of the population's life over the past 35 years, let alone the past three years. My own conviction would be that the NHS's impact has been enormous – if measured in terms of minimising suffering and maximising people's capacity to live actively, rather than of 'saving lives' – but I would find it hard to back that statement with hard evidence.

Lacking any way of measuring the impact of the NHS on the people's health, conventionally there are a number of approaches to the problem of trying to assess its performance: to get some idea of whether things are improving or not, independent of the (inevitably) self-interested views of the providers. The first is simply to look at the inputs of money and manpower into the NHS. Here the assumption is that if more money is spent, if more doctors and nurses are employed, then it seems reasonable to assume that standards are improving. The second is to look at the activities of the NHS. Here the assumption is that if more patients are being treated, if more operations are being carried out, then once again it can be reasonably assumed that things are improving. The third is to look at consumer satisfaction. Here the assumption is that patients will know whether or not standards are adequate. Each approach, as we shall see, turns out to raise some formidable problems of interpretation and to yield only precarious or ambiguous conclusions.

Trying to make sense of public expenditure figures and trends is now a major industry. But there is no reason to doubt the present Government's claim that spending on the NHS has increased in real terms – i.e. after allowing for inflation – since it took office in 1979. The size of the increase is open to question. The Government's claim in the 1983 Public Expenditure White Paper[5] that 'the scope for growth in services', between 1979 and 1983, was about five and a half per cent is almost certainly exaggerated. Indeed the curious language betrays the ambiguity – indeed fraudulence – of the claim. The only reason why the Government can claim a five and a half per cent growth rate is that it includes in its figure the so-called 'efficiency cuts': i.e. the notional half per cent a year which health authorities are supposedly saving through increasing efficiency. Unfortunately the Department of Health and Social Security (DHSS) has never been able to provide evidence that improvements in efficiency – as distinct of savings flowing from reductions in services – have actually been achieved. Still, even allowing for this, there undoubtedly has been an *increase* in the NHS's budget. The average annual rate of increase in public spending is modest by historical standards: it probably represents (taking account also of increased income from charges) a growth rate of about two per cent a year in the NHS's resources. But, given the fact that the economy as a whole has not been growing during this period, even this modest increase represents a significant shift of national resources towards the NHS.

Moreover, this is confirmed by the rise in the number of people working in the NHS: the service's most important resource. In 1979, to quote the 1983 White Paper again, there were the equivalent of 37,000 full-time doctors in English hospitals. By 1982 the figure was 40,000. For nurses the equivalent figures were, respectively, 358,000 and 396,000. Again, the figures need interpreting with care: if the working week is cut, as it has been for nurses, then higher numbers do not necessarily indicate more hours at the bedside. But, once again, the statistics – such as they are – give a lie to the rhetoric of cuts.

Finally the Government can, and does, argue that the evidence of the expenditure and manpower figures is confirmed by the evidence about the NHS's activities. Here the latest available figures are those for 1981; those for 1982 will, in any case, not mean very much because they will be distorted by the effects of the industrial troubles. Thus between 1979 and 1981, the number of acute in-patients treated rose by nearly 300,000, while the number of out-patient attendances rose by over 1,000,000. All this would surely appear to confirm the view that talk about sliding standards and impending collapse is best explained by the internal political dynamics of the NHS, rather than reflecting a deteriorating situation.

Unfortunately, we cannot even derive this conclusion from the evidence that we have got. Figures of activity do not tell us anything about the effectiveness of the NHS or about the quality of the service provided. It is easy enough to increase productivity – and give the impression of improving efficiency – by, for example, taking in less ill patients or by sending them home earlier (so transmuting visible public costs into invisible private costs to the families concerned). Nor do the figures of activity tell us anything about the extent to which the NHS is dealing with specific conditions and complaints: in this respect, even information about waiting lists and times are not very instructive since they are very much an artefact of clinical practice and administrative procedures[6]. When challenged to provide evidence about the quality and scope of services provided by the NHS, the DHSS tends to find itself flummoxed. After years of trying to elicit evidence from the Department on this point, the House of Commons Social Services Committee has still not made any progress[7].

But if we cannot make much sense of the statistics, surely there need be no such problems when it comes to considering the verdict of consumers. Here, at least, we can hope for hard evidence about how people feel about the services provided. Alas, once again we find ourselves in a swamp of ambiguity. On the face of it, the evidence is consistent and conclusive. People love the NHS. None of the talk of deteriorating standards has ever found the faintest echo in polls of public opinion. Over the decades, a remarkably steady 90% or so of those interviewed have declared themselves to be satisfied with the NHS; indeed most of them are 'very satisfied'. But it is not altogether clear as to what such figures actually mean. Do they simply reflect the fact that most people approve of the NHS as an institution? Or does it mean that they approve of the actual quality of the services provided? There is at least some evidence to suggest that overall satisfaction masks considerable dissatisfaction with particular aspects of the service although, predictably, consumers tend to grumble about very different aspects of the NHS – such as poor communications – to those identified by the providers in their laments about falling standards[8].

If the opinions of consumers appear to be somewhat ambiguous, their behaviour is not. Over the last decade there has been a sharp increase in the number of consumers opting out of the NHS and into the private sector[9]. In 1970, just under two million people were covered by private insurance schemes. By 1980, the figures had reached 3,500,000, and was still climbing. Increasingly, people appear to be voting with their feet against the NHS. However, even these figures need to be interpreted with care. One of the main reasons for the sharp increase has been a change less in individual preferences than in collective bargaining strategies: more and more unions – particularly, though not exclusively, those representing white collar workers – have chosen to negotiate for private health care coverage among other fringe benefits.

Perhaps more important still, the private sector offers health care of a specialised and limited kind. By and large, it does not deal with life-threatening illnesses or the degenerative chronic conditions of old age. It tends to deal with the relatively minor complaints of the middle-aged working population. Its growth therefore suggests that the short-comings of the NHS, as perceived by consumers, are of a particular kind: i.e. that the NHS gives lower priority than consumers would wish to dealing promptly with non-life-threatening conditions which, however, may affect the ability of the sufferer to live an active working life. Consumers in the private sector are thus buying prompt treatment, privacy and the right to a consultant's personal attention.

It would therefore be misleading to interpret the rapid increase in the private sector as a broadside criticism of the quality of care offered by the NHS, and thus as confirmation that standards in the NHS are indeed slipping. Not only, as stressed already, does the private sector remain small when set against the NHS. But most of those who use it hedge their bets and do not opt out of the NHS for good: they play the two systems to their own advantage – particularly by remaining registered with an NHS general practitioner[10]. More significantly still, the demand for private health care underlines that the NHS is responsive not to consumer preferences but to the paternalistic decisions of the professional providers. Indeed, given the NHS's own fundamental ethos, it could not be otherwise. The NHS was set up not to meet *demands*, but needs. It rations scarce resources according to *needs* as perceived by the professional providers and, to an extent, by politicians. Inevitably, higher priority will be given to what the professionals see as needs rather than to meeting consumer demands. Predictably, the NHS is not responsive to those consumer demands – such as those for individual attention, speed, privacy and so on – which are met in the private market[11].

The main need to which the NHS is responding, and which has been set out in a succession of policy documents by the DHSS[12], is that posed by an ageing population. More and more the NHS is becoming a health service for the elderly, with 50% or more of the acute beds occupied by pensioners: indeed it may be precisely this 'crowding out' effect which helps to explain the increasing popularity of the private sector. But to make this point is, of course, also to stress that simply to analyse the inputs to the NHS or its activities is to consider only one side of the equation. The other side of the equation is that of the changing demands for health care in Britain. Even if the resources of the NHS have continued to grow, it could still be that the growth has been inadequate to cope with new demands – and that it is precisely this gap between supply and demand which explains the anxieties about the impending collapse of the NHS. The next section therefore turns to considering the demand side of the equation.

The Demands for Health Care

Measuring the demand for health care is, if anything, an even more metaphysical enterprise than trying to assess the adequacy or otherwise of the NHS. Once again, it was Enoch Powell who summed up the dilemma: *'L'appetit vient en mangeant'*, he pointed out. The availability of health care generates its own demand; the scope for raising standards appears to be infinite. Not only is this true of medical technology. But, even more important, it is true of health *care*. In other words, even if we limited spending on medical technology (the fashionable cry) we would still be left arguing for more resources to improve the quality of care for the elderly, the mentally handicapped and so on: the occasional scandal reminds us of how far we still have to go in this direction. There is no sign that even those countries which spend more than three times as much per head of population on health care – Sweden, for example – have reached saturation point, in the sense of exhausting their capacity to discover new demands for spending more.

However, there is general agreement that an ageing population imposes extra pressures on health (and other social) services. The point can be simply illustrated. In 1980/81, the average cost per head of health and social services was £1,000 for those aged over 75, compared to £130 for those in the 16 to 64 age group. Conventionally, therefore, Governments – Labour and Conservative – have assumed that a 0.7% annual increase in the NHS is required to cope with the consequences of an ageing population. Equally, Governments have reckoned that there must be a further increase to cope with the effects of technological drift: the introduction of new drugs and so on. So, in a sense, it can be argued that the NHS requires annual growth of at least one per cent to accommodate new pressures, and that consequently it has for the past few years been surviving on what is little more than a standstill budget.

The point can be conceded. There are, in any case, so many uncertainties about the interpretation of public expenditure figures that it is not worthwhile arguing about the small print. But this leaves us with our initial puzzle unsolved. It may well be that the resources devoted to health care in Britain are inadequate: as the Royal Commission concluded, among many others, there is no way of determining 'adequacy'. Equally, however, there is no evidence that any inadequacy has – in material terms – become *more* pronounced in recent years. So we are still left searching for an explanation for the mounting sense of crisis, and its accompanying rhetoric of decay and disillusion.

Let us return, therefore, to our metaphor and look at the NHS as the theatre of inadequacy. We have already argued that the actors have every incentive to exaggerate any deficiencies in the NHS. Perhaps we should now also ask why the actors perceive there to be such deficiencies in the first place (conceding that they may be perfectly genuine in their perceptions of a widening gap between the attainable and the desirable, even when full allowance has been made for the temptation to theatrical exaggeration for the benefit of the audience). In doing so, we shall also explore the wider problem of adapting inherited Welfare State policies and institutions to a new economic environment[13]: for it is only in this context that the NHS drama begins to make sense.

The Welfare State, as it developed in the 30 years after 1945, grew fat on the dividends of the Growth State. The assumption shaping its policies and institutions was that tomorrow's generation would be better off than today's and that, consequently, we could commit ourselves to policies which depended on continued economic growth for their implementation. In the field of social security, for instance, we committed future generations to paying higher pensions to their parents. In the case of the NHS, to take a symbolic example, we committed ourselves to building hospital Concordes: that is, hospitals which were designed on the assumption that future generations would be able to afford much higher standards and which were thus far more expensive to run than the buildings they replaced.

The assumption that the Growth State was eternal did not survive the oil crisis of the mid-seventies. However, the momentum of the policies forged before the great divide continued. Thus the NHS entered the 'eighties still committed to all the policies forged in the days of optimism about growth. Not only is the aim of policy still to improve services for the deprived groups in the population, such as the elderly and the mentally ill and handicapped. But it is also to improve the geographical distribution of resources within the NHS, to bring the deprived regions of the country up to the national standard of provision. In short, there has been no retrenchment in *policy expectations* in line with the retrenchment in *resource availability* made inevitably by national economic crisis.

It is therefore not surprising that there is a widespread perception of deterioration – although the deterioration is only relative to policy expectations set in a totally different environment. Equally important, the fact that the NHS budget is growing more slowly than expected when the various policies were forged in the 'seventies, means that implementation often becomes a zero-sum game. That is, priorities cannot all be painlessly financed out of the dividends of growth but are at war with each other. If budgets are expanding fast, it's possible to give priority to the expansion of services for the mentally handicapped without necessarily cutting acute services: the former simply expand at a faster rate than the latter. When times get bad, however, it may actually be necessary to cut parts of the service in order to finance expansion elsewhere. And, inevitably, the politics or re-distribution are more bitter than the politics of expansion. To achieve equity in the distribution of resources, it may be necessary to close hospitals in inner London and other areas of declining population in order to finance services for the growing population in other parts of the South East: the result may be to create a misleading impression that services are being cut, when in fact they are simply being re-directed.

The problems of adapting plans based on optimistic assumptions about growth to a new economic environment are accentuated by another characteristic of the Welfare State, of which the NHS offers a particularly developed example. This is the sclerotic rigidity of Welfare State institutions[14]. The Welfare State creates a highly organised political constituency for the preservation of the status quo. It is highly unionised and professionalised. Moreover, when it comes to resisting the closure of a hospital or a school, the professional providers can mobilise the consumers as well (by definition the constituency for the status quo will be stronger than the constituency for those who would benefit from change: the new hospital or school has not yet been opened, and has thus not been able to mobilise its constituency). In this respect, the NHS is not so very different from universities where, once again, the diffusion of veto power makes adaptation to new circumstances difficult, and where the institutional bias is against change. So the paradox is that in a period when new social policy aims can often only be achieved by *re*-distributing resources, our inherited institutions conspire against such a solution. In an institutional sense, the Welfare State is its own worst enemy – guaranteed, in the new economic environment, to perpetuate perceptions of inadequacy.

The NHS not only offers the spectacle of institutional rigidity: a service where over the past decade, the number of interest groups able to veto or at least delay change has increased greatly[15]. But, additionally, there is a reason unique to health care why perceptions of inadequacy should be particularly acute in the NHS. This is that standards of medical care are international, while the resources available for providing health care are national. Medical knowledge knows no frontiers; doctors are highly mobile. It is therefore not surprising that doctors in particular should define the desirable in terms of the 'best' – as defined by the latest technical break-through, the most recent scientific paper – model offered in the global village of medical practice. Inevitably, they will compare, usually unfavourably, what is possible in Britain with what is happening in the United States or elsewhere.

There is a trap in such comparisons. Usually the comparison is between a model of excellence taken from abroad and the average in Britain, which may well flatter the former. But if the NHS is to be compared in terms of peaks of excellence (as distinct perhaps from minimum standards of quality) with countries like the United States or Sweden or Germany, then inevitably there is going to be a growing gap between what Britain's NHS can deliver and what the health services of other nations can afford to provide. The reason for this is simple. Britain happens to be a poorer country. Her income (1979) per head of population is 7,170 dollars, while the equivalent figures for the United States, Germany and Sweden are respectively 10,650, 12,450 and 12,820 dollars. These differences are further compounded by the fact that Britain spends a smaller proportion of a smaller national income on health care than the other countries: in round figures, just under six per cent as against around nine per cent or more for the other countries[16].

Now it may be said that Britain should devote a higher proportion of the national income to health care (although in practice the high spending countries are all trying to reduce the rising bill for health care, and the NHS is often held out as a successful model of cost containment). But it is worth pointing out that if Britain were to attempt to achieve the same *level* of spending per head of population as Sweden, this would mean devoting something like 18% of the national income to health care: treble the present proportion. This is perhaps to exaggerate: the differences in actual spending between Britain and other countries are not as great as the brute figures might seem to imply, since Britain gets more value for money out of every pound spent – a reflection, in part, of the NHS's success in squeezing wages and salaries. Still, the calculation does offer a dramatic reminder that if Britain's system of health care is to be measured by what is done in much richer societies, then there will always be a gap between the desirable and the achievable. If the comparison were to be between the NHS and health services of, say, Spain and Italy – countries much nearer, though somewhat below, Britain's income per head – a very different and more flattering conclusion would be drawn.

Learning to Live with Inadequacy

In the last resort, the arguments advanced in the previous section would suggest the crisis of the NHS is part of a much larger crisis of adjustment in Britain. It is a crisis of adjustment to the fact of economic stagnation. The rigidities of British institutions not only have helped to contribute to the economic problems that now face the country but also make the process of adaptation more painful and more difficult. It is a crisis of adjustment to the fact that British society is now the poor relation of the advanced Western economies. Taking much richer countries as the reference group for comparison is to invite disillusion and to evoke a sense of sliding standards and impending decay. In both these respects, the NHS can be taken as a symbol of British society, mirroring the larger stresses of its environment.

In this situation, there is almost certainly no alternative to learning to live with inadequacy: the extent of the 'inadequacy' being defined by past hopes (based on now unrealisable assumptions about economic growth) and the standards of richer countries (whose economic achievements Britain probably cannot expect to match). In other words, instead of being swayed by the theatrical indignation of the actors, the audience should be asking itself whether the NHS is delivering the best that can be expected in a poor-rich country whose past has left a heritage of exaggerated expectations and social ambitions above its economic station. Given such a question, it may be that the overwhelming majority of the public who declare themselves to be satisfied with the NHS are more realistic in their assessment than the health service providers who translate their own (perfectly legitimate) aspiration to achieve the highest possible standards – as defined by professionals, at any rate – into a denunciation of existing achievements.

Health care, even in the richest countries, is about rationing what will always be inadequate resources[17]. Given this, we should perhaps ask first whether the NHS rations resources in a reasonably fair and socially acceptable way. Here the answer is that the NHS appears to do better than most health care systems. Inequities in the distribution of resources, both as between different parts of the country and different groups of patients, remain: but at least the differences are gradually being narrowed – though, here again, lack of economic growth has inhibited policy implementation[18]. By and large, the NHS has achieved equity in access to health care. If the middle-classes receive better quality medical care than others, it is because they have resources – information and social confidence – which enable them to exploit their opportunities of access more than other social groups[19]. Finally, the NHS is a massive instrument for re-distributing resources to the most vulnerable section of the population: the old.

It is this perceived fairness of the NHS which perhaps explains its greatest achievement: the fact that it has made scarcity and inadequacy socially acceptable. The NHS, as we know, turns away people to die. The best known example of this, though not the only one, is the strict rationing of facilities for treatment of renal failure – where Britain is much less generous than many other countries. In part, the acceptability of such decisions may reflect the fact that decisions about resources are presented as clinical decisions: economic policies are transmuted into professional ones[20]. In part, however, the acceptability of scarcity surely also reflects the more general perception of the NHS as a fair instrument for matching resources to needs.

But public support for the NHS, as an institution for making the best of inadequacy, may turn out to be a wasting asset. For it rests on a particular view of society: a society responsive to needs as well as to demands. In the case of the NHS this means, as argued already, an acceptance of the values of paternalistic professionalism. And both paternalism and professionalism are now under challenge, from both Right and Left. If we want a health service which is more responsible to consumer demands, then the NHS may well not survive in its present form. For its characteristic is precisely that it distributes resources according to professionally defined needs, not in response to the power of organised groups in either the political or the economic market. In this respect, as in others, it is tempting to argue there is no crisis of the NHS. Instead, our confusion and anxiety about health services reflects a wider social crisis, reflecting uncertainty and doubt about the appropriate boundaries between public and private provision of welfare, about the power of professionals and bureaucrats and the limits of altruistic social policies in an age of economic austerity[21].

Notes

1. Enoch Powell, *Medicine and Politics* (Pitman Medical, 1966). Mr. Powell was Minister of Health from 1960 to 1963.

2. Royal Commission on the National Health Service, *Report* (HMSO, 1979, Cmnd. 7615).

3. J.N. Morris, 'Are Health Services Important to the People's Health?'. in *British Medical Journal*, 19 January 1980, pp. 167–168.

4. Thomas McKeown, *The Role of Medicine* (Basil Blackwell, 1979).

5. Chancellor of the Exchequer, *The Government's Expenditure Plans 1983–84 to 1985–86* (HMSO 1983, Cmnd. 8789).

6. See, for example, H.F. Sanderson, 'What's in a Waiting List?', in *British Medical Journal*, 6 November 1982, pp. 1368–1369.

7. Social Services Committee, *Public Expenditure on the Social Services*, Second Report, Session 1981–82 (HMSO, 1982, H.C. 306).

8. See, for example, Janet Gregory, *Patients' Attitudes to the Hospital Service*, Royal Commission on the National Health Service Research Paper No. 5 (HMSO 1978).

9. For the private sector, see Gordon McLachlan and Alan Maynard (eds.) *The Public/Private Mix for Health* (The Nuffield Provincial Hospitals Trust, 1982).

10. I am grateful for this point to David Horne, currently carrying out research into the private sector at the University of Bath.

11. For a critique of the NHS from a market perspective, see Michael W. Spicer, 'The Economics of Bureaucracy and the British National Health Service,' *Milbank Memorial Fund Quarterly/Health and Society*, Vol. 60, No. 4, Fall 1982, pp. 657–672.

12. For example, Department of Health and Social Security, *Priorities for Health* (HMSO, 1976); most recently, DHSS, *Care in Action* (HMSO 1981).

13. Rudolf Klein, 'The Welfare State: A Self-Inflicted Crisis?' *Political Quarterly*, Vol. 51, No. 1, January/March 1980, pp. 24–34.

14. The general problem of institutional rigidity, with particular application to Britain's present economic and political difficulties, is examined in: Samuel H. Beer, *Britain Against Itself* (Macmillan 1982) and Mancur Olson, *The Rise and Decline of Nations* (Yale University Press, 1982).

15. Rudolf Klein, *The Politics of the National Health Service* (Longmans, 1983).

16. Robert J. Maxwell, *Health and Wealth* (Lexington Books, 1981).

17. For an American exposition of this point, see Victor R. Fuchs, *Who Shall Live?* (Basic Books, 1974).

18. Social Services Committee, *op. cit.*

19. For the view that equity has been achieved, see E. Collins and Rudolf Klein, 'Equity and the NHS: Self-reported Morbidity, Access and Primary Care', in *British Medical Journal*, 25 October 1980, pp. 1111–1115. For a different interpretation of the evidence, see Julian Le Grand, *The Strategy of Inequality* (Allen & Unwin, 1981). But note that Le Grand's conclusion that equity has not been achieved depends on assuming that the available statistics of morbidity measure the need for health services, including hospital services: this is a very questionable assumption indeed.

20. Guido Calabresi and Philip Bobbitt, *Tragic Choices* (Norton, 1978).

21. For evidence suggesting that economic adversity makes people less altruistic, see James E. Alt, *The Politics of Economic Decline* (Cambridge University Press, 1979).

50

Acceptable Inequalities

FROM ACCEPTABLE INEQUALITIES.
D GREEN (ED), LONDON IEA
HEALTH UNIT
1988

I. Introduction

Much is made of inequality in health and health care. Inequality, it seems, is always with us. The harder we try, the more we invest in the National Health Service and the more effort we put into health and safety at work, health promotion and all the rest of it, the worse the situation appears to become. Not only is there inequality in the use of health services, but, it is asserted, there is also widening inequality in life expectancy and the experience of ill-health. Such was the theme of the Black Report published at the beginning of the decade.[1] Such has been the message of a succession of reports since, culminating in the last will and testament of the outgoing management of the Health Education Council.[2]

Deeply engrained in the national consciousness, constantly reiterated in the medical press and the media, is the sense of another British social policy failure. From this follow demands for higher spending on the NHS, for greater investment in health education, for more generous income support for poor families and, indeed, for more urgent action to bring

[1] Sir Douglas Black (1980), *Inequalities in Health: Report of a Research Working Group*, London: DHSS.
[2] Margaret Whitehead (1987), *The Health Divide*. London: Health Education Council.

unemployment down. Inequalities in health are perceived, as it were, as the barometer which measures the ills of society in the largest sense as well as the failures of the NHS.

Such, at least, appears to be the consensus. It is, however, a consensus which depends on filtering out dissonant evidence and excommunicating or ignoring those who offer more optimistic interpretations. In what follows I shall briefly review the available evidence, and the various ways in which it can be read, before addressing my main theme, which is to try to break up and analyse the notion of 'inequality' itself. It is a notion which, like equality itself,[1] is more complicated and more multi-dimensional than the current debate would imply. In effect, inequality is a many-threaded tapestry.[2] If (as I shall argue) there are different kinds of inequalities, and different ways of interpreting their significance, it follows that we have to consider which of them we *can* do something about and which of them we *want* to do something about. Some inequalities may be acceptable; others may be intolerable; yet others may be unavoidable. The purpose of this essay therefore is to make a start, no more, on the task of unpicking the threads.

In tackling the theme, I stand as an aesthetic egalitarian, to adopt a phrase thrown out somewhat contemptuously by Joseph and Sumption.[3] My instinctive preference is for more equality rather than less. The extreme kinds of inequality, I would argue, are like the worst kinds of pornography: they corrupt the sensibilities of society as a whole, and make us all less than fully human, by blunting our sense of sympathy (to use Adam Smith's terminology).[4] It is a position which implies that what matters is not so much the degree of inequality in itself (as measured statistically, using Gini co-efficients or whatever) as the degree of deprivation or degradation implied by being at the bottom end of any given distribution of resources; conversely, inequality may be justified to the extent that it improves the lot of the worst-off.[5] But, equally, I would maintain that inequality does not speak for itself in terms of the policy responses that should be made. There are many kinds of inequalities that have always been tolerated, and always will be: more of that below. To pretend that we need not choose policy priorities between tackling

---

[1] D. Rae (1981), *Equalities*, Cambridge, Massachusetts: Harvard University Press; M. O'Higgins (1987), 'Egalitarians, Equalities and Welfare Evaluation,' *Journal of Social Policy*, Vol. 15, Part 3, pp. 293–315.

[2] L.S. Tempkin (1986), 'Inequality', *Philosophy and Public Affairs*, Vol. 15, No. 2, pp. 99–121.

[3] Sir Keith Joseph and J. Sumption (1979), *Equality*, London: John Murray.

[4] A. Sen (1987), *On Ethics and Economics*, Oxford: Basil Blackwell.

[5] J. Rawls (1973), *A Theory of Justice*, Oxford: Oxford University Press.

different kinds of inequalities in health and health care is simply to invite the kind of disillusion that has followed the long campaign to eliminate poverty: the best way of ensuring a global sense of defeat, and total paralysis, is to invent a global policy target. Conversely, the best way of making some headway is to define as precisely as possible what is acceptable and what is not on different assumptions and criteria.

There is also the general question of whether, in discussing health and health care, we are dealing with something different from other spheres of inequality. Are inequalities in health and health care any different from, and less acceptable than, inequalities in income, education, housing and so on? In putting this question, we need to distinguish sharply arguments about the principles that should determine the distribution of health and those which shape the distribution of health care, and the factors that should in each case be taken into account when devising the machinery needed to give effect to any desired distribution. For there are different causes of inequality in health and health care, just as there are different arguments about what implications to draw in each case. The argument for seeing health as different rests on the contention[1] that health is a necessary condition for the achievement of all human potentials, whether as political citizens or as participants in the economic market-place or as family actors. It is precisely this which makes Nozick's response to Williams[2] – that if medical need should be the only criterion for medical treatment then the only proper criterion for the distribution of barbering services is barbering need – frivolously irrelevant: long hair is somewhat less of a barrier to being able to work than, say, an unset broken leg. It would seem, then, that the health needed to function properly (and the health care required to ensure such functioning) is a necessary enabling condition for all human activities.

Health Care – 'Needs' and Preferences

This is, at first sight, a persuasive principle. But some general difficulties about it have to be noted, since they will haunt the subsequent discussion. One is that the argument for the primacy of health, as somehow unique and different, has been developed in the context of claims to the provision of health *care*, i.e. access to treatment. If, however, it turns out that health, seen as the ability to function adequately in different contexts, is

---

[1] A. Weale (1983), *Political Theory and Social Policy*, London: Macmillan; N. Daniels (1985), *Just Health Care*, Cambridge: Cambridge University Press.

[2] R. Nozick (1974), *Anarchy, State and Utopia*, New York: Basic Books; B. Williams (1967), 'The Idea of Equality', in P. Laslett and W. G. Runciman (eds)., *Philosophy, Politics and Society*, Second Series, Oxford: Basil Blackwell.

determined largely by factors other than medical intervention – such as income, education and housing (as well as personal habits such as smoking and drinking) – then does the principle apply equally strongly to all these spheres and any other goods that may be relevant to the production of health? If so, does the argument for equal claims flowing from equal 'needs' for health care inevitably lead to universal egalitarianism? Or should we conclude that inequalities in health and health care are not so uniquely different from, and not necessarily less or more acceptable than, those in other spheres? Furthermore, there is the notorious problem of giving anything like a precise, operational definition of what is meant by the 'health' required to function effectively. This, inevitably, is contingent on occupation, family circumstances and environment. Even with a broken leg, I can probably function reasonably well as a university professor; however, things would be very different if I were a trapeze artist. If my hearing is bad and I am to function effectively as a citizen I probably require a deaf-aid, but do I also need a hip replacement to go to political meetings or should I be pushed there in a wheelchair? What, in any case, is the dividing line between 'needs' (a dangerously abstract concept) and preferences? What distinguishes those conditions which set up a claim against society from those which simply raise a question about an individual's willingness to spend money on his or her health as against, say, opera or holidays abroad?

The other difficulty revolves around the long debate on whether health care is just one more consumer good, and should be treated as such, when it comes to designing the machinery to give effect to any desired distribution. If we examined the distribution of motor cars in a society where a computer infallibly assigned income according to need to every man, woman and child – Egalitaria, let us call it – we would expect to find wide divergences. Some people would have decided to do without a car, others would stick to their old bangers; a few might starve themselves in order to buy a Rolls. On the whole, it would seem reasonable to guess that no one would get terribly excited about, or that an academic industry would develop around, the theme of inequalities in car ownership. We would simply assume that the Egalitarians were following their own preferences. Would we have the same reaction, even in Egalitaria, if some people chose to take out adequate health insurance policies? The answer, surely, is 'No'. We do not treat health care as a market good like any other, for complex reasons: partly because self-neglect may have social spill-over effects and costs, partly because of the problems posed by the imbalance of information as between the consumers and producers of health care, partly because of the contingent nature of health-care needs and the difficulties of switching from one supplier to another (changing consultants is rather more problematic than trading in cars, particularly if the first one called in botched the job).

In considering inequalities in health care provision, then, we assume that a certain degree of paternalism is justified. The problems of an unequal distribution of either health or health care cannot be tackled, as I shall argue, by moving towards a more equal distribution of incomes (highly desirable though that might be for other reasons). Such an approach will always remain inadequate as long as there is an unequal distribution of other resources: the accumulated stock of intelligence, information, social skills and the other abilities developed over time and required to manipulate any given bundle of income, claims or entitlements to the maximum effect.

Are Inequalities the Same as Differences?

A final prefatory remark. The inequalities discussed in this essay must be distinguished from what might be called mere differences. If it turns out that red-haired people have a life expectancy twice that of brown-haired people, this might well be an interesting, researchable difference. If it turns out that people living in parts of the country with hard water have a lower incidence of coronaries[1] than those living in soft-water areas, then again this is a highly significant difference for exploring the causes of cardiovascular disease. In neither case, however, would we talk about inequalities. To invoke this word is to set up the presumption of a *prima facie* case for social concern, perhaps even moral outrage, and policy action. In other words, there has to be an element of perceived social injustice: a pattern of systematic arbitrariness or unjustified discrimination. So if it turned out that red-haired people had a life expectancy twice that of brown-haired people because they were systematically given preferential treatment in the NHS, while the latter were regularly sent to the back of the queue, we might properly invoke the concept of inequality. We might well come to the same conclusion, also, if we found that the poorest people were condemned by their own poverty to living in the soft-water parts of the country, and thus to a higher rate of coronaries.

Indeed, as we shall suggest in the next section, the resurgence of interest in inequalities in health in the 1980s largely represents the semantic tactics of political mobilisation: the use of differences/inequalities in health to mobilise opinion against perceived incqualities in other spheres – income, housing and employment – since these, in turn, are related to differences/inequalities in health.

---

[1] J.N. Morris (1975), *Uses of Epidemiology*, third edn., Edinburgh: Churchill Livingstone.

2. The Debate About Inequalities

The link between low incomes, inadequate housing, a bad environment and poor health has been recognised for a long time. It was this realisation that dominated health policy in the 19th century, starting with Chadwick's 1842 report.[1] It was Chadwick who drew attention to the 'comparative chances of life in different classes' and to the effects of environments on health. He did so not in order to mobilise opinion against the inequalities in social conditions that gave rise to health inequalities but to identify the specific factors amenable to action by government in order to change this situation: notably clean water, good sewers and better housing. It was a tradition of thinking about health that was to be displaced, for the most part of the 20th century, by the myth of scientific medicine as the *deus ex machina*. And while the contribution of scientific medicine has indeed been great – despite the controversy as to precisely how much it has contributed to either the quantity or quality of life (probably more to the latter than to the former) – by the 1970s it was becoming clear not only that excessive hopes had been invested in it but also that it represented an accelerating cost escalator.

The naive assumption of the founders of the NHS – that improved health services would liquidate the demand for medical attention by improving the nation's health – proved a delusion. As Enoch Powell pointed out,[2] in medical care *l'appetit vient en mangeant* if there are no price barriers. Hence the revival of interest, internationally, in the social conditions and individual behaviour which promote ill-health. As the scope (and cost) of medical technology turned out to be ever-expanding, so there seemed an increasingly urgent case for moving from the provision of health care to the promotion of health itself. If the former was not delivering the hoped-for goods (and was getting ever more expensive), why not try the latter strategy? It was in this new intellectual context that the Black Working Group was appointed. Its objectives were:[3]

1. To assemble available information about the differences in health status among the social classes and about factors which might contribute to these.

---

[1]M.W. Flinn (ed.) (1965), *Report on the Sanitary Condition of the Labouring Population of Great Britain, 1842*, Edinburgh: Edinburgh University Press.
[2]J.E. Powell (1966), *Medicine and Politics*, London: Pitman Medical.
[3]Sir Douglas Black (1980), *Inequalities in Health: Report of a Research Working Group*, London: DHSS.

2. To analyse available information about the differences in health status among the social classes and about factors which might contribute to these.

The Black Report and Health Inequalities

However, the reason why the Black Report continues to have political resonance and to be invoked in debate even today reflects the way in which members of the Working Party moved from differences to inequalities, and so translated a diagnostic into a prescriptive role:

> 'Present social inequalities in health in a country with substantial resources like Britain are unacceptable, and deserve so to be declared by every section of public opinion . . . We have no doubt that greater equality of health must remain one of our foremost national objectives and that in the last two decades of the twentieth century a new attack upon the forces of inequality has regrettably become necessary and now needs to be concerted',

they wrote in their preface. Health inequalities were seen, it would seem, as a way of generating more political support in the battle against poverty: a campaign which was otherwise flagging.

At the heart of the Black Report, and of the subsequent debate about inequalities, was the analysis of differences both in health status and the use of health services in terms of social classes, based on the Registrar-General's occupational categories. This, of course, represents the central tradition in British sociology and social analysis, going back to Chadwick and beyond; a tradition which has generated as much intellectual fog as insight. If there is a difference between social classes (so ran the Black Report's implicit assumption), then this in itself represents an inequality in the sense of giving cause for moral or political concern. But social class is a rubber tin opener as far as analysis is concerned. Why should we be concerned if we do not know the precise significance of any finding? And we don't. As the Black Report itself pointed out (only subsequently to ignore its own reservations), there are serious problems about using social class as a tool of analysis: problems which range from the classification of married women under their husband's occupation to the fact that there can be wide variations in resources relevant to health (housing, education and income) within any given social class. If our intention is to try to relate *specific* differences in housing, education and income to *specific* differences in health and healthcare use, then social class is much too blunt a tool. Similarly, if our concern is to identify unacceptable inequalities – systematic patterns of discrimination against particular groups of the population, equivalent to brown-haired people being put at the end of the queue – then, once again, social class is far too broad a concept.

It is, therefore, not surprising that a large literature[1] has developed in the wake of the Black Report, given the ideological overtones of the whole debate. Its interest, for the purpose of this essay, lies as much in the style of the academic debate as in its contents: a style which is much closer to a theological controversy than to a dispassionate scientific inquiry. Any challenge to the Black Report is seen as a betrayal: any article or paper which argues that the differences identified by the Black Report either do not exist or do not merit the status of inequalities brings a flood of attempted rebuttals, with a strong suggestion that anyone who does not agree with its conclusions must be in favour of poverty, slums and illiteracy (or, worse still, a supporter of Mrs Thatcher!). A new industry has developed designed to demonstrate the link between deprivation and poor health, with a not so hidden agenda of trying to prove that Conservative policies are widening inequalities in health, particularly because of the effect of unemployment.

Since no one since the days of Chadwick has ever attempted to deny that there is a link between social conditions and health (the real challenge, rather, is to identify with precision which particular aspects of deprivation are crucial), and since the case for reducing unemployment, getting rid of poor housing and giving everyone a decent education would be just as strong even if none of these factors were linked to ill-health, much of this discussion seems to be redundant. To the extent that the post-Black research industry is addressing the problem of identifying the specific factors linked with ill-health so, ironically, it is casting doubt on the original Black use of social class as the main analytical tool: for example, Townsend's micro-study of health in one NHS region demonstrates significant differences *within* social classes – which might have to do with such environmental factors as pollution, but which are certainly not caught in the catch-all concept of social class.[2] As yet, however, there is no debate about inequalities *within* the working class, and about the need to re-distribute resources *within* it: a point to which we shall return.

Errors in Black Report's Conclusions

In any case, it seems reasonably clear that the Black Report was wrong in some of its most headline-catching conclusions, which have since passed into the conventional wisdom. Most notably, the work of Raymond Illsley and Julian Le Grand has raised very large questions indeed – to

---

[1]M. Whitehead (1987), *The Health Divide*, London: Health Education Council.
[2]P. Townsend, P. Phillmore and A. Beattie (1986), *Inequalities in Health in the Northern Region*, Bristol: University of Bristol.

put it cautiously – against the report's conclusion of widening inequalities in health over time (for a summary, see Illsley (1987)).[1] Again, the flaw in the Black analysis is the reliance on social class. Since social classes change over time both in their composition and in their size, any comparison over time does not compare like with like. Moreover, the Black conclusion rests on an analysis of the working population. It thus excludes, by definition, that part of the population – the over-64s – which has notched up the greatest improvements in health (as measured by life expectancy) over this century.

Lastly, the Black Report brushes aside the evidence that at least some of the differences between social classes reflect selective social mobility: the healthiest move upward, the least healthy drift downward. Not surprisingly, therefore, and entirely in line with the commonsense assumption that the improvements in living standards of recent decades must have had *some* effect, the alternative analyses carried out by Illsley and Le Grand – using individual life expectancies rather than social class mortality figures – show a diminution of differences in the distribution of health over the decades.

Similarly, the Black Report's assertion that access to the NHS is biased against the working classes – once use is related to 'need' as measured by the available, unsatisfactory, indicators of morbidity – has been shot down. There is little evidence of bias in access to general practice, the gateway to the rest of the NHS.[2] Perhaps the most interesting aspect of this study is that, as with Illsley's and Le Grand's work, it prompted an immediate avalanche of attempted rebuttals: inequalities were something to be cherished and defended as political ammunition, and not to be lightly surrendered to the first critic; inequalities have, in effect, become political property. In the event, the finding has been fully supported by subsequent studies.[3] And the strategy of those who continue to defend the original Black thesis has switched to arguing that while, just conceivably, quantitative equity in access to the NHS might have been achieved, this tells us nothing about the quality of care given once access had been obtained. To switch the argument from quantity to quality does, indeed,

---

[1] R. Illsley (1987), 'Occupational Class, Selection and Inequalities in Health', *Quarterly Journal of Social Affairs*, Vol.3, No. 3, pp. 213–223.

[2] E. Collins and R. Klein (1980), 'Equity and the NHS', *British Medical Journal*, Vol. 281, pp. 1,111–1,115.

[3] E. Collins and R. Klein (1985), *Self-Reported Morbidity, Socio-Economic Factors and General Practitioner Consultations*, Bath Social Policy Paper No. 5, Bath: Centre for the Analysis of Social Policy; F. Puffer (1986), 'Access to Primary Health Care', *Journal of Social Policy*, Vol. 15, Part 3, pp. 293–315; Office of Population Censuses and Statistics (1986), *General Household Survey for 1984*, London: HMSO.

raise some important issues about what should or should not be regarded as acceptable inequalities. So, having shown just how problematic and value-laden even the ostensibly neutral exercise of measuring and interpreting differences may be, we turn next to examining which of these differences might be regarded as acceptable or unacceptable inequalities.

3. Which Differences Matter?

Let us return to Egalitaria. This is a country, to remind the reader, where a computer divides out everyone's income according to need: so, for example, someone with severe disabilities will get more money than someone who is fully mobile and active. It is a just society, as far as income distribution is concerned. If we found differences in health and health-care use in Egalitaria, we would presumably simply describe these as interesting differences – possibly relevant for research, but certainly not cause for indignation. There could, in such a society, be no beating of the political drums about inequalities in health. We would therefore be identifying acceptable inequalities, in the sense of differences which (while possibly regrettable) do not call for social and political action.

To start with, we would almost certainly find a continuing difference in life expectancy between men and women. These differences have indeed been widening:[1] in 1950 women could expect to live five years longer than men, but by 1981 this widened to 6.4 years. And this trend is in no way unique to Britain. Conversely, of course, women tend to suffer from more ill-health than men. But it would seem rather odd, certainly in Egalitaria but also in contemporary Britain, to describe this as something unjust or perverse. There would be little cause for the men to take to the streets in protest against such discrimination.

Nor is it totally clear that life expectancy, as such, should be seen as an unmitigated 'good': would even the most dedicated of egalitarians want to argue for an absolutely equal share of 'life expectancy' to go to everyone, irrespective of genetic inheritance, irrespective of the capacity actually to enjoy life? The question needs to be put only because the Black Report, and the literature spawned by it, continues to use mortality as its main analytical tool. This is reasonable enough to the extent that mortality statistics are the only reliable data available over time; it only becomes dangerous when the limitations of using this kind of data are forgotten.

---

[1]M. Whitehead (1987), *The Health Divide*, London: Health Education Council. This is the source of most of the figures that follow.

Geographical Environment, Social Class and Life Expectancy

Similarly, we would find continuing differences in Egalitaria between people living in different parts of the country. Strikingly, geographical differences in life expectancy – and indeed disease patterns – have persisted for more than a century, particularly between town and country. In 1842 Chadwick's researchers found that while the average age of death in Manchester was 38 for professional persons and gentry, it was only 17 for mechanics and labourers; in Rutlandshire, however, the average age of death was 38 for mechanics and labourers and 52 for professional persons and gentry.[1] In other words, the geographical environment often overrode social class in the 19th century. And the same is true today. If we examine standardised mortality ratios, we find that men in social classes IV and V in East Anglia have almost as good a record as those in social classes I and II in Scotland, while women in social classes IV and V in East Anglia have a better record than those in social classes I and II in both Scotland and the North West. This would suggest that, even in Egalitaria and even in a society where social class had been abolished, there might still be large regional differences, just as it suggests that the distribution of income (and all that goes with it, such as housing and education) is only one factor determining health: East Anglia is not the richest region in the country. Once again, then, we would seem to have identified an acceptable kind of inequality.

We might also discover in Egalitaria differences in life expectancy related to specific occupations as distinct from social class. Some occupations are more dangerous than others. In Egalitaria, we probably would not get too concerned about such differences. Given an equitable distribution of income, the choice of occupation could be seen as unconstrained: if some people choose to risk their lives and limbs by climbing chimneys or by working in noxious surroundings, so be it (provided they take out adequate insurance policies and do not impose costs on others). In any other society, however, such differences might well be thought of as unacceptable inequalities, insofar as the choice of occupation is dictated either by lack of income or by lack of alternatives.

This point is to underline the importance, and also the difficulty, of determining when a difference can be ignored because it reflects things which cannot be altered by anyone (such as one's sex or genetic inheritance), or factors which represent personal preferences and decisions freely made (such as the choice of job or smoking). If a difference in health or health-care use falls into either of these categories, then it can surely be described as an acceptable inequality. And in Egalitaria, there

---

[1] M.W. Flinn (ed.) (1965), *op. cit.*, Edinburgh: Edinburgh University Press.

is little problem about making this sort of categorisation. But in a country where, unlike Egalitaria, decisions about health and health-care use are made under often severe constraints, cultural as well as economic, the situation is more complex and more worrying. If health can be seen as an investment good, then we have to ask whether there are unacceptable inequalities in the resources people bring to the investment decisions – which would, in turn, produce unacceptable inequalities in health.

Smoking and Social Class

Smoking provides a classic example for analysing this particular issue. It is related to the incidence of both cancer and heart disease. In Egalitaria, we would presumably not classify the differences in mortality between smokers and non-smokers as inequalities, even though governments might still wish to try to persuade individual smokers to give up their habits because of the discomfort and injuries imposed on others: smoking is emphatically not a self-regarding activity. But in Britain smoking is related to social class. While the middle classes have been giving up their cigarettes in recent years, the working classes and in particular working-class women have been smoking more. If these trends continue, then almost certainly the differences in life expectancy between social classes will widen in future. Should the illness and shortening of life so created be classified as an unacceptable inequality on the grounds that smoking represents pressures – poor housing or unpleasant jobs or low incomes – which make it impossible for people to take wise investment decisions about their health? Or do we regard it as an acceptable inequality on the ground that none of these pressures robs people of their freedom of choice, and that to accept this line of reasoning would inevitably lead one into denying personal responsibility for all sorts of destructive and anti-social behaviour? Indeed, might it not be argued that the pattern of smoking reflects the fact that the rise in incomes is greater than the spread of middle-class behaviour, so that the working classes are now adopting the habits that the middle classes are giving up in pursuit of health?

The answers to these questions are not self-evident, and it may help to shift the argument onto somewhat different if related ground. Let us return to Egalitaria. This is a country, be it emphasised again, which has got an egalitarian income distribution. It need not, however, necessarily be a country with an egalitarian distribution of other kinds of resources (notably education) or other influences (notably family background) relevant to investment decisions about health. The real difference between Egalitaria and Britain lies in the fact that the former's people all have an equal chance to buy themselves a good education. If they choose not to do so, the losses they suffer as a result can be seen as morally neutral.

In Britain today, however, these conditions certainly do not hold. If the wrong investment decisions are taken about smoking – or diet, come to that – because of the inegalitarian distribution of education, we probably should describe the consequent differences in health as unacceptable inequalities. In short, when talking about the distribution of life chances – including health – we should probably first consider the distribution of skills to take any chances that are going.

Social Class Responses to Health Education

Shifting the argument from the distribution of income as an enabling condition for health to the distribution of other resources, such as education, also reveals a paradox and raises a large question. Not only are there differences in the smoking habits between different social classes, but there are also striking differences in their response to health education. The middle classes respond to such education much more readily than the working classes. The paradox, therefore, is that health promotion may eventually widen the differences in life expectancy between the social classes, and that the best way of narrowing the gap between them would have been to encourage everyone to take up smoking! There is nothing as egalitarian as universal self-indulgence.

In turn, this raises the question – to which we shall return in the conclusion – of whether narrowing differences between social classes (or any other groups) can or should ever be seen as an *overriding* policy objective. If, for example, our policy objective were to be to improve the population's health, however defined, by as much as possible, we might deliberately decide to *widen* differences by concentrating on those groups where government intervention is most feasible and cost-effective. Inequalities may be seen as acceptable, to introduce a new consideration into our analysis, if the cost of diminishing them is higher than the health improvements that could be brought about in other ways. In short, we have to consider the social and moral opportunity costs of dealing with inequalities.

Conversely, those committed to the reduction of differences might wish to argue that the distribution of health is like the distribution of income: that it does not matter if those at the top end of the distribution lose some of their health (by being encouraged to smoke or drink?), provided that the gap between them and the bottom of the distribution narrows. If there is a trade-off between social justice, seen as the reduction of inequalities, and the total sum of 'health welfare', difficult choices still have to be made on either approach to the question. Even if we agree that a difference should be classified as an inequality – that is, a cause of social and moral concern – it does not automatically follow that we are obliged to give it urgency, primacy or priority in our actions regardless of other claims on our resources, energies and attention.

Criteria and Determination of 'Need'

Turning to differences in the use of health services, we again encounter a series of difficulties when we start working through the implications of applying seemingly simple principles. Let us start with the 'strong' principle of equality in health care, mentioned earlier. This is the principle that everyone should have an equal chance to get equal treatment for equal 'need'. Not only does this raise the question as noted already, of what is meant by effective functioning. But it also raises the problem of who defines 'need', according to what criteria.

The solution of this problem, in the context of the NHS, is to leave the determination of 'need' to the professional providers. Present policy is to ration resources geographically in such a way as to ensure that, in theory at least and given equal efficiency, people with equal degrees of professionally defined 'need' will have equal chances of getting treatment irrespective of where they live. So an unacceptable inequality is a difference which biases such chances arbitrarily and without justification: a reasonable enough definition, it would seem, and one which allows a feasible policy response in the shape of redistribution policies (RAWP) within the NHS.

But we are still left with some difficulties. The medical profession is notoriously jealous of its autonomy and it is far from clear that there is anything like professional consensus about how to define 'needs' and how to respond to them. Indeed, it is tempting to argue that what the NHS offers is not so much equal treatment for equal 'need' as equal access to consultants who will then apply different criteria of 'need' and different kinds of treatment. This inevitably creates differences which, however, stop short of unacceptable inequalities: if the consultants in my district pursue extremely conservative methods of treatment, and I am thereby denied an equal chance of aggressive intervention, I would be hard put to it to describe it as an unacceptable inequality. More crucially still, my chances of getting *any* treatment may depend as much on my own resources as on the level of NHS resources in my district: in other words, on my own abilities to manipulate the system. If there is a bias in the NHS it is as much in the distribution of the abilities required to make best use of access as in the distribution of the access itself. If I am middle-aged, middle-class, assertive and with high expectations then I will get more out of my doctor, and the NHS, than if I am elderly, working class, deferential and with low expectations. Here, quite clearly, there is a systematic difference, but does it amount to an unacceptable inequality calling for remedial action?

Are There Any Unacceptable Inequalities in Health Care?

So the argument comes back to a central question put at the beginning of this paper. Are there any differences which are unacceptable simply because they happen to be found in the health-care arena? Is the differential ability to shop effectively and claim entitlements aggressively somehow more shocking or objectionable when displayed in health care than in, for example, getting the most out of the education system or exploiting every loophole in the tax system? Depending on our answers to these questions, very different strategies will follow. If differences in the ability to get *health care* are seen as unacceptable inequalities calling for action, then it would follow that more NHS resources should be devoted which discriminate actively in favour of those patients who otherwise do not assert themselves or indeed avoid the health-care system. If so, we may be back to choosing between investing our resources in the reduction of inequalities, as such, and maximising the total supply of health. If, however, we argue that it is differences in the general ability to exploit any situation which represent an unacceptable inequality, then we are left with the problem of how to tackle such inequalities – and we might perhaps conclude that education, rather than health, should have primacy in any strategy.

To emphasise the role of non-financial resources in creating differences in the use of public health care is also to stress a central irony in the debate about private health care. The case against private care, as it is usually put, is that it creates unacceptable inequalities by allowing people to buy quicker and more comfortable treatment. The assumption, in other words, is that the unacceptability derives from the fact that the preferential treatment is *bought* with hard cash: i.e. that it is wrong for health care to be distributed according to the ability to buy rather than 'need'. It is, of course, quite clear that if I have got a health insurance policy, I will do better than my neighbour who has not should I want to get my hernia fixed up or a new hip joint. I am, therefore, buying an advantage by jumping the NHS queue. But is there really anything to choose morally between buying an insurance policy and inviting one's GP to dinner?

There is indeed a certain paradox in the frequently put argument that private health care is undesirable because it allows the middle classes to exit from the NHS, instead of using their voices and political muscle to demand improvements for everyone within it. For, on past evidence, the result of locking the middle classes into the NHS might well be to widen inequalities within the service. By pushing for the expansion of those services, like repair surgery, from which they benefit most themselves (and which they otherwise get in the private sector), the middle classes might well divert resources from those parts of the service used by the politically least effective sections of the population – the chronically sick elderly, the mentally handicapped, and so on.[1]

Political power, like financial power, tends to be lopsided and bureaucratic, and professional biases may be just as important as market biases.

Inequalities in the Health-Care Environment?

The case of services for those who cannot be cured underlines the importance of another, much debated dimension of inequality. In theory, at least, it may be possible to devise neutral, technical criteria for determining the allocation of resources according to 'need' in dealing with specific medical or surgical conditions. But how do we start devising fair or just principles of allocation, which would allow us to decide whether inequalities were or were not acceptable, when it comes to the environment in which care is provided? The point applies even in the case of acute medicine. Few people would argue that being able to have a private room while being treated for, say, a broken leg or a coronary, represents an unacceptable inequality. But the point becomes crucial in the case of, for example, the chronically ill elderly or the mentally handicapped where the environment is, to a larger extent, the care. In this case, it is difficult even to identify the groups who should be compared in the process of identifying differences which, in turn, might or might not be categorised as acceptable or otherwise. They raise, in a particularly strong form, a dilemma identified by Schelling, when he asked which differences should be seen as inequalities in medical care or merely another manifestation of what it means to be poor:

'The poor who are merely sick and in no need of a physician's attention, who spend the day in bed not feeling well, do it in drearier surroundings than sick people who are well-to-do. People who are lame or arthritic or fatigued who have to ride crowded buses are worse off than those who can afford taxis. The sick and injured who have to get out of bed and cook their own meals are noticeably worse off than those who can afford help. And this is truer of those who never feel well, who hurt during whatever they do, who have trouble breathing, who are partly paralysed, or who are so old that even having to remain standing is a mild form of torture. It is not easy to distinguish between those whose discomfort or fear is due to

[1] R. Klein (1980), 'Models of Man and Models of Policy', *Millbank Memorial Fund Quarterly/Health and Society*, Vol. 58, No. 3, pp. 416–429.

the poor surroundings in which they receive medical care and those whose discomfort or fear is due their being poor'.[1]

In short, Schelling concludes, it is crucial to be clear as to whether we are arguing that the poor who are sick should be made better off compared with the sick who are not poor, or whether we are saying that they should be made better off compared with the poor who are not sick. Our definitions of what differences should be categorised as unacceptable inequalities will depend on such judgements.

4. Conclusion

This essay ends, as it began, with questions rather than answers. It does not provide ready-made criteria for distinguishing between acceptable differences and unacceptable inequalities. For the purpose has been to argue that there are no such set-in-concrete criteria: that inevitably the process of deciding which differences should be put on the policy agenda will depend on intellectual argument and political bargaining, with the frontiers changing over time. Even for inegalitarians, there will be some differences which are so shocking as to demand action, but *what* shocks will change over time. Even for egalitarians, there will be many differences where the opportunity costs are too high to justify action, but the nature of these costs will also change over time. And health, it would seem, is not so very different from any other policy arena; differences in health status and health-care use do not carry any privileged status, which justifies their immediate translation into unacceptable inequalities demanding remedial policies. To the extent that differences in health care reflect unacceptable inequalities in society at large, so the case for action should be argued in the larger context and in the currency of argument appropriate to it.

---

[1]T.C. Schelling (1979), 'Standards for Adequate Minimum Personal Health Services', *Millbank Memorial Fund Quarterly/Health and Society*, Vol.57, No. 2, pp. 212–234.

51

From Status to Contract: The Transformation of the British Medical Profession

HEALTH CARE PROVISION UNDER
FINANCIAL RESTRAINT. H L'ETANG ED.
ROYAL SOCIETY OF MEDICINE
1990

From Status to Contract

In at least one respect, the changes that are taking place in the National Health Service (NHS) represent a more radical transformation than its creation in 1948. The 1948 model NHS marked, in many ways, the apotheosis of the medical profession [1]. It preserved the tradition of medical autonomy while handing over to the profession command over publicly-provided resources. There was an implicit concordat between State and profession. The State achieved budgetary control, although at the price of leaving it to the doctors to determine how resources were used at the point of service delivery; the medical profession achieved freedom from control and scrutiny, although at the price of accepting the constraint of working within a fixed budget. The NHS of the 1990s, building on trends already evident in the 1980s, is clearly going to be rather different. The concordat between State and profession is, in a sense, being renegotiated.

In particular, the medical profession's claim to authority, on the basis of its collective status, is being challenged. Increasingly, individual members of the profession are being asked to justify their own performance in terms of explicit criteria such as contracts. Hence the title of this paper, whose theme it is to explore the shift from status to contract; the social, political and financial forces that are driving the changes, the nature of the transformation itself and the longer-term implications for the management of health care in Britain.

Before exploring the reasons for changes, however, it may be helpful to define more explicitly what is meant by the shift from status to contract [2]; Fig. 1 therefore sets out the key words and concepts involved. The notion of status involves, in the first place, a particular view of society which sees it as being composed of corporations or guilds that in turn confer status and authority on their members. Such bodies have leased out to them the powers of the state. They regulate themselves, enjoy a high degree of autonomy and judgment of competence is made by members of the guild, that is professional peers; lastly, but importantly, they operate on trust. Conversely, the notion of contract implies a much more individualistic view of society. It emphasizes not the collective responsibility of corporations or professional bodies but the accountability of individuals for their own performance. The emphasis is not on self-regulation but on public regulation, not on the role of peers but that of hierarchy, not on trust but on review. The contrast has been drawn in deliberately sharp terms for in practice the two models often overlap. However, they are not mere intellectual conceits. If one wanted to characterize some of the main differences between Britain and the United States, both in health care and more generally, they would be caught quite well in the contrast

Status ⟶	Contract
Corporatism	Individualism
Authority	Performance
Self-regulation	Public regulation
Autonomy	Accountability
Peers	Hierarchy
Trust	Review

Figure 1 *Changing perspectives.*

between a status and a contract society, between a society with a bias towards corporatism or collectivism and one centred on the individual.

Forces for Change

The changes in Britain's NHS during the 1980s must be seen as part of a larger social transformation [3] when there was a period of reaction against both collectivism and corporatism. Much of the intellectual inspiration behind the Thatcher government's policies came from economists and others with a highly individualistic, not to say atomistic, view of society. The prevailing diagnosis of Britain's economic ills was that it reflected the sclerosis of a society dominated by corporatist interest groups, be they trade unions or professions. Significantly, Milton Friedman, one of the influential figures involved, was an advocate not only of monetary economics but also of breaking the legal monopoly of the medical and other professions [4], that is, of pursuing the logic of the market and free competition wherever it might lead and whatever it might mean for established institutions. Whereas in the past the professions had been largely exempted from the legislation dealing with monopolies and restrictive practices, the Thatcher government argued that they should be required to justify any claim to immunity [5]; the onus of proof was reversed, as it were. Whereas in the past successive administrations had quailed at the thought of a confrontation with the legal professions the Thatcher government challenged them directly with proposals for ending restrictive practices and strengthening the public regulation of professional bodies [6]. Thus a legal services ombudsman, to review the way in which professional bodies process complaints, is to be set up.

   In all this, the Thatcher government's strategy represented a challenge to the British tradition of clubbability, not surprisingly, perhaps, given that Britain has a prime minister who would not have been admitted to the membership of most clubs until very recently. There has been a realization, reinforced by a series of financial scandals in the City of London, that self-regulation based on trust among gentlemen was an inadequate guiding principle for public policy. Hence the increasing emphasis on public regulation, on accountability and review of individual performance. It is a trend which has, inevitably, affected the medical profession. For example, the General Medical Council has shown itself increasingly sensitive, both under its present president (Sir Robert Kilpatrick) and his predecessor (Lord Walton), to the new pressures; currently, the introduction of machinery for reviewing doctors' professional performance is being considered [7].

In the case of the NHS another force for change has been at work and one pulling in a different direction. The entire history of the NHS, from the moment of its birth onward, has been punctuated by financial crises, assertions that it was underfunded and that standards were threatened by inadequate resources. However, in the 1980s these claims reached a new crescendo and under-funding became a major and highly emotional issue, dominating the media and the political agenda. For a government dedicated to restricting the growth of public spending, in principle if not always in practice, this presented a dilemma. Was there an alternative to spending its way out of trouble? The strategy chosen was to have profound implications for relations between the State and the profession. For it was to switch the emphasis of public policy from inputs to outputs and to argue that the level of the annual expenditure increment was less important than the efficiency with which the total was spent. It was a theme which was being pursued throughout the British government but which was taken up with special energy in the case of the NHS. The result was that the government met every criticism of under-funding by pointing to the increase in the level of activity, the annual increase in the number of patients treated and operations performed. Rapidly growing efficiency was seen as the answer to the charge that expenditure was growing too slowly.

But how was the rapid growth in efficiency, designed to meet the extra demands created by both demographic and technological change, to be achieved? Here the response was not an invocation of the market principle but increasing emphasis on strengthening management. From this there developed yet another challenge to the status model of health care delivery as we shall see in the next section which examines the transformation within the NHS.

The New Agenda

Early in the history of the NHS the profession and the state negotiated the terms and conditions of service which defined the responsibilities of general practitioners. These stated that 'the doctor shall render to his patients all necessary and appropriate medical services of the type usually provided by general medical practitioners'. In this solipsistic universe, the ought was derived from the is; what medical practitioners should do was defined by what they did. This definition was negotiated, as has been aptly pointed out [8], 'on the basis of mutual trust' and represented 'a gentleman's agreement'. If, now, we turn to the terms and conditions of service for general practitioners, imposed on a reluctant and bitterly protesting profession in 1990, we find a different picture [9] for here is the state imposing its own priorities on general practice. There is no question of a gentleman's agreement and most GPs would probably deny the title to the secretary of state for health. The new contract sets specific targets for general practitioners such as the proportions of patients to be screened, immunized and tested. These targets are not compulsory inasmuch as the new contract is based on financial incentives rather than bureaucractic diktat. If we also take into account that family practitioner committees (the managerial bodies responsible for general practice) will also be reviewing referral and prescribing patterns, it is clear that the days of self-regulated autonomy may be drawing to a close. The individual general practitioner will increasingly have to justify his or her own performance according to criteria developed not just by their professional peers but by public policy; a conclusion softened, but not altered, by the fact that the review of performance will be carried out by the FPC's medical advisers rather than lay managers.

Turning to the hospital sector of the NHS, perhaps the best starting point is the 1990 public expenditure white paper [10], the annual document which sets out the British government's spending plans. This neatly illustrates the driving force behind many of the institutional changes introduced by the 1989 Review of the NHS [11]. Here we find, predictably enough given the switch of emphasis from inputs to outputs, not just the spending plans but also activity targets. For example, the White Paper records the following annual targets set in 1986 for achievement by 1990; 14,000 coronary artery by-pass grafts, approaching 50,000 hip replacement operations and 550 bone marrow transplants. Furthermore, the White Paper gives figures of the rates achieved (per million population) by each of the country's regional health authorities. In effect, central government has started to decide what the NHS should actually deliver not just, as in the 1970s, in terms of financial priorities or inputs but of the specific services that should be delivered to the population or outputs. Not only does this imply a managerial transmission belt, which runs through Duncan Nichol's NHS management executive, for translating central decisions into local activity. It also implies a changed relationship between managers and the medical profession, since it is not managers who carry out operations or treat patients. In effect, it means that managers have been made responsible for influencing directly what doctors do; a major challenge to the traditional relationship between the two and to the self-perception of the medical profession as an autonomous, self-regulating corporation. Specifically, they have been charged with increasing medical productivity. In Britain, in sharp contrast to the United States, variations in operating rates [12] tend to be seen as evidence of under-rather than over-performance by the medical profession, and it is the low performers, not the high ones, who give cause for concern.

Increasingly the medical profession is being held accountable for the way in which it is using resources provided from the public purse. The theme is improving value for money. It is, moreover, not only the government which is pushing in this direction but also the national Audit Office (the British equivalent of the General Accounting Office). For example, the NAO has been critical of health authorities for not ensuring that individual consultants do their appropriate share of the work and has argued that their contracts 'should be translatable into schedules of fixed commitments' [13]. In others words, accountability should be based on explicit contracts, not informal gentleman's agreements based on trust. The model of accountability [14] is moving the corporatist to the managerial style (Fig. 2) In the corporatist mode the professional is accountable only to his or her clients and peers. Additionally, the courts have a role in protecting the interests of the client although in the British case, unlike the United States, judges have tended to see doctors as fellow professionals whose collective judgment should not be challenged [15]. In the managerial mode, however, we have a third strand of accountability, a point clearly reflected in the 1989 Review of the NHS and the changes that flow from it.

Perhaps the most significant change, so far as the theme and title of this paper is concerned, is the new-style contract for consultants. Hitherto consultant contracts have been held by the regional, not the district,

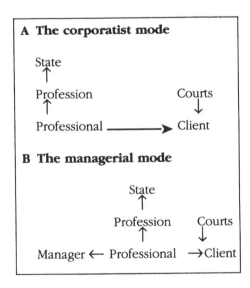

Figure 2 *Accountabilities.*

health authorities in whose area the doctors work and the contracts themselves have tended to be rather general in specifying the duties involved. All this is to change for there is, the government argues [16], 'a need for an improved process of accountability'. Accordingly, contracts will in future include a detailed job description which might, for example, include 'a work programme showing for each morning and afternoon the main duties and their location' and it will be the district general manager, as agent for the region, who will be responsible for monitoring the contract and reviewing it annually. While the government documents stop well short of suggesting that the contract might specify particular output targets, so many operations of a particular kind to be carried out each year, NHS managers have been heard to mutter privately about the desirability of so doing; indeed that would be the logic of making consultants accountable to managers for the way in which they use resources.

The 1989 Review also proposed changes in the distinction award system. At present this conforms very much to the status model since it is left to the profession to decide which of its members deserve extra merit payments which, at the top end, may double a consultant's salary. It is a system which, in a sense, can be seen as a mechanism for reinforcing and expressing the profession's own set of values. It is based on peer judgment and depends on trust within the profession; the procedure for making the award is a reminder that guilds also used to be known as 'mysteries'. In the government's view, however, the system should now be changed in order to achieve two new objectives, 'to reflect the wider responsibilities of consultants for the effective use of resources, as well as the clinical merit of their work; and to ensure that the scheme offers consultants stronger incentives to maintain and improve their contribution to the service'. Accordingly, the government proposed that the criteria for making awards should be changed to require consultants to demonstrate 'commitment to the management and development of the service' as well as clinical skill, and that the committees making the awards should include regional chairmen and managers. Similarly, the review suggested that the composition of the national advisory committee on distinction awards should be changed to 'provide for a stronger management influence on the choice of award holders'. This change is symbolic of the shifting relationship between the State and the profession. The distinction award system was part of the price paid by Nye Devan to secure the co-operation of consultants and no administration had hitherto dared even to question it in public.

There are other elements in the current transformation of the NHS that will affect the position of the medical profession. It is not the purpose of this paper to analyse them except insofar as they bear on its theme.

However, one trend requires noting: that from accepting the authority of members of the profession to requiring justification for their individual performances. The stress on managerial accountability has already been noted. Similarly, there is a new stress on clinical accountability as reflected in the insistence that medical audit should be universalized both in hospital medicine and general practice [17]. It is a trend which was anticipated by some of the medical profession's leadership [18] and present plans will leave the profession itself to run the new audit systems, although it is not clear how, in the long term, considerations of efficiency in the use of resources and of clinical quality can be kept apart. Again there can be no doubt about the general direction of change. It is from status to contract, from autonomy to accountability.

Future Implications

The changes in the NHS have been driven, as has been argued, not only by a particular view of society but also by the dynamics of health care financing. Both factors are likely to outlive the present government. Even though many people repudiate the Thatcher vision of a market society, the language of consumerism has become almost universal. The result is that deference to the authority of professionals is now a rapidly disappearing legacy. Similarly, Britain, despite its success in running what is probably the most parsimoniously effective health service in the world, still faces the problem of how to respond to the pressure for more spending. The emphasis on squeezing out more productivity from any given budget is therefore not likely to diminish. Indeed in both respects, developments in Britain now are simply bringing it into line with other countries, notably the United States. We are therefore not dealing with some passing phenomenon, some sort of political hiccup, but what is likely to prove an enduring trend. It is therefore worth reflecting, in conclusion, on some of the longer-term implications.

From the point of view of the state (and the lay citizen) it may seem self-evidently desirable that clinicians should be accountable for the way in which they use public resources. However, there is a catch in the argument [19]. Health care everywhere is about rationing scarce resources. In the United States rationing takes the form of limiting access to the health care system, in Britain of limiting treatment, in some circumstances when access has been achieved. The 1948 model NHS conceded authority, self-regulation and autonomy to the medical profession but, in return, it also diffused responsibility for rationing decisions. Government decisions about the NHS budget were translated into thousands of clinical decisions by doctors. To put it dramatically, it was doctors, not politicians, who turned people away to die. The new model NHS is likely, however, to change this. If it is government which sets targets for the level of service outputs, and, as already quoted, the number of specific procedures to be carried out annually, then increasingly it will also be ministers rather than doctors who will be seen to be responsible for decisions about rationing. Moving towards public regulation, accountability and performance review may therefore have a perverse outcome. The switch from status to contract is an attempt to lower the political costs of financial stringency by increasing the productivity of the NHS, but it may, conversely, raise the political costs of rationing by converting what were previously seen as clinical into highly visible governmental decisions.

If this argument is accepted then it would seem that the 1989 model NHS may have some in-built tensions. In the short term, the result may well be that the NHS will do much better financially in the 1990s than it did in the 1980s. If Ministers are seen to have a direct responsibility for rationing decisions they may well become more generous. Additionally, of course, the political furore that accompanied the changes has greatly strengthened the secretary of state's ability to extract extra funds from the Treasury. In the longer term, however, it may turn out that the political system is not designed to carry such responsibilities. Pessimistically, it may be argued that certain kinds of decisions, such as deliberately providing less than optimum quality care, can only be taken on the basis of paternalistic authority; that tragic choices are best made by the people whom we hire to make our mistakes for us, namely the professionals [20]. Optimistically, it may be argued that new political institutions and mechanisms will have to be invented, perhaps of the kind now being tried out experimentally in Oregon [21]. Either way, it seems improbable that a stable settlement has been achieved.

Finally, the change from status to contract raises a large question. What will be the effect on the morale of the medical profession and the other NHS service providers? In many respects, the NHS has lived off the dedication of its staff; for example, successive surveys have shown that a high proportion of consultants work far longer hours than required by their present contract [22]. This dedication has, in turn, reflected the medical profession's sense of ownership of the NHS, in many respects the largest syndicalist organization in the world. It was a sense of ownership which always rested on an element of self-deception for the state cannot hand control of a £20 billion tax-financed enterprise to a self-regulating corporation. The challenge for the future will be to see whether the medical profession can be persuaded to identify itself with the NHS, while no longer seeing itself as the owner, and accept the switch from autonomous authority to accountability for performance.

References

1. Klein R. *The politics of the NHS,* 2nd ed. London: Longmans, 1989.

2. The phrase, albeit used in a rather different context, is that of Sir Henry Maine. *Ancient law.* London: JM Dent & Sons, 1917.

3. Day P, Klein R. The politics of modernization: Britain's National Health Service in the 1980s. *The Milbank Quarterly* 1989; 67: 1–35.

4. Friedman M. *Capitalism and freedom.* Chicago: University of Chicago Press, 1962.

5. Secretary of State for Trade and Industry. *Review of restrictive trade practices policy.* London: HMSO, 1988; Cm 331.

6. Lord High Chancellor. *Legal services: A framework for the future.* London: HMSO, 1989; Cm 740.

7. General Medical Council. *Annual Report, 1989.* London: GMC, 1990.

8. Irvine D. Standards in general practice: The quality initiative revisited. The 1989 Gale Lecture 14 October 1989. *Mimeo.*

9. Department of Health. *Terms of service for doctors in general practice.* London: DH, November 1989.

10. Chancellor of the Exchequer. *The Government's expenditure plans, 1990–91 to 1992–93: Chapter 13 – Department of Health.* London: HMSO, 1990; Cm 1013.

11. Secretaries of State for Health, Wales, Northern Ireland and Scotland. *Working for patients.* London: HMSO, 1989; Cm 555.

12. Ham C, ed. *Health care variations.* London: King's Fund Institute, 1988.

13. National Audit Office. *The NHS and independent hospitals.* London: HMSO, 1989; HC 106.

14. For a discussion of the concept of accountability, see Day P., Klein R. *Accountabilities.* London: Tavistock, 1987.

15. Miller FH. Informed consent for the man on the Clapham omnibus: an English cure for the 'American disease'. *Western N Engl Law Review* 1987; 9(1): 169–90. See also Montgomery J. Medicine, accountability and professionalism. *J Law Soc* 1989; 16(2): 319–39.

16. Department of Health. *NHS consultants: Appointments, contracts and distinction awards.* Working for patients – working paper No 7. London: HMSO, 1989. For the final outcome, see Harvard J. A revised consultant contract. *B M J* 1990; 300: 1221–2.

17. Department of Health. *Medical audit.* Working for patients – working paper No 6. London: HMSO, 1989.

18. Hoffenberg Sir Raymond. *Clinical freedom.* London: Nuffield Provincial Hospitals Trust, 1987.

19. Klein R. Health care in the age of disillusionment. *B M J* 1982; 25: 1–4.

20. Hughes E. *Men and their work.* London: Collier-Macmillan, 1958.

21. The Oregon Health Decisions Programme is discussed in Callahan D. *What kind of life: the limits of medical progress.* New York: Simon and Schuster, 1990.

22. Review body on doctors' and dentists' remuneration. *Twentieth report.* London: HMSO, 1990: Cm 937.

52

The State and the Profession: The Politics of the Double Bed

BRITISH MEDICAL JOURNAL
3 October 1990

In retrospect it is clear that those who fought Nye Bevan's plans for setting up the National Health Service were right in at least one important respect. The setting up in 1948 marked a revolution in the relation between the state and the medical profession. But it was not quite the revolution that the critics had anticipated and prophesied. It did not mean the triumph of bureaucracy over professionalism or the subordination of doctoring to ministerial diktat. Instead, it created a situation of mutual dependency. On the one hand the state became a monopoly employer: effectively members of the medical profession became dependent on it not only for their own incomes but also for the resources at their command. On the other hand the state became dependent on the medical profession to run the NHS and to cope with the problems of rationing scarce resources in patient care. The subsequent history of the NHS can, in institutional and political terms, be seen largely as a series of attempts to manage this mutual dependency, to find ways of accommodating the frustrations and resentments of both sides in the partnership, and to devise organisational strategies for containing conflicting interests within the framework of the NHS. My theme, in short, is that it is possible to understand what is happening in the NHS today – and indeed what has happened over the past 40 odd years – only if it is seen as the stage on which the tensions built into its design are acted out. For the drama to conflict between state and profession is not an accidental byproduct of Britain's health care. It is the inevitable outcome of the financial and institutional framework that was set up in 1948. The puzzle is not that there has been so much conflict but that it has, so far, been possible to cope with it in such a way as not to destroy the NHS.

Symmetrical Frustration

For 40 years the state and profession have been engaged in a repetitive cycle of confrontation. The issues have changed over time (though some constant themes are evident), and so have the personalities, as Labour secretaries of state have yielded to Conservative ones in the demonology of the medical profession (the special place of Mr Kenneth Clarke in this respect mainly reflects a lack of collective memory). Yet despite 40 years of bickering and recrimination the NHS has survived. Despite decades of denouncing the inadequacies of the NHS the medical profession remains dedicated to its defence. Despite the political costs of being regularly pilloried in the media for its stinginess the government proclaimed its loyalty to the principles of the NHS in the 1989 review. Despite the frequent protestations that the NHS is on the point of collapse public support remains undiminished. Consensus about the desirability of the NHS has survived and contained the conflict within it. How has this been achieved? What are the prospects of maintaining the balance in the coming decades?

One answer may be that there is a neat symmetry of frustration in the relationship between the state and the profession. In the case of the state it is its control over money that makes the NHS such an attractive proposition; in the international context the NHS is quite clearly the "best buy" model for delivering comprehensive universal health care at the lowest price and in a reasonably equitable way.[1] But it is, of course, precisely this control that frustrates the medical profession – in Enoch Powell's words: "The unnerving discovery every Minister of Health makes at or near the outset of his term of office is that the only subject he is ever destined to discuss with the medical profession is money."[2] If the medical profession is not engaged in wrangles over its own pay it is battling for more funds for the NHS. Conversely, the NHS provides a setting in which the medical profession can exercise its skills with almost complete autonomy: within the limits of the available resources NHS

[1] Organisation for Economic Cooperation and Development. *Financing and delivering health care*. Paris: OECD, 1987.
[2] Powell JE. *Medicine and politics*. London: Pitman Medical, 1966.

doctors have been more free to exercise their professional judgments than their peers in the United States and in most other Western countries. But it is, of course, precisely this autonomy that frustrates the government. If ministers are to achieve their priorities they are sooner or later driven to question medical practices and to search for ways of achieving some sort of influence over clinical decisions on such matters as, for example, lengths of stay or expenditure on drugs.

There are other factors also. In the case of the state, to concede autonomy to the medical profession is also to delegate responsibility for rationing: the NHS allows political decisions about resources to be disguised as clinical decisions about individual patients. In the case of the medical profession the system allows it largely to control entry and thus to assure employment for its members: the fact that doctors (like every other group) frequently consider themselves to be underpaid should not disguise the fact that the NHS guarantees them an income linked to the going rate of the professional middle classes. In the past the medical profession has done well out of the intervention of the state in medical care: a profession that had a sizable proletariat of insecure and poorly paid practitioners before 1911 has become collectively more secure and wealthier with each step in the evolution of the state system. Above all the NHS commands loyalty that transcends self interest, whether political or professional. It is because there is a general perception that the NHS is an admirable instrument for distributing health care fairly – that it is preferable to have a system where the incentives are to do too little, even if this means more queues, rather than do too much – that consensus has hitherto contained conflict and that the individual discontents have not led to a repudiation of the 1948 settlement.

Once we recognise, however, that these discontents are not just accidental aberrations but are built into the design of the NHS it follows that we cannot simply take the comfortable view that the future will be like the past. Having lived with these tensions for the past 40 years why should the NHS not accommodate them in coming decades? Given the certainty that conflict will continue and the possibility that the NHS may be living off an inherited but not necessarily renewable capital of commitment and loyalty, is it possible to devise better strategies for managing the resentment generated by the mutual dependency of the state and the profession? What, in particular, can be learnt from past efforts to do so?

Economy Before Logic

One option, clearly, is to try to transmute political into technical issues: to fly on automatic pilot instead of engaging in a constant dispute about the route. Here the most obvious example is the attempt, stretching back to the early days of the NHS's history, to devise a formula for determining medical pay by analysing data rather than by engaging in a power struggle. It was to achieve precisely this aim that the government set up the Royal Commission on Doctors' and Dentists' Remuneration in 1957[3] – the independent review body that devised both the notion of and the mechanism for comparing medical incomes with other professional incomes; the mechanism still survives today. As Professor John Jewkes pointed out in a dissenting memorandum:

> The responsible Government Departments are in the extraordinary, and perhaps unique, position that they largely control the demand for, the supply of, and the price offered for the services of the medical and dental professions. . . . It is this grip of the Government which explains why the profession has spent so much time, inevitably without success, in search of a formula which would in perpetuity protect it against arbitrary action on the part of the State. For the same reason it is only to be expected that, in any new major settlement with the professions, doctors and dentists will not be wholly, nor perhaps even primarily, concerned with the new level of earnings established. They will also be vitally interested in the light thrown by these decisions, in terms of works not of words, upon the view which the Government holds as to the place of the medical profession in society. . . .

Subsequently, however, both Labour and Conservative administrations, including the present one, have shown their belief that the logic of national economic management must override the logic of the NHS pay determination machinery. Most dramatically the first review body – originally appointed in 1962 – resigned in 1970 because the government was prepared to implement only half the 30% increase recommended. It was this which precipitated a major confrontation between the government and the profession, with the BMA advising its members not to cooperate in NHS administration or to sign national insurance medical certificates in protest against what was seen as "arbitrary action" by the state. The successor body was appointed on the understanding that its recommendations would not be rejected or modified by the government "unless there were obviously compelling reasons for so doing."[4] In the event, Britain's stormy economic history has provided quite a few such compelling reasons. The experience of pay determination therefore warns against optimism about the scope for insulating the NHS from political or eco-

---

[3]Royal Commission on Doctors' and Dentists' Remuneration. *Report*. London: HMSO, 1960. (Cmnd 939.) (Chairman: Sir Harry Pilkington.)
    [4]Review Body on Doctors' and Dentists' Remuneration. *Report*. London: HMSO, 1971. (Cmnd 4825.)(Chairman: Lord Halsbury.)

nomic pressures by means of technical fixes, whether by devising formulas for pay or formulas for determining its budget by allocating a fixed proportion of the national income.

Engineering Consensus

Inevitably, it would seem, the management of mutual dependency and the resulting conflict depends on the political system – that is, political context, style, and conventions that shape the relationship between the state and the profession. Here it is possible to identify some important changes that distinguish the past decade from the previous 30 years. From the 1950s to the 1970s the NHS provided perhaps the most convincing text for those who argued that Britain had a corporatist policy making system, with policy emerging from a process of negotiation and bargaining between Whitehall ministries and interest groups like the medical profession, industry, and the trade unions.[56] It was a system in which differences might on occasion erupt into open conflict – as was indeed the case with the NHS – but where all participants were constrained by the knowledge that they had a shared interest in maintaining the framework. In the words of Sir George Godber, one of the main architects of change at the time,[7] it was a period in which progress was largely made within the NHS by a process of engineering consensus.

In the 1980s, however, the Conservative government has explicitly challenged and repudiated the notion of a corporatist approach to policy making. Corporatism has been identified as a source of stagnation, institutional sclerosis, and the pursuit of self interest at the expense of the public interest. Consensus became the enemy instead of being the objective. It is a view of politics that sees a strong state dealing with strong citizens (strong because they are empowered by the giving of more resources and more say over their lives, whether in housing or education) rather than with interest groups like professions, which act as the agents of their members. It therefore implies a quite different political style; the old conventions have been related to the history books. It also implies a different view of the "place of the medical professional in society": like other professions, such as law, it becomes increasingly regarded as just one more lobby or pressure group rather than carrying some special

[5]Eckstein H. *Pressure group politics*. London: Allen and Unwin, 1960.
[6]Beer SH. *Britain against itself*. London: Faber and Faber, 1982.
[7]Godber G. *Change in medicine*. London: Nuffield Provincial Hospitals Trust, 1975.

imprimatur deriving from the nature of its expertise or its claims to represent a particular set of values.

Exclusion in 1989

The contrast can be illustrated by comparing the 1974 reorganisation of the NHS with that now being implemented. In 1974 corporatism as interpreted by the secretary of state, Sir Keith (now Lord) Joseph, ruled supreme. The new design of the NHS was hammered out in consulation with the professions. The product of committees, it spawned yet more committees in an attempt to ensure that every interest in the NHS would be represented.[8] In doing so it universalised veto-power and by seeking to satisfy everyone managed to please no one. Indeed, it seemed to show that corporatism led only to rigidity and inflexibility. Conversely, the 1989 review seemed to be based on the belief that it would be possible to avoid repeating the mistakes of the past by not trying to consult or satisfy any of the NHS interest groups. It was the first time in the history of the NHS that the medical profession was systematically excluded from the decision making process leading up to the review; an exclusion which may perhaps explain the subsequent bitterness rather more than actual policy content. Indeed, the BMA's subsequent advertising campaign served largely to advertise the fact of the profession's exclusion. It drew attention to the profession's loss of privilege: in happier, corporatist days the profession had its own direct and private links with civil servants and ministers – an iron triangle of consultation that turned out to be made of cardboard in the 1980s.

Looking to the future, therefore, it seems clear that the way in which the relationship between the state and the medical profession is managed will depend not on what happens within the NHS but on what happens to Britain's political system. If the 1980s turn out to be an interregnum – if the assault on the role of interest groups proves to have exhausted itself – then there may well be a return to the politics of the double bed: peace between partners through propinquity. The emphasis might then once again be on trying to engineer consensus through the participation of professions, trade unions, and other interest groups in the policy process – the European rather than the American model. It seems unlikely, however, that memories of the 1970s and earlier decades will disappear entirely or that the risks of corporatist stagnation will be quietly accepted. If the professions are once again to be seen as partners in the policy

---

[8]Klein R. *The politics of the NHS*. 2nd ed. London: Longman, 1989.

process rather than pressure groups exclusively pursuing their own interest it may mean that they will also have to show their willingness and
capacity to adapt and change and, above all, to recognise that they are
accountable as much to the society that grants them their privileged status
as to their own members. If such a new political settlement cannot be
achieved, however, it seems unlikely that the NHS will survive long into
the twenty first century.

53

Risks and Benefits of Comparative Studies: Notes from Another Shore

THE MILBANK QUARTERLY
Volume 69, Number 2, 1991

One of the characteristics of the *Milbank Quarterly* under the editorship of David Willis was its intellectual cosmopolitanism. On the one hand, Europeans like myself were given an opportunity to display their wares to an American audience, once we had survived the ordeal of being edited more rigorously and more intensely than ever before. For being edited by David Willis *was* an ordeal, one that left the author feeling both exhausted and exhilarated. No one has ever been more intolerant, surely, of either intellectual or verbal sloppiness; no one, too, has had such a willingness to invest his own time and ideas in improving other people's work; no one could be so inexorably and innocently exasperating, yet leave his authors with a sense of total gratitude. On the other hand, the *Quarterly* has consistently, over the years of his editorship, put the issues of American health care into an international context. In doing so, it has provided its readers with an antidote to the dangers of ethnocentric overexplanation: the temptation to explain all the health care problems of one's country in terms of its own very special institutions and circumstances. It has thereby illuminated the question of what is – and is not – so very special about the United States, and delineated more precisely the nature and limits of American exceptionalism.

For if we are to understand what is special to the United States, or any other country, there is no alternative to adopting a comparative approach.

In what follows, I shall therefore elaborate on this theme, without in any sense attempting to review the field or the literature comprehensively. This has been done elsewhere (Atteveld, Broeders, and Lapré 1987). Nor shall I analyze the advantages and disadvantages of different strategies of comparison, a topic that has already received ample attention (Marmor 1983). Instead, I shall concentrate on a subspecies of comparative studies: the literature generated by the enduring fascination with each other's systems demonstrated by American and British students of health care over the decades. It is, in a sense, a perverse intellectual love affair. No two countries could be more different in terms of their geography, wealth, and political institutions; only a common language unites them, creating the illusion that understanding words must necessarily lead to comprehension of meaning. In what follows, I shall therefore reflect on this experience, before drawing out some general implications for comparative studies – and concluding, however tentatively, with some speculations about convergence in policy outcomes.

A One-Way Traffic in Ideas?

In the 1950s when Britain was beginning to realize that it was no longer an imperial or world power, the Prime Minister – Harold Macmillan – described its future role as being Greece to America's Rome. By this he meant, buttering up the national ego, that Britain would provide the intellectual drive, while the United States would supply the brute power. In fact, as the health services literature confirms, things have turned out rather differently. Perhaps the most significant aspect of the trans-Atlantic traffic in ideas is also the most simple and obvious: there is an intellectual imbalance of trade in favor of the United States, with Britain running a large deficit. A series of American scholars have, over the decades, made a remarkable contribution to our understanding of the origins and dynamics of Britain's National Health Service (NHS) (among them Eckstein 1958, 1960; Fox 1986; Marmor and Thomas 1972) as well as illuminating specific policy issues and options (Enthoven 1985; Fox 1978). There is no similar reciprocal literature of British scholars writing about the United States. Both quantitatively and qualitatively, the health care literature on the two countries speaks with a strong American accent.

Perhaps this is neither surprising nor significant. The imbalance could well be a function of the difference in the size and resources of the two academic communities. Much the same comment could, in all probability, be made about most other areas of scholarship. If comparative studies in all fields are, in part at least, the product of academic tourism, it is not after all astonishing that publications reflect the general scale and direction of the tourist trade. Add linguistic accessibility as an additional factor drawing American scholars to Britain, and it may be that further reflection on the imbalance in trade is redundant. The health care literature may simply be one more example of American dominance in the international marketplace of intellectual goods and cultural phenomena.

The puzzle revives, however, if we take account of the content of the literature. The authors I have mentioned contributed to an understanding of the British situation precisely because they were driven chiefly by disciplinary curiosity, by a desire to comprehend the dynamics of health care systems. Yet, in other cases, the driving force – as in so much of the comparative literature – was not so much the desire for understanding, but rather the search for arguments to use in domestic policy debates. In other words, the British experience was viewed as a laboratory for experimenting with a particular formula for financing and organizing health care, from which it would be possible to draw lessons for the United States about the applicability or otherwise of the model being tried out.

The "what can we learn from Britain's experience" literature produced some distinguished work, but its focus shifted in line with the domestic concerns of the United States. If one knew nothing about the evolving U.S. debate on health care, it would be possible to reconstruct it to a large degree by looking at what American scholars were writing about the National Health Service in different epochs, always allowing for the lag between research and publication. Thus, in the still optimistic early 1970s, when radical reform of the American health care system seemed a distinct possibility, the focus was on the achievement of equity in Britain (Anderson 1972). In the pessimistic 1980s, when the American obsession was with cost containment above all other issues, the interest in the NHS shifted to its ability to ration scarce resources (Aaron and Schwartz 1984). When planning and consumerism were on the U.S. agenda in the 1970s, these were the issues that interested American scholars working in Britain (Rodwin 1984). When attention shifted to such problems as malpractice suits and defensive medicine, again they were the topics that brought American scholars across the Atlantic (Rosenthal 1987). Similarly, the growing interest in health promotion in the 1980s produced an Anglo–American comparative study (Leichter 1991). In many of the studies cited, Britain was paired with Sweden, logically enough given that the two countries have the same model of universal, tax-financed health care, if with significant variations in the organization of the delivery system.

The interest in the NHS was, however, not just driven by an intellectual desire to seek illumination in the search for solutions to America's health care problems. It was also impelled by a determination to find political texts for sermons, that is, to use the experience of the NHS as evidence that particular solutions would or would not work in the United States. The resulting literature would suggest that selective perception is the original sin of comparative studies. For those in the United States who opposed anything remotely resembling "socialized medicine," Britain's waiting lists could be held out as dire warning of things to come if America moved in the direction of a national health service. In particular, the NHS provided a rich text for public choice economists, eager to demonstrate the dangers inherent in state bureaucracies; it meant, they argued, an underfinanced system employing underpaid doctors in under-capitalized hospitals (Buchanan 1965; Lindsay 1980). Conversely, those pushing for some system of national insurance in the United States tended to fasten on to the NHS's successes – notably its ability to provide a universal service with reasonable equity and remarkable parsimony – as evidence of the advantages of such a system. Both views caught important insights, if at times also perpetuating myths (British doctors, for example, are not underpaid by local standards). Neither interpretation caught the complex reality.

Looking at the much sparser British literature on the United States, there is no such neat symmetry. American experience provides a simple text. It demonstrates the dreadfulness of leaving health care to the market-place and thus, by implication, underlines Britain's triumphant good sense in creating the NHS. America's failure was thus taken as proof of Britain's success: a conclusion flattering to national self-esteem, if somewhat lacking in logic. The classic, and best known, text expounding this view is, of course, Titmuss's *The Gift Relationship* (1970): an eloquent disquisition on the advantages of a health care system based on altruism and mutual help, freely given, over one where financial considerations corrupt even the blood supply. It was a book that had, and continues to have, considerable resonance in Britain, despite evidence that its analysis of the American situation is in many respects inaccurate and misleading (Drake, Finkelstein, and Sapolsky 1982): a reminder, once again, that much of the comparative literature represents a search for evidence that will bolster stereotypes resistant to both argument and evidence. The point would emerge even more strongly from any more general analysis of the British health care literature, let alone political debate. The evocation of American experience is used to make the flesh creep. The assumption is that any development that can be presented as an invasion of American ideas or practices will automatically be rejected with horror. Indeed, as I will discuss below, this was very much the reaction in the 1980s when American ideas were filtering through, albeit selectively, and even influencing government policy. American ideas were widely perceived as tainted by their source, rooted as they were in a health care system that excluded the poor and revolved around the profit motive.

What conclusions, if any, can we draw from this rather brutal and summary review of the Anglo–American comparative literature? It is, of course, a caricature, and meant as such. It leaves out many valuable studies that have examined details of the two systems. However, it does indicate, I think, that comparative studies can distort as well as illuminate; that they bring risks as well as benefits. The fault line does not run simply between the discipline- or curiosity-driven and policy-concern-driven studies. There is no inherent reason why an interest in policy issues – or even a strong bias toward a preferred policy solution – should necessarily lead to selective perceptions, and there are plenty of scholarly studies to prove the point. However, it is clear that the temptations are stronger in the latter case; so is susceptibility to the occupational disease of comparativists, which is a highly developed capacity to find what they were looking for.

This is not to argue against comparative studies; far from it. Comparisons are essential if one is to achieve an understanding of one's own national health care system. Logically, as argued at the start, it is impossible to make a statement about cause and effect within a national system without checking it out against the experience of another country. So, for example, it could be said – looking only at Britain – that rationing is the inevitable price to be paid for a parsimonious national health care service operating with a capped budget. If I then look at the United States, however, I would discover that rationing is also apparent there – albeit in a different form, by exclusion from the system of coverage – even though there is no national health service, no capped budget, and spending levels are twice as high as in Britain. I might therefore be tempted to conclude that rationing is inevitable in all health care systems – a conclusion that, however, then requires to be tested against the experience of yet more countries. The necessity of comparative studies therefore hardly needs laboring. What my perhaps somewhat mischievous caricature of the Anglo–American comparative literature suggests, however, is that we should pay more attention to those characteristics of comparative studies calculated to enhance understanding, as distinct from buttressing preconceived notions. These are twofold, as I shall argue in the next section. First, comparative studies have to be explicit about the criteria being used: the spheres of analysis, as it were. Second, analysis has to be anchored in an understanding of the specific historical origins of national institutions, and of their economic, social, and political context.

Spheres of Analysis

If one of the driving forces behind comparative studies is the attempt to understand the advantages and disadvantages of different systems –

perhaps even to devise, with the aid of intellectual and institutional transplants, the perfect health system – then it is clearly crucial to have clearly defined and agreed currency of evaluation. The point is so obvious that it would scarcely require mention were it not for the fact that it is usually ignored. In a sense, we take our criteria of evaluation for granted most of the time. They can probably be summed up in terms of the three *E*s: equity, economy, and effectiveness. These are the kind of generally accepted, common-sense, assumptions that seem to underlie much of the comparative literature, with only a rarely felt need to make them explicit – and, by making them explicit, set them out for critical scrutiny of what they mean, and how they are interrelated.

Yet, to take the last point first, it is clear, from even the most superficial run through the comparative literature, that the relative weight attached to the three criteria has shifted over time, and appears to be strongly related to changes in the economic and political environment. As already noted, the comparative literature of the 1960s and the early 1970s was largely shaped by a concern about equity, with strong emphasis on comprehensive coverage of the population and the rational planning of services as necessary (if not sufficient) conditions. It was a literature that accurately reflected the optimistic assumptions of an era in which continued economic growth was taken for granted in the Western world – and with it, the continued expansion of the welfare state. Conversely, the decade of economic turmoil that followed the oil shock to the world economy in the mid-1970s led to a rather different focus, reflecting the more pessimistic (or realistic, depending on one's point of view) assumptions about likely economy growth and the role of the welfare state. The emphasis was very much on comparing the performance of different health care systems in terms of their ability to contain costs.

In this, the role of the Organisation for Economic Co-operation and Development (OECD) is of particular interest. As part of its more general interest in economic management and public expenditure, OECD published a series of comparative analyses of health care systems (OECD 1977, 1985, 1987), which not only helped to set the terms of debate, by focusing on cost-containment issues, but also encouraged scholars generally to use its currency of evaluation by supplying the necessary statistics. All scholars interested in comparative health studies are deeply indebted to OECD for its heroic efforts in pulling together disparate national data and providing accessible and (reasonably) accurate time series. OECD data have informed countless comparative studies and policy arguments (see, e.g., Maxwell 1981 and Pfaff 1990). However, by generating these data OECD was, of course, also subtly helping to shape the nature of comparative inquiries by focusing on health inputs: spending levels, the number of beds, manpower figures, and so on. This is not to imply deliberate intent or to suggest that a conspiracy of economists and statisticians were trying to dictate the terms of comparative studies. There was no need for a conspiracy. The economic stringencies of the period were, in any case, leading to an inflation in the influence of economists in the field of health care research (Fox 1990). Rather, it is to argue that the focus and methods of those engaged in comparative studies are inevitably influenced by the nature of the available data. It is a general point: witness the epidemic use of public expenditure statistics in the comparative literature on the development of the welfare state (such data have the further advantage, apart from their easy availability, of not requiring the chore of learning foreign languages). It applies with special force, however, to comparative health care studies, perhaps because of the famine of other data, notably about the impact of different types of health care systems on the populations being served.

It is a gap that the OECD reports have recognized from the start. Indeed successive reports have attempted ever more strenuously to fill it, particularly in the late 1980s when the emphasis switched from economy to effectiveness. Thus, the latest report (OECD 1990) reviews evidence on international differences in medical care practices and in health service utilization. Yet, in doing so, it underlines the problematic nature of the comparative task. In part this springs from the sketchiness of much of the data, and the difficulty (and expense) of generating comparable cross-country information. The most ambitious attempt to do so on the basis of population surveys in seven countries (Kohn and White 1976) remains a monument to the dangers and frustrations of the enterprise. It has never made the contribution to the comparative health care debate that might have been expected from its scale, cost, and sophistication, largely, I suspect, because the complexity of the data defies easy comprehension and yields few direct policy conclusions. There are, of course, more successful examples of international information collection (i.e., Glaser 1970 and 1978). In any case, the real difficulty of comparison may derive less from the inadequacy of information than from the deficiencies in our conceptual framework for using and evaluating it, to return to my argument at the start of this section.

Consider the 1990 OECD report, which seeks to pull together a variety of evidence from different sources. This suggests, for example, that the United States has (by international standards) a poor record in the birth control of technological innovation. Similarly, it shows that the American rate for certain procedures, notably hysterectomy, is far above most other Western countries – although Canada and New Zealand are not far behind. Conversely, it demonstrates that, predictably, Britain tends to come out at the parsimonious end of the spectrum. All of this simply confirms that a country that spends twice as much as another is likely to provide rather more in the way of medical activity. How much of that extra activity is superfluous, in the sense of yielding no benefit to the patient, is a different question to which we have no satisfactory or complete answer. We do know (because we have the appropriate statistics) that there is little link between health service spending and mortality; we do not, however, know (because we lack the relevant statistics) whether different levels or patterns of spending affect the quality of life of the population concerned – although this may be a much more important criterion. Indeed we do not even know the extent to which particular phenomena or outcomes are inherent to specific health care systems in a causal sense. Wide variations in practice *within* the United States – and other countries, even Britain (Ham 1988) – suggest that it is all too easy to be overly deterministic in assuming that system characteristics are necessarily the decisive factors. The fact that large variations in practice patterns seem to be general across health care systems might suggest that other factors – such as the culture of the medical profession and the uncertain nature of medical knowledge – are equally important. This is to come back, once more, to one of the most valuable functions of comparative studies, which is to guard against ethnocentrism in explanation by identifying similarities in different systems (Fox 1986; Marmor and Thomas 1972).

To sum up the argument so far, the source of the confusion (in which we all share) is that much comparative health care research is data rather than question driven. This may well be the inevitable result of the costs of collecting comparable data in different countries; of necessity we are forced to make the best of what is available, even though the information is usually generated by national concerns and by specific disciplinary or clinical interests, rather than by asking what we would need to know in order to answer specific questions. Hence, the difficulty of comparing different systems in terms of all three dimensions – economy, equity, and effectiveness – and exploring the relationships and tradeoffs among them. The assumption of the 1990s seems, increasingly, to be that assuring effectiveness – by eliminating unnecessary, redundant, or low-yield forms of treatment – is a necessary condition for reconciling the demands of economy and equity. The question remains, is it a sufficient condition, in the absence of full knowledge about which medical interventions are actually effective?

Moreover, when moving into the learning or prescriptive mode of comparison, does it make sense to compare health care systems in isolation from the societies that have created them? How transferable is experience? There is, for example, some evidence that political support for state welfare programs, including health, depends in large measure on the extent to which the middle classes benefit from them (Baldwin 1990;

Goodin and Le Grand 1987). This, in turn, implies that some degree of inequity may be a necessary condition if national health care systems are to flourish: if the system is perceived to be mainly redistributive, it may lack political support – although the extent to which this limiting condition applies will vary in different political systems. Thus, Sweden has a higher tolerance of explicit redistributive policies than, say, the United States.

In the next section, therefore, I will address the question of the extent to which it is useful to compare health care systems without also comparing the way they have been shaped, over the decades, by their political, social, and economic environments. Such understanding, it is argued, is a necessary condition for the transfer of experience or ideas. In other words, the two modes of comparative studies – those of understanding and of prescription – may be complementary rather than antithetical. If prescription does not rest on the kind of research produced by discipline- or curiosity-led research, then it is likely to offer quack remedies.

Learning from What Experience?

At this stage in the argument it may be useful to return to the starting point of this paper: the American fascination with Britain's National Health Service. While proposals for a comprehensive system of national health insurance were still on the political agenda in the United States, in the 1960s and early 1970s, there was a steady procession of scholars, health professionals, and politicians who came to inspect the NHS as a possible model for imitation; in their wake they brought their opponents, who came in search of evidence to use against the import of the British system. Both parties seemed, however, to share the view that the British model was in some sense exportable. From the British perspective, this always seemed a puzzling assumption. Indeed, it seemed positively perverse for Americans to be looking for inspiration for reform in a country that differed so radically in a number of highly relevant respects.

The NHS, like the British welfare state generally, is the product of a tradition of bureaucratic paternalism and a monument to professional rationality (Fox 1986; Klein 1983). It is a tradition going back to Chadwick's 1834 Poor Law Report, which was nurtured by the Webbs and which informed many of the post-1945 reforms. It is the product, moreover, of what, until recently at least, has been a homogeneous society – divided by class rather than by race – and of a highly centralized political system in which governments are virtually guaranteed automatic majorities for their policies in parliament. Britain, too, is a small country – it would fit into California with something left to spare – where it has always appeared to make sense to talk about national policies, national standards, and national services, although in recent years the Scots have increasingly begun to question this inherited piece of wisdom. Thus, long before we begin to examine the institutional characteristics of the NHS, it should be obvious that its foundations rest on peculiarly British soil. Even if the institutions could be exported, the soil could not.

Yet in practice the NHS has always depended on – and exploited – an inherited legacy of attitudes, and it may well be that it is the gradual depletion of this legacy that accounts for the growing sense of crisis and the search for new solutions in the 1980s (Day and Klein 1989). The point hardly needs laboring. One of the triumphs of the NHS, it is conventionally held, is that it manages to provide a comprehensive service both reasonably equitably and extremely parsimoniously. What is much more rarely recognized is the extent to which this achievement depends on the public's acceptance of the medical profession's definition of needs: political decisions about resources are, in effect, disguised as clinical decisions. In return for conceding an extraordinary degree of clinical autonomy to the medical profession, the state in fact delegated to it the responsibility for rationing – and thus made it socially acceptable. It is precisely this implicit contract or bargain that is now in question, given the recent changes in the NHS introduced by the Conservative government (Klein 1990). In turn, the public's acceptance of rationing decisions by doctors may well reflect deep-rooted attitudes of deference to professional expertise. These, however, are gradually being dissipated: witness the semantic revolution in public debate that is transforming patients (those to whom things are done, essentially a passive concept) into consumers (those who go out to buy things for themselves, essentially an active concept). To the extent that Britain is becoming more like the United States, so in fact there may be scope for convergence, a point to which we shall return in the next and final section.

Even this short, and overly simple, account should underlie the importance of putting health care institutions into their context: the exportability of systems (or parts of them) depends crucially on the comparability of the societies concerned. Note the emphasis on the comparability of the societies, rather than of the health care institutions themselves. By the 1980s it was becoming clear that the United States was unlikely to adopt anything like a national health service, that Britain's NHS offered an inadequate and implausible model. Attention in the American comparative literature switched to Germany (e.g., Light 1985; Wysong and Abel 1990) and Canada (e.g., Barer, Evans, and Labelle 1988; Marmor and Mashaw 1990) as possible models: countries with a federal political system, pluralistic health care systems based on insurance and fee-for-service payments to physicians that yet manage to contain costs. Indeed, these offer far more plausible models than Britain's NHS. It is still worth noting, however, the political limitations on their possible import into the United States. Consider, in particular, the case of Germany. Its example may appear particularly seductive in American eyes because of its success in containing spending. Yet this success depends less on the finance and organization of the health care system (precisely those characteristics that might, in theory, be transferable) than on the willingness of the medical profession to administer the cost-containment policies themselves (Iglehart 1991a,b). It draws on a century-old tradition of corporative policy making in Germany (Stone 1980) that is quite incompatible with America's political culture and institutions (Morone 1990), and is thus not exportable.

All of this would suggest that comparative studies should not be in the export–import business – selling ready-to-install models – but that they can extend national ideas about what is possible. They may be at their most useful when they prompt questions about how a particular approach to health care organization or finance could be translated, conceptually and practically, into a different context. The point is neatly illustrated by the transformation in the Anglo–American traffic in ideas that took place in the 1980s. From having been virtually a one-way stream of traffic in the previous decades, this became very much more of a two-way flow, with American ideas actually influencing British policy. On the face of it, this was a perverse and paradoxical development: the most successful health care system in the advanced industrial countries (at least in terms of economy, and perhaps also equity) importing ideas from the least successful. In conclusion, therefore, we briefly examine this reversal in the intellectual terms of trade in order to explore its implications.

Reversing the Roles

When in 1989 Mrs. Thatcher's government announced sweeping changes in the NHS, based on the notion of creating an internal market and introducing general practitioners in the role of budget holders (Day and Klein 1989), the predominant reaction was one of outrage and horror. Not only was the very idea of introducing competition into the NHS sacrilegious: an insult, as it were, to the memory of the founding fathers and their faith. Perhaps worse still, it was American in origin, and there was no shortage of American scholars to point out that competition had not been very successful in solving America's own health care problems (Light 1990). Britain seemed about to become a case study in the folly of learning too eagerly and too naively from the experience of other countries: a warning against importing foreign ideas.

In the event, it seems set to become a case study of a very different kind – of the sea change that ideas may undergo while crossing the Atlantic, and the way in which they develop in a new kind of habitat. For the direct influence of American ideas about the organization of the national health care system was limited. True, the notion of an internal market clearly reflected the proposals by Enthoven (1985) in a much discussed analysis of the British situation. However, the reason why the idea of competition found resonance was that it fitted neatly into the ideology of the government and followed the logic of the diagnosis made by the policy makers themselves. This ran along the following lines. The NHS had proved its worth. It ensured financial control and enjoyed great political popularity. However, there was a rising demand (largely orchestrated by the medical profession) for extra funds. If this was to be resisted, as it was by a government anxious to limit the rise in public spending, then something had to be done to squeeze more productivity out of the system. Moreover, the NHS was notoriously insensitive to consumer demands. Again, then, something had to be done – within the existing framework – to compel providers to take more heed of consumer preferences.

The logic of this line of reasoning led to the interest in competition – among both hospitals and general practitioners – as a way of introducing incentives to efficiency and responsiveness into an overrigid, provider-dominated system, a line of reasoning that Sweden now appears to be following as well (Saltman 1990). Moreover, the government had already applied much the same kind of logic to the education system several years before the NHS reforms; school budgets now depend on the number of pupils they can attract.

If the government wanted to look for tools to improve efficiency, where better to look than the United States? The NHS had been largely able to ignore questions of microefficiency for 40 years precisely because of its success in controlling total costs. It was parsimoniously effective in general, even though wasteful in detail. Conversely, the United States had desperately searched for ways of promoting microefficiency in the doomed hope that this would control total costs. It was wasteful in total even though striving for efficiency in detail. In the process, however, the United States had developed information systems, review processes, and managerial skills whose sophistication and quality dazzled the British visitors who, increasingly through the 1980s, flocked to America in search of tools and ideas.

The paradox is, then, perhaps not as perverse as it may seem. Competition in the British context will have a very different meaning from what it has in its country of origin. It will be limited in scale and scope. It will, above all, be contained within a rigid framework of regulation and financial control. It will therefore serve mainly to provide incentives to individual producer units and to give greater transparency to what the NHS actually does. The main result of the internal market so far has been to give visibility to the great inequalities in both performance and pricing of health authorities. There has not been a transplant of American policies; rather, some ideas from America have become naturalized and, in taking out British citizenship, have adapted to and become absorbed in the native health care culture.

Just conceivably, a similar process may be taking place in the United States. The United States appears to be moving hesitantly and falteringly toward embracing the key principle of the NHS, and indeed of all health care systems that have been successful in controlling their costs: a central, capped budget. This is the theme that appears to be emerging increasingly from the babble of competing proposals that, even from across the Atlantic, now suggests that health care reform is back on the U.S. political agenda. There are many variations of this theme (e.g., Aaron 1991; Marmor and Mashaw 1990), but widespread agreement on the need for a single payer. The United States may thus be moving toward adopting a framework of financial regulation within which competition can flourish, just as Britain has introduced an element of competition within the already existing framework of regulation. The U.S. system of regulation will be very different from Britain's, just as competition means something very different in the context of the NHS. However, there may be convergence – not so much in the institutions as in the ideas that shape those institutions – for which those engaged in comparative studies can, perhaps, take at least some of the credit.

References

Aaron, H.J. 1991. *Serious and Unstable Condition.* Washington: Brookings Institution.

Aaron, H.J., and W.B. Schwartz. 1984. *The Painful Prescription.* Washington: Brookings Institution.

Anderson, O.W. 1972. *Health Care: Can there be Equity?* New York: John Wiley.

Atteveld, van L., C. Broeders, and R. Lapré. 1987. International Comparative Research in Health Care. A Study of the Literature. *Health Policy* 8:105–36.

Baldwin, P. 1990. *The Politics of Social Solidarity.* Cambridge: Cambridge University Press.

Barer, L.M., R.G. Evans, and R.J. Labelle. 1988. Fee Controls as Cost Control: Tales from the Frozen North. *Milbank Quarterly* 66(1):1–64.

Buchanan, J.M. 1965. *The Inconsistencies of the National Health Service.* London: Institute of Economic Affairs.

Day, P., and R. Klein. 1989. The Politics of Modernization: Britain's National Health Service in the 1980s. *Milbank Quarterly* 67(1):1–33.

Drake, A.W., S.N. Finkelstein, and H.M. Sapolsky. 1982. *The American Blood Supply.* Cambridge, Mass.: MIT Press.

Eckstein, H. 1958. *The English Health Service.* Cambridge, Mass.: Harvard University Press.

———. 1960. *Pressure Group Politics.* London: Allen & Unwin.

Enthoven, A.C. 1985 Reflections on the Management of the National Health Service. London: Nuffield Provincial Hospitals Trust.

Fox, D.M. 1986. *Health Policies and Health Politics.* Princeton, N.J.: Princeton University Press.

———. 1990. Health Policy and the Politics of Research in the United States. *Journal of Health Politics, Policy and Law* 15(3):481–99.

Fox, P.D. 1978. Managing Health Resources: English style. In *By Guess or by What?*, ed. G. McLachlan. London: Nuffield Provincial Hospitals Trust.

Glaser, W.A. 1970. *Paying the Doctor.* Baltimore: Johns Hopkins University Press.

———. 1978. *Health Insurance Bargaining.* New York: John Wiley.

Goodin, R.E. and J. LeGrand. 1987. *Not Only the Poor.* London: Allen & Unwin.

Ham, C. Ed. 1988. *Health Care Variations.* London: King's Fund Institute.

Iglehart, J. 1991a. Germany's Health Care System: Part 1. *New England Journal of Medicine* 324(7):503–8.

———. 1991b. Germany's Health Care System: Part 2. *New England Journal of Medicine* 324(24):1750–6.

Klein, R. 1983. *The Politics of the National Health Service.* London: Longman.

———. 1990. The Political Price of Successful Cost Containment. In *Health Care in the '90s: A Global View of Delivery and Financing.* Los Angeles, Calif.: Blue Cross of California.

Kohn, R., and K.L. White. 1976. *Health Care: An International Study.* London: Oxford University Press.

Leichter, H.M. 1991. *Free to Be Foolish.* Princeton, N.J.: Princeton University Press.

Light, D.W. 1985. Values and Structure in the German Health Care Systems. *Milbank Memorial Fund Quarterly/Health and Society* 63(4):615–47.

———. 1990. Learning from Their Mistakes? *Health Service Journal* 100(5221):1470–2.

Lindsay, C.M. 1980. *National Health Issues: The British Experience.* Santa Monica, Calif.: Hoffman–LaRoche.

Marmor, T.R. 1983. *Political Analysis and American Medical Care.* Cambridge: Cambridge University Press.

Marmor, T.R., and D. Thomas. 1972. Doctors, Politics and Pay Disputes: "Pressure Group Politics" Revisited. *British Journal of Political Science* 2:421–42.

Marmor, T.R., and J.L. Mashaw. 1990. Canada's Health Insurance and Ours: The Real Lessons, the Big Choices. *American Prospect* 3:18–29.

Maxwell, R.J. 1981. *Health and Wealth.* Lexington, Mass.: Lexington Books.

Morone, J.A. 1990. American Political Culture and the Search for Lessons from Abroad. *Journal of Health Politics, Policy and Law* 15(1):129–144.

Organisation for Economic Co-operation and Development. 1977. *Public Expenditure on Health*. Paris.

———. 1985. *Measuring Health Care, 1960–1983*. Paris.

———. 1987. *Financing and Delivering Health Care*. Paris.

———. 1990. *Health Care Systems in Transition*. Paris.

Pfaff, M. 1990. Differences in Health Care Spending Across Countries. *Journal of Health Politics, Policy and Law* 15(1):1–68.

Rodwin, V.G. 1984. *The Health Care Planning Predicament*. Berkeley, Calif.: University of California Press.

Rosenthal, M.M. 1987. *Dealing with Medical Malpractice*. London: Tavistock.

Saltman, R.B. 1990. Competition and Reform in the Swedish Health System. *Milbank Quarterly* 68(4):597–618.

Stone, D.A. 1980. *The Limits of Professional Power*. Chicago: University of Chicago Press.

Titmuss, R.M. 1970. *The Gift Relationship*. London: Allen & Unwin.

Wysong, J.A., and T. Abel. 1990. Universal Health Insurance and High-risk Groups in West Germany: Implications for U.S. Health Policy. *Milbank Quarterly* 68(4):527–60.

54

Rationing in Action – Dimensions of Rationing: Who Should Do What?

BRITISH MEDICAL JOURNAL
31 July 1993

Priority setting is a complex interaction of multiple decisions at various levels in the organisation and constrained by history. There is no self evident set of ethical principles or analytical tools to determine what decisions we should take at various levels, nor is there an obvious or easy way to resolve the clash of claims on resources. To make priority setting more "rational" we should concentrate on the processes and structure of decision making and the relation of macro and micro decisions. The debate should promote reasoned, informed, and open argument, draw on a variety of perspectives, and involve a plurality of interests. The aim must be to build up, over time, the capacity to engage in continuous, collective argument.

My starting point is the all pervasive nature of priority setting in all health care systems. Decisions about how to allocate resources – what we call, if we want to raise the emotional level of the debate, rationing – take place at all levels of the organisational hierarchy and the delivery system. Everyone in any health care system is (to exaggerate only a little) taking decisions about how best to prioritise resources all the time. The process starts from the moment I enter my general practitioner's surgery.

The receptionist takes a decision, when I ask for an appointment, about how urgent my case is: what Roy Parker called, in a seminal article published 25 years ago, rationing by deterrence or delay.[1] When I eventually get to see my doctor, he or she will decide whether to give me five minutes or ten. Next will come a decision about whether or not to refer me to hospital (unless I shortcircuit the whole process by having a heart attack). Then I may or may not be put on a waiting list, and eventually – if I survive rationing by delay and depending on the priority rating I get – I may get to be treated in hospital. While I am there, doctors will take decisions about just what resources to throw at me – rationing my dilution, in Parker's terminology – and just how many tests and investigations to order. Finally, there will be decisions about how long to keep me in hospital: rationing by termination of treatment.

Two things need to be noted about this process. Firstly, all the microdecisions about priority setting are constrained by macrodecisions about resource allocation taken at superior levels in the organisational hierarchy: decisions in the Cabinet about how much to allocate to the NHS, decisions by the Department of Health about what priority targets to set to health authorities, and finally decisions by purchasers about what services to buy. Secondly, all the microdecisions are taken in terms of "need" as interpreted by the professional providers, notably the medical profession – that is, the perceived level of severity and urgency. Need, we have to recognise, is both an imprecise and an elastic concept, variously interpreted by different practitioners[2]: hence, of course, the frequently observed and much commented on variations in referral and operating rates.[3]

Multiple Decisions for Allocating Resources

So when we talk about priority setting we are really discussing the complex interaction of multiple decisions, taken at various levels in the organisation, about allocating resources. The secretary of state for health, Mrs Bottomley, could doubtless make the task of priority setting for doctors somewhat easier if she winkled out more funds for the NHS, though it is dangerous to assume that there would be no need for rationing if only Britain spent a higher proportion of the national income on health care. The case of the Netherlands provides a warning on this point: the Netherlands spent 8% of its gross domestic product on health care in 1990, in comparison to the United Kingdom's 6.2%,[4] yet it is currently debating what should and should not be included in the services provided – witness the publication of the Dunning report.[5] Conversely, the medical profession could make Mrs Bottomley's life much more pleasant by putting fewer people on the waiting lists (not a self evidently absurd proposition, given that there are no nationally agreed criteria for treatment and considerable evidence of variations in thresholds used by different consultants). To exaggerate only a little, demand for health care is what the medical profession chooses to make it: the pace at which it introduces new technologies, the rate at which it adopts new procedures, and so on.

Moreover, we are talking about decisions constrained by history: the inherited pattern of distribution between different sectors of the NHS and between different specialties. Priority setting is, inescapably, an incremental process. It involves decisions about how to spend the annual budgetary increment or how to react to budget cuts. In theory it may be possible to reallocate exisiting resources – to start from a clean slate and adopt a strategy of zero based budgeting – but in practice institutional resistance makes it difficult to do so on a large scale or in the short term. The constituency for the status quo tends to be powerful in health care, as in other services. Those who benefit from the existing pattern of service provision, whether as providers or consumers, tend to be concentrated and organised advocates for maintaining it, while those who stand to gain from the reallocation of funds are, by definition, a diffuse and difficult to identify group. The point is well illustrated by an analysis of the 1992–3 purchasing plans carried out at Bath[6] as part of a larger study of resource allocation policies in the NHS funded by the Nuffield Hospitals Trust. This showed a general reluctance to choose between competing claims on resources, with little evidence of explicit rationing (in the sense of limiting the menu of services offered by the NHS) or of any willingness to make dramatic changes. To the extent that the purchasers were prepared to modify the existing distribution of resources, it was very much at the margins. They tended to pursue a policy of "spreading the money around" – that is, of keeping as many people as possible happy by giving them some funds – even if this meant giving them only token amounts.

There is nothing surprising about such findings. They are very much in line with what would be expected on the basis both of theory and of the NHS's practice over the past 40 years. But it may be possible to draw out some less obvious implications. My starting point in doing this is the contention that there is no self evident set of ethical principles or of analytic tools which allows us to determine what sort of decisions we should take at different levels in the organisation. Consider, first, the question of what priority the government should give to health care when considering competing claims on resources. No one has yet come up with a convincing method for determining how much should be spent on the NHS. Much has been made of the famous 2% formula, the contention that the NHS needs an annual increment of 2% in its budget to cope with demographic and technological change. But this is based on extrapolating past trends and does not tell us anything about the adequacy or otherwise of the baseline from which the calculations start. Nor do comparisons with other countries help much. If another country spends a higher proportion of the national income on health care it may be because it is providing more health care or because each unit of service produced is more expensive or, come to that, because it is spending too much on ineffective procedures. And some nations – notably Denmark and Japan – spend much the same proportion as Britain without seemingly perceiving their health care systems to be underfunded and suffering from the kind of periodic crises that have afflicted the NHS since its birth.

Distributing the Budget

Moving, next, to decisions about how to distribute the total budget among services, there is once again no obvious or easy way of resolving the clash of claims on resources.[7] Quality adjusted life years (QALYs), as even the advocates of this decision making tool concede, are at best aids to decision making, providing an input of information. They are beset by methodological problems about the valuation of different states of health, by lack of data about outcomes, and by the problem of patient heterogeneity (the fact that the benefits of any given procedure may vary greatly among patients). Public opinion surveys are extraordinarily sensitive to the way in which questions are put and raise worrying issues about what weight should be put to answers given without any contextual information. Moreover, "the public" is a complex notion. As consumers of health care we may well have different priorities from those we have as citizens, just as there may well be differences between the consumers and the providers.[8] We could say, of course, that priority should always be given to procedures that are demonstrably effective over those that are not. It is difficult to disagree with the proposition, but I am not sure how far this gets us given the extent of our ignorance about effectiveness. Similarly, we could say that priority should follow need. But, again, how far does this get us, given the ambiguity of the concept? Moreover, if it is difficult to devise acceptable principles for prioritising medical interventions (the curing or repair function of the NHS), the problem is compounded when we address questions about allocating resources to the caring function of any health care system and the management of chronic conditions.

Making Priority Setting More "National"

All this may suggest that the argument is moving towards the despairing conclusion that there is no "rational" way of determining priorities: that, like it or not, we are still left with priorities emerging from pluralistic bargaining between different lobbies, modified by shifting political judgments made in the light of changing pressures. To an extent, indeed, that is my conclusion. But I would like to argue, firstly, that such a conclusion is not as negative as so often assumed and, secondly, that there is scope for making the process of priority setting more "rational."

My first contention is that, given the plurality of often conflicting values that can be brought to any discussion of priorities in health care, it is positively undesirable (as well as foolish) to search for some set of principles or techniques that will make our decisions for us: the idea of a machine for grinding out priorities is absurd. What is so often wrong about pluralistic bargaining is that it is not pluralistic enough: that discussion is dominated by some voices (notably those of the medical profession). Similarly, pluralistic bargaining often tends to confuse arguments based on interests with those based on values (although most of us have a highly developed capacity for translating our self interest into the high flown language of values).

From this follows a second point, which is that if we are concerned to make priority setting somehow more "rational" (a dangerous word, anyway), we should concentrate on the process of decision making. Rationality, from this perspective, lies in creating a situation in which there is open dialogue, in which opportunities for taking part in debate are widely distributed, in which arguments can be tested against evidence and the conflicts between different values or preferences can be explored. It is a concept of rationality which goes back to Aristotle[9] and which puts the emphasis on finding "good reasons" to justify decisions. And it is an approach which, I would argue, leads us out of the dead end of searching for some overarching formula for determining priorities by directing our attention to the *structure* of decision making.

The Structure of Decision Making

Taking this approach, the question then becomes: how far does the present structure of decision making allow rational argument (in the sense of reasoned and open discussion) about priorities? So we might start at the top of the decision making hierarchy and ask how the secretary of state and her department reach – and can justify – their priorities. We might further ask what criteria and evidence are used to come to such decisions about the allocation of resources: the balance between political expediency, cost-benefit considerations, and other factors. Next we might probe the extent to which other actors – such as the House of Commons health committee – can challenge and test the way in which the department formulates its policies. Are there enough opportunities for putting the department on the rack of cross examination and exploring alternative options?

Moving down one step in the organisational hierarchy, we might ask much the same sort of questions about purchasers. What assumptions, evidence, and criteria shape the policies about priorities? Which interests are represented in the decision making arena and, equally important, who is excluded? If public opinion surveys do not necessarily make much of a contribution of reasoned argument, although they may contribute some raw material, are there other ways in which purchasers test out their own plans and offer an opportunity to others to challenge their arguments and presumptions? Is the process of priority setting transparent enough?

Similarly, moving to the micro level of decision making, we can ask about the processes by which clinicians prioritise between the competing claims on resources and on their time. What criteria do they use in determining entry to, and progress up, waiting lists? What are their definitions of "need," and what weight do they give to different considerations – such as the age of the patient, the costs and effectiveness of different types of treatment, or the social implications of delay? And, again, we might ask to what extent such decisions are open to challenge: whether, for example, medical audit is an adequate instrument for testing different clinical policies and priorities. Should clinicians have to justify their judgments about priorities – about whom to treat, at what level of intensity – to a wider audience?

Finally, we should be concerned about the relationship between macro and micro decisions: in particular the feedback between the different levels in the organisational hierarchy. It is not self evident that at present there is adequate information about how broad macrodecisions about priorities, taken at the top of the hierarchy, translate into clinical decisions at the bottom about who should be treated and how. Again, waiting lists provide a classic example: lacking any evidence about the criteria used for giving priority to different patients, we simply do not know whether lengthening queues mean that the threshold of admission has been lowered or whether they imply that access is being delayed or denied to patients who previously would have been treated. Yet, in the absence of such information, how can there be rational argument about the government's priorities?

The Structure of the Debate

My argument then, to sum up, is that there is no technological fix, scientific method, or method of philosophic inquiry for determining priorities. Of course, the three Es – economists, ethicists, and epidemiologists – all have valuable insights to contribute to the debate about resource allocation and rationing, though none of them can resolve our dilemmas for us. But what really matters is how that debate is structured: how far it promotes reasoned, informed, and open argument, drawing on a variety of perspectives and involving a plurality of interests. The debate about priorities will never be finally resolved. Nor should we expect any final resolution. As medical technology, the economic and demographic environment, and social attitudes change, so almost certainly will our priorities. And we have to recognise that much of medicine is about the management of uncertainty, where research may roll back the frontiers of ignorance but is never likely to eliminate totally the need for clinical discretion and the use of judgment in interpreting the evidence about efficacy and outcomes.

Our aim must therefore be to build up, over time, our capacity to engage in continuous, collective argument. This means, in turn, devising institutions that encourage, rather than discourage, challenge, allow the implications of pursuing different priorities to be tested out, and provide the information required for reasoned debate. In short, we should be at least as much concerned with the structure of our institutions, and the way in which they work, as with the development of techniques. The politics of priority setting (in the widest sense) matter as much as the methodologies used.

This is very much a recipe for the long haul, but it is one that acknowledges the multidimensional complexity of priority setting, for it is precisely this complexity which does not allow any easy or quick solutions and which forces us to accept (however reluctantly) that this is a voyage of discovery where we will never reach a final destination. To put it another way, this is an argument that will never be finally settled, but in which we can try at least to ensure that it is conducted with due concern about openness, the appropriate use of evidence, and attention to what counts as good currency in the debate.

Notes

1. Parker R. Social administration and scarcity. In: Butterworth E, Holman R, eds. *Social welfare in modern Britain.* London: Fontana, 1975:204–12.

2. Cooper MH. *Rationing health care*. London: Croom Helm, 1975.

3. Ham C, ed. *Health care variations*. London: King's Fund Institute, 1988.

4. Organisation for Economic Cooperation and Development. *The reform of health care*. Paris: OECD, 1992.

5. *Report of the government committee on choices in health care*. Risjwijk: Ministry of Welfare, Health, and Cultural Affairs, 1992. (A J Dunning, chairman.)

6. Klein R, Redmayne S. *Patterns of priorities*. Birmingham: National Association of Health Authorities and Trusts, 1992.

7. Hunter D. *Rationing dilemmas in health care*. Birmingham: National Association of Health Authorities and Trusts, 1993.

8. Groves T. Public disagrees with professionals over NHS rationing. *BMJ* 1993;306:673.

9. Beiner R. *Political judgment*. Chicago: University of Chicago Press, 1983.

55

The Goals of Health Policy:
Church or Garage?

HEALTH CARE UK
ANTHONY HARRISON (ED)
KING'S FUND INSTITUTE LONDON,
1993

In discussing the evolving goals of health policy, from the foundation of the National Health Service to the present, there is one difficulty which faces the analyst right at the start. This is how to set a boundary around the notion of 'health policy' and, by so doing, making the task manageable. For about three decades after 1948, the notion of 'health policy' was in effect defined by the National Health Service. Health policy was NHS policy; the goals were those explicit or implicit in the NHS. However, one of the most striking developments of recent years has been the growing elasticity of the concept. It has become stretched to cover almost every aspect of public policy. Only consider the implications of the revival of the public health tradition, with its emphasis on social engineering rather than medical intervention. The new goal, as expounded in *The Health of the Nation* is promoting good health, rather than dealing with ill health.

In what follows, however, this analysis will not attempt to deal with this expanded, ambitious definition of 'health policy'. Instead, the strategy will be to use a narrower definition of the concept and to concentrate on the goals of the health care delivery system, as they have changed over time, by examining both the aims of those actually responsible for designing and running the NHS and the criteria used in judging its performance. In doing so, the theme will be that, increasingly, the goals of health care policy have shifted from a quasi-religious to a more instrumental approach: from viewing the health care system in terms of a church – all embracing in its social role and embodying certain moral values – to seeing it as a garage responsible only for the repair and maintenance of bodies. The two conceptions still co-exist, with the result, it will be argued, that there are contradictory expectations, which in turn explain why Britain's health care system is likely to change even more in the next decade or so than it has in the past 10 years.

Improving Health Care or Changing Society?

This restriction of the scope of analysis needs justification. The first reason for resisting the temptation to explore the new, enlarged definition of 'health policy' is that this analytical path leads in too many directions. If we say that the promotion of good health, and the prevention of ill-health, should be our goal, we are in effect putting forward a criterion for judging a whole range of public policies. There is a long tradition for such an approach, going back at least to the time of Chadwick. Two examples neatly illustrate the implications of adopting this wider definition of health policy.

In 1876 Benjamin Ward Richardson published his vision of a society shaped by health policy *Hygeia – A City of Health*. Both the design of his ideal city and the lives of its inhabitants were to be ruled by the health imperative: the goal was to root out all habits and practices that might promote ill-health:

> And, as smoking and drinking go largely together, as the two practices were indeed original exchanges of social degradation between man and the savage, the savage getting very much the worst of the bargain, so the practices largely disappear together. Pipe and glass, cigar and sherry-cobler, like the Siamese twins who could only live connected, have both died out in our model city.

Richardson was a utopian visionary. However, much the same emphasis on social engineering is evident in the submission by the British Medical Association to the 1925 Royal Commission on National Health Insurance. In this the BMA argued that:

> . . . the organisation of a National Health Insurance scheme is not necessarily, or even probably, the best means of utilising limited resources for the promotion of national health. It is more than likely that there are a number

of other directions in which severally, or collectively, a corresponding expenditure would produce an even more satisfactory return. Such are (1) proper housing (2) town planning with the proper provision of open spaces and recreation facilities (3) smoke abatement (4) a pure milk supply (5) public house reform and the reduction of the sale of alcoholic beverages (6) the destruction of vermin (7) education (8) the aiding of medical research.

The list of desirable changes could, of course, be extended. So, for example, one could argue for full employment and income redistribution as necessary conditions for improving the nation's health. However, there are a number of problems about this line of argument. Reducing the scale of unemployment and poverty are, surely, important goals in their own right. Why should the production of 'health' be wheeled on as an argument for promoting policy goals which are desirable in themselves? Would we be less concerned about trying to reduce unemployment if there was no link between joblessness and the population's health? Would we stop worrying about poverty if it was demonstrated that there was no connection with disease? If the notion of 'health policy' is not to become an all-purpose banner to rally social reformers – thereby losing all precision and meaning – it might be better to see improvements in health as the by-product of policy goals which should be pursued in their own right.

The second problem about using an all-embracing definition of 'health policy' is linked to this. One of the most striking phenomena of the past decade or so has been the process of institutional blame diffusion. Once we saw education as the key to social transformation: as the way forward to producing a more equal society. Now the dominant view is that we asked too much of our schools and that they cannot carry this weight of social expectations: that examination results do not mean much because they are the product not of the school's performance but merely reflect its social environment. Once we thought that it was the responsibility of the policy to deal with crime. Now Chief Constables are vying with each other to point out that they cannot be held responsible for soaring crime rates, since these are the product of social conditions: that the police cannot be expected to cope with the consequences of social dislocation. The same could be said of public housing, where high expectations of its social engineering potential have turned to sour disillusion. And the same, of course, is now being said about the NHS.

There is truth in all these defensive assertions. But there is also a danger. This is that, in our recognition of social complexity and the interdependence of a multiplicity of policies, we may lose sight of what can and cannot be expected of individual institutions: that blame diffusion will lead to a blurring of responsibility. If everything is dependent on everything else, how are we to define the goals of specific institutions like the NHS? Another way of putting this would be to ask: what should be the policy goals of the NHS, recognising that the contribution of any health care system to 'health' – at least as conventionally measured by mortality and life expectancy – is very limited.

Hence the case for concentrating on the goals of health care policy in the narrow sense: to focus on what can and should be expected from a health care system. Even with this restriction on the scope of analysis, difficulties remain. Should the goals be defined in terms of the objectives that policy makers have set themselves over the years? Or should they also include the prescriptive policy aims which have been or might be used to assess the performance of the NHS? The distinction is important. If we look at the academic literature, we find that Britain's welfare state is frequently criticised for its failure to achieve greater equality. Yet if we look at the intentions of the policy makers, we find that the achievement of greater equality rarely, if ever, figured among their policy goals. There is a risk, therefore, of retrospectively condemning policy makers for failing to achieve goals which they never set for themselves.

In what follows, the analysis deals with both descriptive and prescriptive policy goals, while trying to distinguish between them as much as possible. Knowing what the goals of the NHS's founding fathers were, and what it is actually trying to do, is important if we are to assess its performance. Discussing what the policy goals should be is crucial if we are to develop any criteria for judging the institutional design of health care systems. If we assume that the NHS is very much in a state of evolution, we need criteria for assessing the way in which Britain's health care system develops, which are independent of the historical legacy of assumptions and ambitions built into existing institutions.

The Church and its Founding Fathers

In analysing the goals of the NHS, as perceived by the founding fathers, the metaphor of a church is helpful in illuminating one of its defining characteristics. Its creation rested on an act of faith. Like most of his contemporaries, Aneurin Bevan had no doubts about the powers of medical science to improve health. On this doctors and politicians spoke with one voice. The challenge was to spread the word: to make health care accessible to all by eliminating financial barriers. The aim was to 'universalise the best', to quote from Bevan's speech introducing the NHS bill in 1946. It was however, a church for rationalists: the element of missionary conviction lay precisely in the belief that it would only be possible to 'universalise the best' by creating an institution which would make it possible to plan rationally, purposefully and comprehensively. Medical science and managerial rationality went hand in hand. From this flowed the emphasis on efficiency and effectiveness: words which were to be used with ever increasing frequency in the 1980s but which, nevertheless, already formed part of the vocabulary used by the founding fathers. Witness Bevan's remark, in the same speech, that 'I would rather be kept alive in the efficient and cold altruism of a large hospital than expire in a gush of warm sympathy in a small one'.

If the metaphor of the NHS as a church seems too farfetched, consider this quotation from Barbara Castle – one of Bevan's disciples and SECRetary of State for Health in the 1970s – speaking at the time of the dispute over paybeds:

> Intrinsically, the National Health Service is a church. It is the nearest thing to the embodiment of the Good Samaritan that we have in any aspect of our public policy. What would we say of a person who argued that he could only serve God properly if he had pay pews in his church.

In other words, the NHS was seen to have a moral, as well as a scientific, mission. It was not just saving bodies. It was also saving souls by embodying certain values of mutual help: very much the view taken by Richard Titmuss in *The Gift Relationship,* his celebration of the NHS as an instrument for promoting communitarian values. From this perspective, then, the goal of a health care system should be, to switch to the prescriptive mode of analysis, to promote social cohesion. The universality of a health care system is not just a means of ensuring access for all but a celebration of the common humanity of all citizens: rich and poor are treated alike in the cancer ward. Similarly, the stress on providing services free of charge is not just a way of ensuring access for all but a declaration of faith that medical care is somehow 'special' and must be distinguished from goods sold in the market place.

From this alliance between belief in medical science and faith in the social healing powers of a universal health care system, there flowed another policy goal – which still dominates today. This is that health care must be allocated according to need. The reason why Bevan rejected a health care system run by local authorities (medical resistance apart) was that this would inevitably perpetuate a distribution of resources based on the differential ability of councils to pay for it. How could the best be universalised, if there was diversity of provision? While the achievement of equity – *ie* allocation according to need, whether to geographical units or to individuals – was never explicitly spelt out by the original designers of the NHS, it was implicit in their whole approach. It has thus provided a prescriptive goal, or benchmark, for subsequent analyses of health care policy.

There is a further twist to this story. One of the implicit aims of policy has been, at least since 1950, to contain spending on health care. It was in March 1950 that the Cabinet decided to cut the NHS budget. And ever since the NHS has been an instrument of public expenditure control. The point is so obvious that we take it for granted. But it is worth stressing, if only to remind ourselves that it marked a repudiation of the idea that spending on health care should be driven by demand. The goal of achieving equity based on need thus came to be translated into a principle for rationing scarce resources within the NHS, rather than a way of determining what its budget should be: we have never, despite the famous two per cent formula, devised a satisfactory way of designing a needs-driven formula for allocating resources to the NHS. Hence, of course, the never-ending dialogue of the deaf about the 'under-funding' of the NHS. If we reject meeting demands as our policy goal, and if we cannot design a needs-based formula, then we are in trouble when it comes to discussing the appropriateness or otherwise of the NHS's budget.

Two other points need stressing in this context. First, the goal of equity, as defined in practice, was essentially paternalistic in character. Need was something that was defined by epidemiologists and other experts: the invention of the resource allocation formula for the geographical distribution of NHS funds is a case in point. And it was the medical profession who determined which demands ranked as needs in deciding whom to treat. Needs, in short, always trumped demands. Taking equity as the guiding policy goal therefore implied – certainly in practice, if not in logic – downgrading responsiveness to demand as a possible policy objective. Second, using equity as the guiding principle for resource allocation has proved unhelpful when it comes to determining priorities between client groups or between different specialties. The drive to steer more resources to the Cinderella services, which started in the 1970s, did not spring from any statistical or scientific demonstration of inequity but from a gut instinct based on revelation of inadequacy. There was need, for sure. But there was, and still is, no scientific way of weighing this need against competing ones.

If we want to sum up the consensus view about the goals of the NHS, as it evolved through its first three decades, there is perhaps no better way than to quote the report of the 1979 Royal Commission on the National Health Service. This summed up the objectives of the NHS as follows:

- To encourage and assist individuals to remain healthy
- To provide equality of entitlement to health services
- To provide a broad range of services of a high quality
- To provide equality of access to these services

- To provide a service free at the time of use
- To satisfy the reasonable expectations of its users
- To remain a national service responsive to local needs

Like many such mission statements this definition of policy goals begged as many questions as it answered. What are reasonable expectations? Who determines responsiveness to local needs? Is providing a free service an objective in its own right or simply a means of achieving equality of access? Above all, though, there is little or no sense that different goals might conflict. Yet it is precisely emerging confict that characterises the years that followed the Royal Commission's report – the era of secularisation – and it is to this theme that the analysis turns next.

Consumers and the New Secularism

Moving to the 1980s, there is a transformation. To a large extent the goals of health policy, in previous decades, were expressed in the language of inputs. In the 1980s the emphasis switched increasingly to outputs, as the Government put increasing emphasis on activity figures in response to criticisms about under-funding, and then to outcomes, the language of the *The Health of the Nation*. There is, moreover, no shortage of explicitly stated policy goals. On the contrary, there is an embarrassment of choice. So, for example, the Department of Health's 1992 Annual Report has an appendix setting out four major policy goals, broken down into 45 subsidiary policy aims. Some of these goals are internal to the Department, such as to make best possible use of staff and other resources, and treat all staff fairly and responsibly. Others are more general in character, such as to develop policies to improve the health and well-being of the population and prevent illness.

But before discussing this richness of policy goals, it is worth reflecting on why there has been this explosion. In part, no doubt, it reflects the style of the new public management thinking that has swept through Whitehall over the past decade. Hence the insistence on explicitly stated aims, against which policy performance can be measured. Hence, too, the recurring emphasis on economy, efficiency and effectiveness in the litany of policy aims. The rhetoric of value for money may not be new; indeed it has been used for 40 years or more. However, it has risen to a crescendo as a result of the new Whitehall fashions.

More important, the new style and the new language reflect a different view of the health care system: a move from seeing it as a church to seeing it as a garage. There are a number of components to this change.

Faith in medical science is no longer as blind as it was in 1948. The role of the medical care system has changed: the old killer diseases such as tuberculosis have been conquered while the new ones such as cancer and cardiovascular conditions have proved stubbornly resistant to the efforts of medical science. As a result, health care is increasingly concerned with repairing or maintaining people who cannot be cured. The AIDS epidemic is a case in point. Moreover, the medical profession's own concern with techniques – with designing ever more sophisticated gadgetry for intervention – invites the comparison with mechanics, (as indeed does the increasing emphasis put on trade-union activities). Lastly, there has been a more general growth of distrust in experts and professionals.

This process of secularisation is reflected in a linguistic revolution: the transformation of the patient into the consumer. This has enormous implications for the way in which we talk and think about the NHS's policy goals. The patient is someone to whom things are done. It implies a passive role, totally at harmony with the paternalistic traditions of the NHS. The consumer is someone who goes out to satisfy his or her wants, an active role challenging the NHS's needs-based distributive goals. The emphasis has switched from seeing the NHS as an instrument for promoting broad social goals, such as social cohesion, to seeing it as satisfying individual expectations: specifically, expectations that people will get an efficient repair and maintenance service.

It is important not to exaggerate by making the contrast with the past too neat or pat. But the evidence of a radical shift in the way we talk about the NHS, and its policy goals, seems overwhelming. The notion of consumer rights is creeping, albeit timidly, into the debate about policy goals: the obvious example is, of course, the Patient's Charter. There has been a rapid growth in consumer groups within the health care policy arena, just as there has been a growth of consumerism in society at large. Political competition has forced the Government to make the reduction of waiting lists one of its main policy goals: *ie* to make responsiveness to demands the test of its policies. There is more emphasis, at least at the level of rhetoric, on giving people greater choice of the services available, as *Working for Patients* puts it.

Views will differ about this process of secularisation: personally, I would rather see the NHS as a garage than as a church. However, whatever view one takes, the important issue is whether the new goals are compatible with those inherited from the founding fathers. The next, and final, section therefore explores the tensions and strains inherent in the co-existence of two very different sets of policy goals.

Conflicting Policy Goals

Consider the whole question of choice as a policy goal. If consumerism is to be more than a rhetorical invocation then choice is essential. It is, surely, the ability to choose between different garages which distinguishes a consumer from a patient or a client. To use the word is to repudiate paternalism. More crucially, surely, it is also to repudiate the goal of meeting need as defined by the experts. *Working for Patients,* as noted above, defined its policy goal as giving people greater choice of the services available. But what if the available services are not those judged to be appropriate or adequate by the consumers? What if the demands of the consumers do not match expert-defined needs? Do we then stick to the traditional view that needs always trump demands? Or do we reverse the doctrine, and argue that demands should have precedence over needs?

There are other ways in which the new policy goals are at odds with those we have inherited. Choice implies redundancy. There must be some spare capacity. But how are we to square that with the goal of limiting spending on the health care system, of seeing empty beds as a sin against the Trinity of economy, efficiency and effectiveness – the conventional, though not necessarily right, view? Similarly, if we put consumer demands in the saddle, is this compatible with a capped budget?

Most important perhaps, what if consumer demands run counter to the policy goals of trying to bias resource distribution to the most vulnerable groups, *ie* those least able to articulate their case, least able to exercise choice and least able to act as 'consumers' in the full sense. What is the point of improving the garage service to those without cars? What if, as moral citizens, we disapprove of the choices made by the consumers of health care? The question is not just rhetorical. As a consumer, I may well give preference to the kind of repair and maintenance services from which I benefit directly: this is what the evidence of the private sector would suggest. But as a moral citizen I may give more weight to providing compassionate care to those who are beyond repair, those whose bodies cannot be improved by medical intervention but whose life can be made more pleasant and whose death can be made more easy by sympathetic and kind care.

There is no clear cut answer to these questions. But one response might well be to say that by invoking the language of the market, we are striking at the principles of the NHS: that the church should not be turned into a garage. So, moving to the prescriptive mode, can a principled case be made for consumerism and choice in health care? Indeed it can: the case for choice rests on the same set of arguments used to justify State provision of health care in the first place: the argument of autonomy put, for example, by Albert Weale in *Political Theory and Social Policy*. Put simply, this runs as follows. Provision of health care is necessary because, without it, people cannot function as fully autonomous human beings, making their own life plans. It is this which distinguishes it from other goods supplied by the market. Taking this line of argument one step further, we can then ask: how is it possible to be a fully autonomous human being without having choice? It is surely the ability to choose between different, alternative courses of action that distinguishes an autonomous individual from someone who is merely the creature of circumstances without any independent volition.

Certainly the evidence of the private sector suggests that choice is an essential part of autonomy. People using the private sector are more autonomous than those using the NHS: in the sense of being in command of things, as distinct from being treated like a passive object. There are, of course, other reasons for using the private sector: notably queue jumping. And choice is often inhibited by the asymmetry in information between consumers and providers that characterises health care – although it may sometimes be exaggerated. So the private sector shows the limits of consumerism in health care, as well as its advantages.

One final conflict between the traditional goals and the emergent ones – between those of the church and the garage – requires mentioning, since it has very considerable implications. The moral vision of the ecclesiastical model is centered on the notion of equality. The goal of the secular model is centred on the notion of maximising the output of health, or at least, the production of health care interventions: witness the emphasis on meeting demand as expressed through waiting lists. It cannot necessarily be assumed that the two goals are compatible. The first objective would mean concentrating resources on those who are most difficult and expensive to reach and treat. The second objective would suggest concentrating on those who are most amenable and accessible to treatment – so maximising the health gains for any given resource input but also increasing inequalities.

These, then, to vary our metaphor, are some of the tensions between the Old Testament and the New Testament views about what the goals of health care policy should be. They suggest that the last set of health care reforms will not be the last. If the NHS is to meet demand as articulated by consumers – instead of need as defined by the experts – then some other policy goal may have to be sacrificed: notably, that of designing the health care system with cost-control as a primary objective.

56

Labour's Health Policy: A Retreat from Ideology

BRITISH MEDICAL JOURNAL
8 JULY 1995

The NHS presents the Labour party, as the next government in waiting, with a particularly difficult political challenge. On the one hand, the party's apocalyptic prophecies about the consequences of the changes in 1991 have been betrayed by events: the NHS has not disintegrated, nor has it been privatised. On the other hand, the party's commitment to financial austerity, should it be returned to office, inhibits it from buying support by making any promises about more generous funding. In the circumstances, the Labour party's manifesto on health, *Renewing the NHS,*[1] is a remarkably skilful document. It signals a retreat from dogmatism and an acceptance of the need for a pragmatic policy under a smokescreen of ideological rhetoric.

The rhetoric is designed to reassure the party faithful. The manifesto evokes a mythical past when everything was splendid in the NHS. It describes a demonised present in which the Conservative government is corrupting the NHS's ideals. But the proposals are designed to reassure the public and the professionals working in the NHS. They turn out to be surprisingly modest, often building on the much denounced changes of recent years, largely cosmetic in character, and designed to allow scope for negotiation and experiment in the process of implementation.

Consider, for example, the commitment to ending the internal market. There is less to this than meets the eye. The split between commissioners and providers is to remain. But instead of "year-on-year competition for contracts" there would be long term agreements. But, of course, this is simply to acknowledge reality. The government has never succeeded in bringing about genuine competition and has perhaps never wished to do so. Moreover, commissioning authorities, as an analysis of their five year strategic plans shows,[2] are increasingly moving towards relying on a restricted number of preferred providers. In part this is because the commissioning authorities want to cut the transaction costs of contracting, which have rightly been identified by Labour as one of the debits of the internal market. In part it is because yesterday's purchasers are turning into today's planners intent on shaping the pattern of services to the needs of their populations.

So, oddly enough, *Renewing the NHS* cites the rundown of St Bartholomew's Hospital as an example of "this government's contempt for rational planning." Yet, whatever one may think of this decision, it was the outcome of a major planning exercise involving a review of the provision of the specialities and of records of research across all the London teaching hospitals.[3]

More radical is the proposed phasing out of fundholding. Wisely, no deadline has been set for this. A prolonged deathbed scene is likely, and it could just be that the patient will turn out to be alive at the end. Not only is the evidence about the success or otherwise of fundholding more finely balanced than *Renewing the NHS* concedes[4] but if the document's welcome aim of ensuring that general practitioners continue to have a powerful role in determining local priorities is to be realised – for example, through locality commissioning – then it may be necessary to reinvent fundholding under another name.

GPs' Increased Influence

Before 1991, general practitioners had little influence on planning by health authorities or on hospital practice. Since 1991 their influence on both has increased greatly.[2] Fundholding has been a major factor in this transformation: it has given general practitioners sanctions. If there were no such sanctions would they retain the influence they now exert? Would it be enough, as the document suggests, to give them "shadow budgets"? Or would it be necessary to put financial flesh on these shadows, so, in effect, reinventing a form of collective fundholding? And might not such cooperatives of general practitioners evolve over time into something remarkably like the competing health maintenance organisations envisaged by Alain Enthoven?[5]

The document prompts other questions as well. For example, the very welcome commitment to restoring to general practitioners the freedom to refer would seem, on the face of it, to be incompatible with the requirement for health authorities to control their own budgets if money followed patients. But if money did not follow patients, would hospitals have any incentive to treat them? The membership of supervisory boards of health authorities and the governing boards of the relabelled trusts would be designed to make them "representative" of the community. But does not the experience of authorities before 1991 suggest that this may weaken rather than strengthen accountability?[6]

The NHS's funding problems would be dealt with by attacking bureaucracy, cutting administrative costs, and increasing efficiency. Does this recipe not recall the general election manifestos published by the Conservatives in years gone by? Lastly, *Renewing the NHS* rightly acknowledges the crucial importance of economic and social policies in improving public health and makes a welcome commitment to health promotion in the widest sense. But how seriously can this commitment be taken when the paragraph on smoking pledges Labour to ban tobacco advertising but makes no mention of increasing taxes?

Policy Fudge

The questions multiply. For *Renewing the NHS* is, in many ways, a policy fudge. And this, paradoxically, is its greatest strength. It seems designed to allow any future Labour government freedom of manoeuvre. Its emphasis on the scope for experimenting with different solutions rather than setting a particular model in concrete is a recipe for flexibility in the design of policy. Its publication has been marked by an emollient emphasis on cooperation with the professions.[7] Should a Labour government be returned to power, the stage could therefore be set for the creation of a new consensus on the NHS rather than a simple reversal of the policies pursued by the Conservatives.

The 1991 model of the NHS has many achievements to its credit.[8] But it has also produced some perverse side effects. The real trick, therefore, will be to build on the achievements of the new model while dealing with its shortcomings. *Renewing the NHS* raises the hope, if no more, that a Labour government might at least embark on such an enterprise.

Notes

1. Labour Party. *Renewing the NHS: Labour's agenda for a healthier Britain*. London: Labour Party, 1995.

2. Redmayne S. *Reshaping the NHS: strategies, priorities and resource allocation*. Birmingham: National Association of Health Authorities and Trusts, 1995.

3. James JH. *Transforming the NHS: the view from inside*. Bath: Centre for the Analysis of Social Policy 1994.

4. Glennerster H, Matsaganis M, Owens P. *Implementing GP fundholding*. Buckingham: Open University Press, 1994.

5. Newman P. Interview with Alain Enthoven: is there convergence between Britain and the United States in the organisation of health services? *BMJ* 1995;310:1652–5.

6. Day P, Klein R. *Accountabilities: five public services*. London: Tavistock, 1987.

7. Delamothe T. Margaret Beckett's third way: cooperation and partnership. *BMJ* 1995;311:13–4.

8. Klein R. *The new politics of the NHS*. London: Longmans, 1995.

Index